DATE DUE

NOV 1 0 1994	
NOV 2 4 1994	
MAR - 1995	
SEP 2 5 2003	

The
Nurse's
Guide
to
Marketing

The Nurse's Guide to Marketing

Ruth R. Alward, EdD, RN

President, Nurse Executive Associates, Inc.
Washington, DC

Caroline Camuñas, EdM, RN

Doctoral Candidate, Teachers College
Columbia University
New York, NY
Associate, Nurse Executive Associates, Inc.
Washington, DC

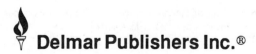 Delmar Publishers Inc.®

NOTICE TO THE READER

Delmar Staff
Senior Administrative Editor: Barbara Norwitz
Developmental Editor: David Prout
Project Editor: Christopher Chien
Production Supervisor: Larry Main
Design Supervisor: Susan C. Mathews

COPYRIGHT © 1991
BY DELMAR PUBLISHERS INC.

Printed in the United States of America

Published simultaneously in Canada
by Nelson Canada,
a division of The Thomson Corporation

10 9 8 7 6 5 4 3 2 1

Library of Congress Cataloging-in-Publication Data

Alward, Ruth R.
    The nurse's guide to marketing / by Ruth R. Alward and Caroline Camuñas.
        p. cm.
    Includes bibliographical references.
    Includes index.
    ISBN 0-8273-4203-9
    1. Nursing services—Marketing. I. Camuñas, Caroline.
II. Title.
    [DNLM: 1. Marketing of Health Services. 2. Nursing Services—
organization & administation. WY 105 A477n]
RT86.7.A37   1990
362.1'73'0688—dc20
DNLM/DLC
for Library of Congress   90-3322
                                                                            CIP

DEDICATION

To Sam and Jorge for their love and patience
throughout this endeavor

CONTENTS

CONTRIBUTORS

Sharon P. Aadalen, PhD, RN
Director of Nursing Education
and Research
United Hospital
St. Paul, MN

Constance M. Berg, MBA, RN
Executive Editor,
Today's Executive Nurse Magazine
Principal, CMB CONSULTING
San Francisco, CA

Nancy Ann Sickles Corbett, EdM, RN
Director of Education
Rancocas Hospital
Willingboro, NJ
Doctoral Candidate, Teachers College
Columbia University
New York, NY

Susan J. Costello, BSN, RN
Patient Educator
Zurbrugg Hospital
Riverside, NJ

Mary Ann Crawford, MSN, RN
Vice-President for Patient Care
Support Services
Akron General Medical Center
Akron, OH
Doctoral Candidate,
Kent State University
Kent, OH

Faye D. Davis, MSN, RN
Executive Director
New York Regional Transplant Program
New York, NY

Maryanne P. Doran, BSN, RN
Staff Development Instructor
Rancocas Hospital
Willingboro, NJ

Anne DuVal Frost, PhD, RN
Co-Founder of the Nurses Network
of Pelham
Project CHILD Director and
Principal Investigator
Associate Professor, Graduate Nursing
Program Director
College of New Rochelle
New Rochelle, NY

Mary L. Fisher, PhD, RN, CNAA
Associate Professor
Associate Dean for Administration
Assistant Campus Dean, IUPUI
Indiana University
Indianapolis, IN

Marsha E. Fonteyn, MSN, RN, CCRN
Doctoral Student
The University of Texas at Austin
School of Nursing
Austin, TX

Christine M. Galante, MA, MSN, RN
Lieutenant Colonel, Army Nurse Corps
Doctoral Candidate, School of Nursing
George Mason University
Fairfax, VA

Janet Gear-Wolfe, BSN, RN
Staff Development Instructor
Rancocas Hospital
Willingboro, NJ

Sharon E. Hoffman, MBA, PhD, RN
Dean and Professor, College of Nursing
Medical University of South Carolina
Charleston, SC

Phillippa F. Johnston, MS, RN
Assistant Administrator
Capitol Hill Hospital
Washington, DC

Karen J. Kelly, MS, RN, CNAA
Associate Director of Nursing for
  Education and Research
Greater Southeast Community Hospital
Washington, DC

Adina Kolatch, MBA
Director of Community Affairs
Visiting Nurse Service of New York
New York, NY

Carol Kronick-Mest, MSN, RN
Patient Educator
Rancocas Hospital
Willingboro, NJ

Rebecca S. McAnnally, RN
Divisional Director of Nursing
Ambulatory Care Services
The Children's Hospital of Alabama
Birmingham, AL

Kathryn M. Mershon, MSN, RN, CNAA
Senior Vice President—Nursing
Humana Inc.
Louisville, KY

Eileen O'Riordan, MS, MBA, RN
Managing Editor, *Today's Executive
  Nurse Magazine*
Systems Manager, Washington Hospital
Fremont, CA

Rebecca M. Reynolds, MSN, RN
Director of Marketing and Resource
  Development
Instructor, Department of Psychiatry
  and Behavorial Sciences
Medical University of South Carolina
Charleston, SC

Reba Stephan Scharf, BSN, RN
Patient Educator
Rancocas Hospital
Willingboro, NJ

Lorraine C. Shoenly, MSN, RN, C,
  CCRN, CEN
Staff Development Instructor
Rancocas Hospital
Willingboro, NJ

Mary F. Spencer, MN, RN
Program Nurse Specialist
Department of Psychiatry and
  Behavorial Sciences
Medical University of South Carolina
Charleston, SC

Gail W. Stuart, PhD, RN, CS
Chief, Division of Psychiatric Nursing
Department of Psychiatry and
  Behavorial Sciences
Associate Professor, College of Nursing
  Graduate Program
Medical University of South Carolina
Charleston, SC

Nancie J. Thole, EdD, RN
Professor
Lewis University—College of Nursing
Romeoville, IL

Elizabeth L. Torresson, MSN, RN
Former President, Penn Recovery
  Systems, Inc.
Director of Medical Surgical Nursing
Rancocas Hospital and
  Zurbrugg Hospital
Willingboro and Riverside, NJ
Doctoral Candidate, Teachers College
Columbia University
New York, NY

Joan Trofino, EdD, RN, CNAA
Vice President, Patient Care Services
Riverview Medical Center
Red Bank, NJ

Ernestine B. Ware, BSN, RN
Head Nurse, Eating Disorder Program
Washington Hospital Center
Washington, DC

REFERENCES TO CASE STUDIES IN CHAPTERS 1–8

CHAPTERS

CASE STUDIES	1	2	3	4	5	6	7	8
1				X	X	X		
2					X			
3			X		X		X	
4	X	X				X		
5						X		
6	X	X				X		X
7		X						
8				X	X	X		
9	X		X	X	X	X		
10				X	X			
11			X	X	X			
12		X	X	X	X	X		
13			X		X	X		X
14			X		X			
15	X	X			X	X		
16	X							
17			X		X			
18		X	X			X		
19					X	X		
20				X				

FOREWORD

As economic factors have moved to center stage in health care delivery, nurses have found that they need more business acumen. Sometimes it seems that nurses spend more time talking budgets, productivity, and risk management than care, comfort, and concern for patients. One problem that nurses face when dealing with the new business orientation is that their education has so little prepared them for the task. In the best of all possible worlds, nurses would only need to know how to nurse; others would tend to the management side of health care provision. Whether the best of all possible worlds will ever exist is a moot question; today the nurse needs to learn the basics of business.

As nurses study the nature of health care as a business, they are quick to perceive the underlying value system: those who bring profits to the system are most valued. This idea is not really new; nurses have always known that physicians are valued because they bring paying patients to the institution. What is new is that nurses have realized how the system underappreciates their own contribution to fiscal solvency. Patients come to the institution, at least in part, because they need nursing care. Recognition of this factor has made nurses take a new look at their own contributions to the profitability of health care institutions.

In addition to seeking recognition for their contributions to the financial well-being of the health care business, nurses have come to see that, with a little initiative, their potential for income production can be enhanced. It was inevitable that nurses—as well as schools of nursing—would develop an interest in marketing.

While there are numerous excellent marketing texts available, few meet the special needs of nurses. Even those marketing texts directed toward the service sector or the health care sector tend to focus on problems of and models for other managers. Alward and Camuñas overcome that deficit with this book, specifically designed for the nurse marketer. This text provides the basic marketing terminology and concepts in a nursing context.

The nurse for whom marketing concepts are new will be assisted in application of the concepts by studying the case studies in the second half of this book. The cases demonstrate application of marketing principles in nursing projects, and range from excellent exemplars to good tries. The nurse can learn from the successes and even from the missed opportunities that may be recognized in the cases. They will help the reader to answer that hard question: "Yes, but what would it mean in a nursing situation?"

The book presents many different illustrations of nursing marketing. Indeed, the reader may be surprised to see the unique and creative ways in which marketing notions are being applied by practicing nurses. Perhaps the greatest service the book will provide is that of stimulating readers to think about previously unconsidered marketable skills, programs, or projects that exist or can be created in their own situations.

Barbara Stevens Barnum, PhD, RN, FAAN
Editor, *Nursing and Health Care*
Chairman, Barnum Communications, Inc.

ACKNOWLEDGMENTS

This book is the result of our effort to make marketing come alive as a nursing managment process that all nurses can use to enhance their practices. It would not have been possible without the assistance of others. We wish to acknowledge the important contribution to this book by the authors of the case studies. Their applications of marketing principles, through a variety of strategies and tactics, illustrate how useful the marketing process can be to the profession of nursing.

Our warmest thanks to Dr. Jorge Camuñas, whose assistance with the preparation of the manuscript was invaluable.

Ruth R. Alward
Caroline Camuñas

INTRODUCTION

Marketing can be thought of as a social and management process in which something of value is exchanged with another party. Many of the concepts of marketing theory and practice are familiar to nurses. Meeting patients' needs and individualizing service are basic values of the profession. Throughout our careers in clinical nursing practice, nursing administration, and nursing education, we have been applying marketing principles, although they were seldom identified as such. In the 1970s, we began to realize that marketing management was part of our professional environment, as the hospitals with whom we were affiliated began to develop marketing strategies.

It has been almost ten years since we were formally introduced to marketing concepts and their value to the nursing profession. Our appreciation for that excellent introduction goes to Barbara Stevens Barnum, who developed and taught a course entitled "Marketing Nursing Expertise" in the nursing graduate program at Teachers College, Columbia University, New York.

What has happened since then? Has the marketing process been accepted by our colleagues in administration, education, research, and clinical practice? What do we need to know about marketing and the management of this process to make it valued by the nursing profession in general? How is marketing being used by nurses throughout the country? This book is our answer to these important questions.

Marketing has become an accepted activity for administrators and practitioners in health care. This has occurred because of the constraints of a shrinking economy, scarce resources, prospective payment, technological innovations, and in general, having to do more with less. Led by business and the federal government, the public has said clearly that less of the nation's goods and services are to go to health care. Cost-containing measures such as prospective payment and managed care systems have mandated that administrators carefully assess the marketplace. Health care practitioners and administrators now look to see if they can use marketing not only more effectively than in the past, but also better than the competition.

Nurses must be able to apply marketing strategies to their daily practice. They must be able to do this well to benefit their organizations, themselves, and, ultimately, consumers of health care, both individually and collectively. In the long run, society as a whole will benefit from cost-effective health care and services that suit the needs of more people.

Basic marketing texts are written for marketing managers primarily in for-profit consumer goods industries, although recent editions generally have a chapter devoted to service and nonprofit organizations. Nurses are required to make an extra effort to translate the concepts presented in these texts, not only to nonprofit organizations, but also to nursing service organizations. It is time-consuming for the nurse to generalize, see relationships, and translate concepts to health care and nursing. This should not be required of the nurse, who is so busy and at the same time eager to learn and use what marketing offers. This book is an appropriate resource for applications of marketing theory and strategies to health care and nursing.

Nurse executives, middle and first-line managers, staff educators, nurse entrepreneurs, and practitioners in hospitals, community agencies, long-term care facilities, and private practice will find marketing concepts useful. The concepts will also be applicable by nursing school deans and faculty, for their recruitment and faculty practice programs. The book can also be used as a text for graduate students in nursing administration programs: as a basic textbook for a marketing course and as a supplemental text for administration courses. Other health care managers without knowledge of marketing theory and strategies may also find it useful.

The book is divided into two parts. In Part 1, marketing as a nursing management process is discussed. Chapter 1 describes the necessity of marketing management for the nurse in today's health care environment. Basic marketing concepts and philosophies are presented in Chapter 2. A discussion of nursing's customers follows in Chapter 3. An introduction to marketing research was included (Chapter 4), although consultants and advanced research skills may be necessary in many situations. Several chapters (5, 6, and 7) are devoted to marketing strategies. No nursing marketing book would be complete without addressing the issue of ethics (Chapter 8). Throughout Part 1, marketing philosophy, as well as the concepts and tools necessary for this management process, are presented. This provides the foundation necessary to become a successful nurse marketer.

Part 2 is marketing in action. Examples of how nurses and allied professionals have used marketing concepts for solving marketing problems are presented by contributing authors. For example, marketing theory and strategies are used to address challenges in recruitment and retention, social marketing, community health, ambulatory and inpatient services, staff development, and nursing education. A few examples of the use of market research methods are included. Case studies are not segregated by the markets they address, because in most cases several markets were targeted rather than only patients, only physicians, or only nurses. We refer to the marketing cases throughout Part 1. A chart of case studies that illustrate concepts in each chapter is located on page xii.

The cases have strengths and weaknesses in their design and execution. Although they are not perfect models of the marketing process, they can be used for discussion and evaluation in many nursing service and education forums. They serve as units of analysis for the student of marketing. It is clear from the variety of applications that the use of marketing strategies is an important addition to the nurse's knowledge base and skills.

Ruth R. Alward
Caroline Camuñas

PART I

Marketing Theory
and Techniques

CHAPTER 1

The Necessity of Marketing Management for Nursing

Why is there increasing pressure on nurses to know about marketing? Marketing has been around for a long time, but only recently have marketing strategies been used by nonprofit organizations and health care organizations. By necessity, hospitals began using marketing heavily in the early 1980s. In nursing, Alward (1983a, 1983b) published articles urging nurse administrators to use marketing theory to the good of the patient, the nurse, and the organization. Effective marketing is necessary whenever there is a highly competitive, resource-constrained environment. These terms certainly describe nursing and health care today.

Kotler (1988, p. 3) quotes a marketing scholar who defined *marketing* as "the creation and delivery of a standard of living." By applying marketing theory, the nurse manager can meet patient needs in a cost-effective way. The problems confronting nursing and health care are deep, difficult, and prevalent throughout the system. None of the problems are going to go away by themselves, nor are they amenable to quick-fix solutions. Marketing is not fad management. It is a combination of social, economic, and management theory applied in special ways to meet needs. With skillful application, marketing can help raise the standard of health care by its emphasis on consumer needs, patient outcomes, and quality of service.

As early as 1969, Kotler and Levy were advocating the use of marketing by nonprofit organizations. They maintained that marketing goes beyond sales, influence, and persuasion to the meeting of needs. In order to meet consumer needs, organizations must have a consumer orientation. An organization cannot avoid marketing; whether to do marketing well or poorly is the choice.

Subsequently, Kotler published *Marketing for Nonprofit Organizations* in 1975. By the time of publication of the third edition (Kotler & Andreasen, 1987), it was no longer necessary for him to proselytize. Health care organizations, along with higher education, had recognized the benefits of marketing. Today, 91% of all United States hospitals have marketing programs and spend a total of $1.6 billion ("Ailing Hospital Ads," 1989). There is now competition among these institutions to use marketing effectively. In health care throughout the world, marketing is

3

now seen as an essential management process. As a significant part of health care organizations, nursing must meet this challenge and use the concepts, functions, and tools of marketing on a daily basis—and must use them effectively.

HISTORICAL PERSPECTIVE

A widely held belief is that marketing is a recent phenomenon, dating from the 1950s. This belief maintains that major developments occur suddenly and have few antecedents. It describes a progression from the production era (1870–1930), to the sales era (1930–1950), and finally to the marketing era in 1950.

Fullerton (1988) presents convincing evidence of the untenability of this framework. Marketing did not develop out of the blue. For example, during the so-called production era, Henry Ford, an innovator of mass production, insisted on offering only black cars. This is often cited as indifference to consumers' wants. However, it was an effort to keep production costs down in order to meet the market's strongest need, which was an affordable, reliable automobile. Ford was aware that there were other tastes; in 1920, he bought the Lincoln Motor Company to satisfy them. Likewise, successful businessmen of the so-called sales era survived the Depression because they knew that it was more important than ever to understand and satisfy buyer wants and needs. They had to be oriented to the consumer. Buyer orientation was the foundation of the two most significant marketing innovations of the 1930s. These innovations, the supermarket and the "consumer engineering movement," had lasting effects on marketing. The consumer engineering movement meant meeting consumer needs by first carefully researching consumer needs and then either designing new or redesigning existing products to meet those needs. Supermarkets attracted customers with low prices, a benefit of self-service. See Exhibit 1.1 for the eras of the development of modern marketing posited by Fullerton.

Today, marketing is of interest in all kinds and sizes of organizations and in political systems. Marketing is used by service industries as well as by those producing goods and ideas. It is used by for-profit, nonprofit, and public agencies. Communist countries are adopting and increasing marketing to revive their stagnant economies and meet their citizens' needs and wants. Socialized health care systems are turning to marketing to increase efficiency and effectiveness (Lohr, 1988).

In general, for-profit industries and companies invested heavily in marketing earlier than did the nonprofits. Marketing was begun first and spread fastest in consumer packaged goods industries. Companies such as Proctor & Gamble, Coca-Cola, General Electric, and General Motors were among the leaders. Commodity industries such as steel, chemical, and paper turned to marketing much later. Many of these companies are still not using marketing as well as they could. Consumer service firms, especially airlines and banks, are now using marketing

EXHIBIT 1-1   Development of Modern Marketing

The Era of Antecedents

Began about 1500 in Britain; 1600s in Germany; with settlement in North America.

Characteristics: The idea of capitalism was just beginning. The dominant value system had little respect for commerce. Most of the population (75–90%) was self-sufficient, rural, and resistant to any increase in low levels of consumption. However, businesspeople did find markets for luxury goods among the nobility and the small middle class (10–25% of the population), for armaments among governments, and for textiles and a few staples. As capitalism gained form and spread, profit-making commerce became respectable. Early forms of important distribution channels developed, such as retail shops, wholesale trade, and traveling salespeople. Banks and stock exchanges, with their equities, paper money, and credit instruments, also appeared.

The Era of Origins

Britain about 1750–1850; Germany and the United States about 1830–1870.

Characteristics: The Industrial Revolution, coupled with highly aggressive attitudes of capitalism, brought pervasive attention to stimulating and meeting demand among nearly all of society. Improvements in production and transportation, as well as tradition-breaking migration, brought increased marketing activities.

The Era of Institutional Development

Britain 1850–1929; Germany and the United States 1870-1929.

Characteristics: Previous eras' changes in production and transportation called for changes in marketing practices. By now, most of the major industries had formed. Mass production required stimulation of demand. Advertising, market research, improved distribution, and expanded retailing made marketing prevalent in society.

The Era of Refinement and Formalization

From 1930 to present in Britain, Germany, and the United States.

Characteristics: Development, refinement, and formalization of industries and marketing practices took place. Distribution became more sophisticated. Market research used improved methods of gathering, measuring, and evaluating information. A large body of marketing data became available. Evidence of lapses in the use of marketing is seen in the German camera industry, and in the United States and British auto industries. Marketing in nonprofit organizations is a phenomenon of the last two decades, with widespread use by hospitals in the 1980s.

Source: Adapted with permission from "How Modern is Modern Marketing? Marketing's Evolution and the Myth of the 'Production Era,' " by R.A. Fullerton, 1988, *Journal of Marketing, 52* (1), 108–25.

extensively, although this has occurred during the past 10 years. Insurance and stock brokerage companies are beginning to use marketing, but, like commodities, they are not yet applying marketing as effectively as possible.

Many foreign companies are now using marketing more effectively than are United States firms. Multinational firms are spreading the use of marketing throughout the world. Smaller companies are finding it necessary to employ these strategies in order to compete in their domestic markets.

Traditionally, marketing has had a bad reputation in socialist countries. Marketing runs counter to their economic theories. However, in the 1970s, the USSR had over 100 state-operated marketing research and advertising firms (Greer, 1973). Under Mikhail Gorbachev's policies of *perestroika* and *glasnost*, marketing is now undergoing broad expansion. Many types of marketing strategies are being used extensively. In Eastern Europe, Romania and Hungary have used marketing for some time (Naor, 1986). Several socialist universities teach marketing.

Nonprofit organizations are facing major problems. Institutions of higher learning, health care, and culture are all turning to marketing for help in survival and for finding answers to their major problems. Less than a decade ago, fewer than 1% of hospitals had directors of marketing. Now, over 40% have a marketing director. Government agencies are also using marketing. Both the United States Postal Service and Amtrak have extensively researched marketing plans to gain customers. The United States Army spends large sums on its marketing program. Other government agencies are using social marketing for antismoking and antidrug campaigns. Unfortunately, their budgets fall short of the money needed or the billions spent by the cigarette companies.

In the late 1970s, the courts struck down professional associations' prohibitions on member advertising to solicit clients. As a result, professionals, including physicians, dentists, lawyers, and nurses, are now allowed to price competitively and to advertise aggressively. This has awakened the interest of these service providers in the use of marketing strategies and tactics. Some health care providers are now using marketing very effectively to improve their relationships with consumers and to increase their share of the available market.

FACTORS AGAINST THE WORKING OF THE MARKETPLACE IN HEALTH CARE

The free market usually produces high-quality goods and services efficiently. However, in health care, four factors militate against the forces of the free market, and have led to regulation of health care. These factors are: (1) imperfect information; (2) third-party payers; (3) gatekeepers; and (4) forced purchase.

Imperfect Information

Optimal solutions to resource allocation problems are brought about in markets when consumers have complete and accurate information about the products they are purchasing. In particular, they must know about the quality and how it compares with similar products. Purchasers of health care generally have limited, inaccurate, or misleading information about the kind and quality of service available and required. Frequently they are forced to make decisions about the purchase while under stress, and have no time to compare services. For instance, when a person has a heart attack on the way to work in the morning, instructions to the ambulance driver will be to go to the nearest emergency room. Little thought is given to the kind or quality of medical or nursing care provided at the nearest hospital. The patient assumes that the hospital will be able to provide the necessary care. In other situations, the patient may have no choice, because there is only one facility in town. Rarely does the consumer of health care have the necessary information to make a discriminating and rational choice.

It is for this reason that people are urged to find a health care provider—physician or nurse practitioner—before they have an acute illness. Because stress levels are not as high, they are better able to evaluate the performance of the provider, and this helps them to make more rational choices. An added benefit, of course, is that the provider gets to know them too.

Third-Party Payers

A major factor in decisions about purchase in the general, free marketplace is price. Price influences when, where, and how a product or service will be bought. This does not occur as directly in health care. Seventy percent of health care costs are paid for by government or private insurers. Because of these third-party payers, the consumer and the provider have less incentive to keep costs down. However, federal, state, and local governments, as well as employers, are now leading the way to control health care costs. Prominent mechanisms are to use preferred provider organizations (PPO), health maintenance organizations (HMO), and prospective payment programs based on Diagnostic Related Groups (DRGs).

Gatekeepers

In a typical market transaction, the consumer decides when to buy a product, how much to buy, and for how long to continue buying it. This is not the case in health care. It is often the providers (physician, nurse, case worker) and insurance policy provisions that determine the quantity, quality, and duration of service. The *gatekeeper* is a person or organization that limits options available but does not make the decision for the consumer. The law of supply and demand that characterizes other markets is not widespread in health care.

Forced Purchase

Purchasing health care is often not an elective decision. Many, if not most, of the purchases of health care are made under much duress, because of the nature of the condition requiring attention. Persons who sustain a head injury, a heart attack, or a diabetic coma require immediate health care. There is little choice; they need health care whether or not they can afford it.

THE RISE OF CONSUMERISM

Since the late 1950s, when the rise of consumerism began, American businesses have had to pay attention to demands for product safety, information, choice, and the opportunity for consumers to voice their concerns. The environmental changes that brought about the movement included better educated consumers, more complex and hazardous products, and disillusionment and dissatisfaction with American institutions. Packard (1957), Galbraith (1958), and Carson (1962) wrote popular books accusing big business of wasteful, dangerous, and manipulative activities. Congressional investigation led to indictments and the passage of legislation to protect consumers. Ralph Nader became the leader of the movement. Since then, many private consumer groups have been formed, and state and local offices of consumer affairs have been created. The movement is international. Scandinavia, Belgium, and The Netherlands have strong advocate groups; those in France, Japan, and Germany are growing.

Kotler (1988, p. 142) defines *consumerism* as "an organized movement of citizens and government to strengthen the rights and power of buyers in relation to sellers." Consumerism has an impact on virtually every business activity, from starting the business to marketing, consumer purchase, product use, and post-purchase satisfaction. A company is forced to see things from the consumers' point of view. Consumerists have proposed and achieved much protection for buyers. Some achievements include: truth-in-lending laws, ensuring the opportunity to know the true interest cost of a loan; unit pricing, requiring the posting of the true cost per standard unit; ingredient and nutritional labeling, listing basic ingredients and the nutritional quality of food; open dating, ensuring the freshness of products; and truth-in-advertising laws, requiring the accurate representation of products.

In health care, consumerism has had a major effect on the quality of care. Ombudspersons serve to protect patients in hospitals. It is now mandatory that the Patients' Bill of Rights be shared with every patient on entry into a health care facility. The government, through the Food and Drug Administration (FDA), assesses medical products and drugs to screen out those that are potentially hazardous, and penalizes companies that do not comply or meet standards.

Most companies have, in principle, accepted consumerism. Many recognize and accept the consumer's right to information and protection. Kotler (1988, p. 143) maintains that consumerism "is actually the ultimate expression" of the marketing orientation. It forces companies to be more consumer centered. Overlooked consumer needs and wants can be identified by consumerist scrutiny. The manager who chooses to look for opportunities as a result of consumerism will find them.

Special Interest Groups

Special interest groups are defined by Adrian and Press (1969, pp. 208, 209) as "a collection of individuals who on the basis of one or more shared attitudes . . . makes certain claims upon other groups in society for the establishment, maintenance or enhancement of forms of behavior that are implied in the shared attitudes." They are capable of exerting political pressure. The rise of consumerism brought about the general public's, the media's, and the politician's skeptical perception that special interest groups look out for themselves.

Professional associations are perceived by the public as special interest groups. Some well-known special interest groups are the National Organization for Women (NOW), the Gray Panthers, the National Association for the Advancement of Colored People (NAACP), the American Medical Association (AMA), and the American Nurses' Association (ANA). Most, if not all, of these associations have political action committees (PACs) to promote their interests. During the past two decades, PACs have increased in number and power. PACs lobby government officials on areas of special concern to them, such as consumer rights, women's rights, minority rights, and so forth. Some industries, such as tobacco and defense, have powerful PACs; the AMA and the ANA also have PACs in Washington to influence legislation. There is increasing concern about possible undue influence of PACs on legislation. As a result, contributions to PACs are not tax-deductible. The amount of money PACs can spend supporting politicians has also been limited to some degree.

Environmentalism

"*Environmentalism* is an organized movement of concerned citizens and government to protect and enhance people's living environment" (Kotler, 1988, p. 152; emphasis added). Environmentalists are concerned with land erosion, strip mining, forest depletion, factory emissions, acid rain, the ozone layer, billboards, litter, and radioactive fallout; and with the health problems caused by food sprayed with chemicals and polluted or contaminated earth, air, and water. They are concerned with life quality now and for future generations.

Considered by some to be more critical of marketing than consumerists, environmentalists complain of too much wasteful packaging. Developed societies produce so much trash that we are running out of ways to dispose of it. Countries are exporting trash! Recall the New York garbage barge that wandered for weeks in the summer of 1987 looking for a place to unload. In 1988, an Italian ship had a load of toxic waste and no place to leave it. France, Germany, and Switzerland are sending hazardous waste to Africa for disposal.

A major problem is that much of our trash is not biodegradable. Plastic is man-made, and nothing in nature will change or decompose current plastics (Sadun, Webster, & Commoner, 1990). Much of the plastic we make—our pens, fast-food containers, syringes, blood bags, and IV tubings—will be found intact in trash heaps by anthropologists in 10,000 years. Consider how much nonbiodegradable trash is generated by one operating room in one day, or even the amount caused by the insertion of one indwelling catheter. Although hospitals have begun to use disposables because of the savings in central supply costs of cleaning and preparing sterile supplies, the societal costs on the environment are ignored.

Improper disposal of wastes is also a problem. Worldwide, our trash is killing fish and animals in our oceans. Beaches are strewn with international as well as local litter. During the summer of 1988, many East Coast beaches were closed because of hazardous medical waste that had come in with the tides. Private haulers were at fault in most cases. However, a few of the problems started in the laboratories or units where needles, syringes, blood tubes, and blood bags were disposed of improperly. Nurses must be aware that failure to follow established procedures can have an impact that is not readily imagined.

THE CHANGING ENVIRONMENT

Until the recent past, nurses have been ardent proponents of social change. Seeing the often horrendous conditions under which people lived and worked, nurses such as Lillian Wald, Lavinia Dock, Harriet Tubman, Margaret Sanger, and Florence Nightingale fought for political, social, and environmental change. Now nurses witness the negative effects of all aspects of the environment on society every day and do too little to influence change. Chopoorian (1986) suggests that nurses must now reconceptualize the environment and develop strategies to modify it. Marketing strategies can help all nurses manage the environment for societal good.

Economic Change

Because of the profession's origins in the military and the church, nurses have not, until recently, been overly concerned with many aspects of nursing economics. Nursing has been seen by society as women's work; this resulted in low pay for long, hard work. Dedication was a hallmark. As a calling, nursing consistently put society's needs ahead of its own. For example, the movement of the patient from the home to the hospital during World War I, the development of functional nursing during World War II, and the creation of the licensed practical nurse (LPN) and associate degree (AD) programs were all aimed at providing more nursing care at less cost.

In the 1960s and early 1970s, the economy was expanding. Management in health care was significantly easier than it is now. All of the disciplines, including nursing, were expanding with little difficulty. Efficient and inefficient systems were rewarded in the same way; that is, by cost reimbursement of usual, customary, and reasonable charges. By 1980, over 10% of the gross national product (GNP) was going to health care as a result of the runaway expense of the system. Rigorous constraints were placed on the system by federal government in 1983; the American taxpayer had said, "Enough." The health care system had to control its costs.

Prospective payment systems have changed the way hospitals view the services they provide. Using DRGs, the price of an individual patient's hospital stay is predetermined and, within specified parameters, varies little according to resource consumption. DRGs encourage decreased length of hospitalization. As a result, patients in hospital are sicker, are discharged earlier than ever before, and require more care at home. This places stress on community nurse services as well as on hospital nursing staffs. Hospitals are financially stressed because some DRG reimbursement rates do not cover full costs, particularly for those who receive the most care (generally, these are the oldest and the sickest patients). There are patient segments that are universally problematic because of the financial burden they place on hospitals. Yet, ethically we must find some way to provide needed care.

Hospitals are experiencing a decline in inpatient revenue because of a combination of the following factors. The average revenue per patient day has gone down, due to the dramatic growth of HMOs and PPOs, a decrease in hospital-based diagnostic tests as a result of cost-containment measures, and prospective payment policies (DRGs). There has been a drop in the number of admissions per year, because of managed care systems. To drive down hospitalization, presurgical second opinions and preadmission approvals are required prior to admission by HMOs, PPOs, and other third-party payers. The declining size of certain patient segments, such as obstetrics and pediatrics, has also reduced revenues. In addition, the average length of stay has declined, because of federal and other third-party payer initiatives that penalize hospitals for keeping patients longer than statistical guidelines suggest. Under DRGs, hospitals are looking to strike a balance between profitable and unprofitable categories of patients.

With less money available, competition for the scarce health care dollar is increasing dramatically. Nursing must be able to compete in a newly pricesensitive world. The medical profession no longer dominates health care, although it remains a primary gatekeeper. The buyer, who most often is a third-party payer, has a predominant role through reimbursement in the selection of health care providers. This distinction is critically important (McNerney, 1988). Nurses must learn to create and develop systems that meet the needs and wants of customers. There is not a purely financial bottom line; nurses must successfully manage quality, ethics, and finances.

The economic changes that have occurred over the past 10 to 20 years have had profound, world-wide effects on health care. No longer can third-party payers, whether governments or insurance companies, afford to provide unlimited care whenever and wherever it is desired. Marketing can help determine some of the aspects of health care most important to the consumer and help provide information needed to make informed decisions.

Demographic Change

Demography is concerned with the internal and external dynamics of population. Marketing, using a demographic perspective, goes beyond characteristics of population by connecting demographic change with marketing decisions (Pol, 1986). Nurses must be able to deal with these factors in developing useful, effective programs to meet these varied needs.

The characteristics of the American population are undergoing changes that will have profound effects upon the delivery of health care. Aging of the population is one change that has major consequences. In 1980, 25 million people, or 11% of the population, were over the age of 65 in the United States. The United States Department of Health and Human Services, Health Care Financing Administration (US DHHS, HCFA, 1981) projects that by the year 2030, 55 million people, or 22% of the population, will be over the age of 65.

As the size of the over-65 population increases, the number of people 80 and over also increases. In the next 15 years, there will be a 67% increase in this group (see Table 1-1). The significance of this is that the very old use the health care system more, because of their great incidence of chronic disease and functional impairment. They also are more likely to require assistance because of limited income, death of a spouse, or lack of family.

Coupled with the aging of the population is a long-term health care system that is inadequate to meet the needs of the elderly, disabled, mentally ill, retarded, or chemically dependent. Creative and innovative solutions must be found to meet these long-term care needs. Marketing management can help to find answers, such as day care centers for the elderly and ambulatory care for substance abuse patients. Torresson discusses marketing an ambulatory substance abuse program in Case Study 16.

TABLE 1.1   The Aging Population with Functional Disability

Age Group	Percentage with some functional disability	Number of persons in age group
65-74	38.6%	14,259,000
75-84	48.4%	6,652,000
85 & older	63.2%	1,354,000

Source: United States Department of Human Services, Health Care Financing Administration (1981). *Long-term care: Background and future directions.* Washington DC: Author.

There are other demographic trends that portend a need for marketing. Because of the low birth rates since the end of the baby boom in the 1960s, demographers are now predicting a shortage of workers at all levels. Schools of higher education are already faced with declining enrollments. Educators as well as those in other professions will have to work harder and smarter to recruit students. In Case Study 15, Thole gives an example of the marketing strategies used by a nursing school to increase enrollment by targeting a specific registered nurse population.

Most women work. This is not going to change. The demand for child care is rising, and certainly was already an issue in the 1988 presidential campaign. Because 97% of nurses are women, lack of affordable child care has an impact on the profession. Eli Ginzberg (1987), in stating that nursing lacks professionalism because of the number of nurses working part-time, forgets that child care is a problem for nurses and women. Marketing strategies are needed to develop good and affordable child care programs, such as day care for sick children, that will encourage nurses to remain employed.

Yet another change is seen in the country of origin for the 600,000 immigrants who enter the United States each year. Most immigrants are now from the Third World countries of Latin America and Asia. What are the ramifications for health care? On the whole this is unknown. These population segments are a vast resource from which to recruit students for nursing schools and workers for hospitals.

Political Change

Any environment that is fraught with competition for scarce resources is bound to be highly political. Marketing research can assist nurses in dealing with highly political situations by providing a strong, factual base for coping with this competitive environment. These facts can suggest potent strategies and tactics for effective marketing plans.

Inequities and difficult access to care are common criticisms of the health care system. The majority of Americans want a free enterprise system. A minority are calling for socialized medicine, as they have been since the 1950s. The characteristics of the present health care system already lie somewhere between these two extremes. Because of the failings of the current system, a new format should be developed. It will take great creativity and much political skill to devise a system capable of meeting the needs of all Americans that can still meet economic and ideological requirements.

Institutional politics are another fact of life. Nursing has had to deal with the political clout of medicine for years. However, this is becoming more difficult, as medicine is being threatened by increased regulation to control costs and quality. No longer can the physician merely request the latest in technology and see it appear. Although expenditures for health care are still growing, physicians' portions are endangered. In fact, AMA's poorly conceived plan to relieve the nursing shortage by creating the registered care technologist (RCT) may be an attempt to assert power. Creating a low-level worker could be seen as a way to put off giving up any of the physicians' share of the total health care dollars to upgrade nurses' salaries.

The recent plethora of books on power and politics attests to the importance of politics as a fact of life for nurses. (A list of books and readings on power and politics in nursing can be found at the end of this chapter.) Nurses must develop skills to cope constructively with this aspect of the environment. They and their managers have the responsibility to negotiate with *savoir faire* in order to meet the needs and wants of consumers. In Case Study 9, Johnston successfully managed institutional politics to the good of all concerned.

Technological Change

Much is written on technology in the professional and lay presses, and much appears on television about this subject. Advances in technology have profound effects upon our lives, and the chances are that the growth of technology will not slow.

It is incumbent on society, and nursing, to apply marketing to technological advances for the benefit of society. However, Hayes and Abernathy (1980) disagree that marketing is useful, stating that "inventors, scientists, engineers, and academics in the normal pursuit of scientific knowledge gave the world in recent times the laser, instant photography, and the transistor. In contrast, worshippers of the marketing concept have bestowed upon mankind such products as newfangled potato chips, feminine hygiene deodorant, and the pet rock" (p.70). Sanchez (1985, p.72) counters that "scientists . . . have also given us nuclear weapons, environmental pollution, and ICBM's. Marketers also have given us fresh fruit and produce during the winter, products we can afford, and access to goods produced all over the world." The very important point that Sanchez makes is that the marketing process guides technology and the use of other resources to satisfy consumers. We agree that the impetus to produce new products comes from identifying the needs, wants, and preferences of buyers.

Advances in technology literally changed nurses' work and the care patients receive. This is very obvious in the care of the surgical patient. For instance, thirty years ago patients having a cataract extraction had to endure two weeks of bed rest; sandbags were placed around the patient's head to restrict movement, and both eyes were covered. Any movement could cause stress on the suture line; complications leading to loss of vision could result. Recovery was an extremely difficult time for the patient. Today, because of technological advances, cataract extraction is routinely done on an outpatient basis. Most patients prefer the minimum time spent in a health care facility, and the new approach was marketed successfully because of this preference.

Technological changes in health care often require modification in managerial systems as well as in nursing care. The implementation of outpatient surgery programs, and the model for a kidney transplant program described by Davis in Case Study 4, are examples of management systems changed because of technology. Without the technology, the programs could not have been developed. Marketing is needed to make the most of these advances.

In addition to planning health care programs based on the needs of clients, the nurse also is a patient advocate. In the role of an advocate, nurses help patients become aware of the proliferating choices in the health care marketplace to satisfy needs and wants. With the use of marketing, these programs can also be cost-effective. For example, a nurse might help a patient with an eating disorder or substance abuse problem choose between inpatient and outpatient treatment.

Legal Change

Legislation affecting business and marketing has been enacted for three major reasons: to protect companies from one another; to protect consumers from unfair business practices; and to protect the public interest. Similarly, health care legislation has been passed to protect health care providers from unfair competition, to protect consumers from unscrupulous professional practices, and to protect the public interest.

Competitiveness is the underlying force that brings about the need for legislation to protect business from itself. Some firms, if unregulated, would make shoddy products, advertise falsely, and cheat through their pricing and packaging. Definition and prevention of unfair competition, and protection of consumers, are the goals of legislation in this area. The laws are enforced by the Federal Trade Commission, the Food and Drug Administration, and the Antitrust Division of the Justice Department.

Governmental protection of the interests of society against detrimental business practices exists in order to maintain an acceptable quality of life. Examples of business behavior necessitating protective laws are frequently in the news, with firms illegally dumping toxic wastes in neighborhood dumps and landfills, or hazardous hospital wastes in the ocean. The Love Canal situation is a prime example of pollution by industry and a government-enforced cleanup. Businesses must take responsibility for social costs of all goods and services produced, and in fact most routinely do so.

Government regulations are essential information for marketers in all fields. They must have this information when planning products and programs. Regulations and their enforcement, especially in health care, will continue to increase.

Social Change

The social environment has undergone fundamental changes in the past 30 years. Consider the statistics that one hears so frequently: the high incidence of divorce; single-parent households; child, spouse, and elder abuse; hunger; homelessness; unemployment; sexism; racism; ageism; and the lack of schooling and health care. Nurses value highly the health and welfare of all people, yet they exert little influence on the development of economic, labor, foreign, health, education, and other policies. An emphasis in nursing has been placed on the person's psychosocial response to these problems, not on the root causes of the problems. Social problems are indeed massive, and may seem overwhelming. Marketing theory can enable nurses to effect social change for the good of both patients and society. Two examples of social marketing are found in Case Studies 4 and 6, in which Davis discusses marketing strategies in an organ donation program, and Frost describes how society's understanding of nursing was improved through a Down Syndrome respite program.

CRITICISMS OF MARKETING

For many people the very term *marketing* conjures up negative scenarios. Marketing is often equated with high-pressure sales, manipulation, and the promotion of low-quality products. We think this is a limited and narrow view; marketing is more than the promotional efforts of persuasion and sales. The major criticisms of marketing are described below.

Waste of Money

A common criticism of marketing by health care providers is that it wastes scarce health care dollars. This is especially true in relation to nonprofit organizations. Health care professionals are very wary of hospitals spending money on advertising. They point out that hospitals, especially large medical centers, functioned well in the past without marketing or advertising. The need is not seen as a priority because hospitals seem so busy. Staff physicians, nurses, and others at The Mount Sinai Hospital in New York felt that the television campaign was a waste of money because their beds were filled. Promotion of outpatient clinics and the physician referral service were not seen as vital to the organization's well-being, nor was promotion of the hospital's image thought to be important. People working at an institution often forget the need to keep a positive reputation before the public in order to remain attractive.

O'Connor argues that marketing is best applied to inexpensive, frequently purchased basic products such as soap, staple foods, pet food, and the like. He believes that marketing is "irrelevant or not applicable" to hospitals (O'Connor, 1985, p. 53) other than for marketing research and new product development. Others counter that marketing strategies helped these products meet customer needs and thus produce successes (Anderson & Near, 1985; Sanchez, 1985). While it is true that research and new product development have been the most visible functions of marketing, they are not the only strategies that can be used successfully. As marketing in health care matures and develops, other marketing processes, including those of promotion, pricing, and distribution, will grow in visibility and importance (Anderson & Near, 1985; Droste, 1988; Sanchez, 1985).

Intrusion

Many people are critical of marketing because it intrudes upon their lives. One route of intrusion is through market research. In any industry, marketing research invades individuals' lives by asking about personal characteristics, beliefs, values, attitudes, likes and dislikes, needs, and wants. The linkage of marketing research with health care is likely to increase the perceived personal nature of the questions. In addition, people are wary because computers facilitate easy access to such information, and can contribute to breaches of privacy, anonymity, and confidentiality.

Questions perceived as intrusive may be necessary when doing market research for a health care service. It is easy to see a source of concern in questions concerning sexual history, alcohol and controlled substance use and abuse, and communicable disease history, especially concerning AIDS, hepatitis B, and venereal disease. This information has the potential to ruin personal lives and shatter careers. The more sensitive the material, the more reluctant the participant in market research.

Promotion is another very intrusive part of marketing. The public complains consistently about its constant exposure to promotional materials in both electronic and print media, and in junk mail. Especially offensive are some of the health-related commercials seen on television, for example, those for over-the-counter hemorrhoidal preparations. Often the content, format, and timing are objectionable.

The American Cancer Society's early promotion of breast self-examination was met with high resistance. Women did not want to acknowledge that breast cancer was a possibility, and so reacted negatively. On the other hand, the social marketing done by antismoking groups still triumphs over the marketing of cigarettes by tobacco companies in this country.

Manipulation

Some feel that marketing is manipulative, especially social marketing (see Chapter 2). Initially, many smokers felt that the antismoking campaign mounted by the American Cancer Society was manipulating them through fear. However, this has abated, as social changes in American society increasingly make smoking an unacceptable behavior to an ever-growing majority. The change has been so fundamental and so pervasive that laws limiting smoking to specific areas passed without difficulty, and require little or no enforcement ("New York," 1988).

Health care organizations generally develop programs that serve the public good. However, nurses and others must be aware of the possibility of program marketing being seen as manipulative. They must be attuned to manipulation and avoid its use in promoting programs. In the long run, manipulation will hurt the organization.

Low Quality

Another concern is that marketing will lower the quality of health care. Until recently, hucksters, quacks, flim-flam artists, and peddlers of snake oil and cure-alls advertised; professionals and hospitals did not. The connotation is that health care providers who advertise are deceptive and incompetent. If they were other-wise, they would not need to advertise. These are real concerns. However, using marketing is not a test of competence. Safeguards must be in place to deal with incompetence whether or not marketing is employed.

Deceptive advertising in health care must be dealt with in the same way other industries have handled it. Promotional efforts must be monitored for truthful and fair representation of services and products offered. There are systems in place to deal with this problem: witness the FDA's intervention in the advertising of cosmetics purporting to reverse aging.

Competition

Some have criticized marketing because it increases competition in the health care field. However, factors other than marketing have influenced this increase. Competition, although present, was less overt in health care until the early 1980s. Health care providers—nurses, physicians, and administrators—often denied that there was even a possibility of competition among them. Financial constraints changed this stance when DRGs were implemented, beginning October 1983. A reduced length of stay for inpatients led to decreasing occupancy rates and increased competition among health care providers. Now health care institutions and professionals aggressively compete.

Nursing is faced with increased competition on all levels. The current nursing shortage is a result, in part, of competition for students. Women are no longer restricted to nursing and teaching for careers. Schools of nursing must compete for the brightest and most talented, along with other professions. No longer do nursing schools have a captive audience from which to recruit. Compounding the difficulty of recruitment are some of the socioeconomic problems of nursing, including image, status, and salaries. Further increasing the competition for students is the decrease in the number of college-age students. Competition is so acute that some schools of nursing have had to close because of low enrollments. Nurse educators have to market their programs aggressively (see Case Study 15 for one example). Sophisticated marketing strategies are essential to develop and promote innovative programs in both nursing service and education.

Hospital nursing departments must also market aggressively to recruit nurses. Competition is so keen in recruitment and retention that we had difficulty finding contributors who were allowed by their institutions to write case studies on the subject! Based on demographics and on the increase in technology, the need for nurses is going to continue, as will the competition for them. Nurses must have marketing skills to cope with, and make the most of, these problems and opportunities.

The competition for patients is also in earnest. Patients bring scarce dollars to an organization. Therefore, institutions must keep their beds filled, or their services used, in a way that will maximize reimbursement. However, it is shortsighted to focus only on census. Skillful marketing can increase effective use of resources by maximizing the level of consumer satisfaction.

Because of the proliferation of options, patients are now able to make more informed choices in health care than ever before. If a given institution does not provide services that the patient wants, the patient can, and will, go elsewhere. An institution can no longer assume that the patient will stay out of loyalty or because of the physicians on staff. Patients are choosing organizations based on the perception of the quality of care delivered (Boscarino, 1988). Major portions of their assessments are grounded in the quality of nursing care.

Although it was rarely acknowledged, competition was widespread even before marketing was used. For example, funding for research and for programs such as dialysis and renal transplant centers, neonatal intensive care units, and burn units was highly competitive, as was attracting philanthropists, nurses, and patients. Marketing can assist nurses in developing effective and efficient competitive strategies. It should also help to determine when to discontinue a service, thus preventing use of resources for activities that will not achieve the nurse's or organization's goals.

Unnecessary Demand

Some fear that the use of marketing will create a demand for unnecessary services. Unnecessary use of health care services already exists, however. Excessive surgeries on many patient segments are well documented, as are other abuses in health care. In fact, unnecessary usage is so widespread that utilization review,

Peer Review Organizations (PROs), second opinion programs, and DRGs have been established to cope with the problem.

In the general marketplace, price is the prime regulator of demand. Requiring the patient to pay for a larger portion of health services (other than for catastrophic illness) has been found to decrease unnecessary use. This is already occurring in Medicare and private insurance programs, through increasing deductibles and premiums. Unfortunately, some patients who should seek care will hesitate because of cost, and thereby suffer serious consequences.

BENEFITS OF MARKETING

Marketing helps manage the exchange of goods and services in a more effective and efficient manner. Kotler and Clarke (1987) cite three major benefits of marketing for health care organizations and their publics: increased satisfaction of consumers, improved attraction of resources, and improved organizational efficiency. Because marketing stresses satisfaction of consumer needs and wants, it tends to produce increased satisfaction and higher quality of service.

Improved attraction of resources is important to the survival of health care organizations. The current nursing shortage, which has caused many hospitals to close units, is a striking example of the difficulties brought on by failure to attract nurses. Other resources a health care facility must attract include physicians, other employees, volunteers, funds, and public support. Without them, as without nurses, a hospital cannot function.

A sterling example of using marketing strategies to attract volunteers, as well as funds, is demonstrated in the Nurses Network of Pelham Project CHILD (see Case Study 6). The use of marketing theory enabled the NNP to develop a needed program and to sustain the growth of the program for societal good. Marketing provides an organized, disciplined method for attracting needed resources.

Health care organizations have limited budgets. Available funds are often inadequate and undependable. Frequently, health care executives make decisions that are, in fact, marketing decisions. They make decisions about opening and closing units, starting new programs and services, and deleting services every day. Making these decisions with insufficient knowledge often results in poor use of scarce resources. The application of marketing theory helps an organization to become effective and efficient while increasing patient satisfaction.

CONCLUSION

Marketing is a nursing imperative for the 1990s. The very rapid changes in our world and the diverse needs and wants of people, coupled with increasingly scarce resources, require that new and effective answers be developed for society not only to cope, but to grow and flourish. Nursing, with the use of marketing strategies, can help solve our problems and lead health care services into the 21st century.

REFERENCES

Adrian, C.R., & Press, C. (1969). *The American political process* (2nd ed.). New York: McGraw-Hill.

Ailing hospital ads need intensive care. (1989, July 31). *Wall Street Journal*, B1.

Alward, R.R. (1983a). A marketing approach to nursing administration—part I. *Journal of Nursing Administration, 13*(3), 9–12.

Alward, R.R. (1983b). A marketing approach to nursing administration—part II. *Journal of Nursing Administration, 13*(4), 18–22.

Anderson, D.C., & Near, R. (1985). Something may not be working in the hospital—But is it marketing? In P.D. Cooper (Ed.), *Health care marketing: Issues and trends* (2nd ed.) (pp. 61–68). Rockville, MD: Aspen.

Boscarino, J.A. (1988). The public's rating of hospitals. *Hospital & Health Services Administration, 33*, 189–99.

Carson, R. (1962). *Silent spring*. Boston: Houghton Mifflin.

Chopoorian, T.J. (1986). Reconceptualizing the environment. In P. Moccia (Ed.), *New Approaches to theory development*. New York: National League for Nursing.

Droste, T. (1988). Good training key to marketing success. *Hospitals, 62*(7), 47, 48.

Fullerton, R.A. (1988). How modern is modern marketing? Marketing's evolution and the myth of the "production era." *Journal of Marketing, 52*(1), 108–25.

Galbraith, J.K. (1958). *The affluent society*. Boston: Houghton Mifflin.

Ginzberg, E. (1987). Facing the facts and figures. *American Journal of Nursing, 87*, 1596-1600.

Greer, T.V. (1973). *Marketing in the Soviet Union*. New York: Holt, Rinehart & Winston.

Hayes, R.H., & Abernathy, W.J. (1980). Managing our way to economic decline. *Harvard Business Review, 58*(4), 67–77.

Kotler, P. (1975). *Marketing for nonprofit organizations*. Englewood Cliffs, NJ: Prentice-Hall.

Kotler, P. (1988). *Marketing management: Analysis, planning, implementation, and control* (6th ed.). Englewood Cliffs, NJ: Prentice-Hall.

Kotler, P., & Andreasen, A.R. (1987). *Strategic marketing for nonprofit organizations*. Englewood Cliffs, NJ: Prentice-Hall.

Kotler, P., & Clarke, R.N. (1987). *Marketing for health care organizations*. Englewood Cliffs, NJ: Prentice-Hall.

Kotler, P. & Levy, S.J. (1969). Broadening the concept of marketing. *Journal of Marketing, 33*(1), 10–15.

Lohr, S. (1988, August 7). British health service faces a crisis in funds and delays. *The New York Times*, pp. 1, 12.

McNerney, W.J. (1988). Nursing's vision in a competitive environment. *Nursing Outlook*, *36*, 126-29.

Naor, J. (1986). Towards a socialist marketing concept—the case of Romania. *Journal of Marketing, 50*(1), 28–39.

New York no-smoking law: Echoing society's "no more!" (1988, July 24). *The York Times*, pp. 1, 21.

O'Connor, C.P. (1985). Why marketing isn't working in the health care arena. In P.D. Cooper (Ed.), *Health care marketing: issues and trends* (2nd ed.) (pp.52–60). Rockville, MD: Aspen.

Packard, V. (1957). *The hidden persuaders*. New York: Pocket Books.

Pol, L.G. (1986). Marketing and the demographic perspective. *Journal of Consumer Marketing, 3*(1), 57–64.

Sadun, A.G., Webster, T.F., & Commoner, B. (March 14, 1990). *Breaking down the degradable plastics scam* (Report for Greenpeace). Flushing, NY: Queens College, CUNY, Center for the Biology of Natural Systems.

Sanchez, P.M. (1985). Marketing in the health arena: some comments on O'Connor's evaluation of the discipline. In P.D. Cooper (Ed.), *Health care marketing: Issues and trends* (2nd ed.) (pp. 69–75). Rockville, MD: Aspen.

United States Department of Health and Human Services, Health Care Financing Administration (1981). *Long-term care: Background and future directions*. Washington, DC: Author.

SUGGESTED READINGS IN POWER AND POLITICS

del Bueno, D.J., & Freund, C.M. (1986). *Power and politics in nursing administration: A casebook*. Owings Mills, MD: National Health Publishing.

MacPherson, K.I. (1987). Health care policy, values, and nursing. *Advances in Nursing Science*, 9(3), 1–11.

Mason, D.J., & Talbott, S.W. (1985). *Political action handbook for nurses*. Menlo Park, CA: Addison-Wesley.

Stevens, B.J. (1985). *The nurse as executive* (3rd ed.). Rockville, MD: Aspen.

Wieczorek, R.R. (1985). *Power, politics, and policy in nursing*. New York: Springer.

CHAPTER 2

Basic Marketing Concepts

MARKETING DEFINED

In order to discuss marketing and its use as a nursing management process, some basic concepts must be defined. What comes to mind when you hear the word *marketing*? Is it selling, advertising, public relations, or other promotional activities? These seem to be the functions that are most often confused with marketing. Although they are part of marketing, much more is implied by this term. A dictionary may define *marketing* as the act of buying or selling in a market; however, in this book, we use marketing in a broader context. Our definition clearly identifies nurses and nurse managers as participants in the marketing process on a daily basis.

Kotler (1988, p. 3) formulated the definition of marketing that helps nurses readily to identify their involvement in marketing activities: "Marketing is a social and managerial process by which individuals and groups obtain what they need and want through creating and exchanging products and values with others." Calling marketing a process means that it is a series of systematic events or activities that lead toward an end or goal. In his definition, Kotler does not limit marketing by calling it a management process used only by organizations; he also describes it as a social process through which society's needs and wants can be met.

Although much marketing literature is oriented toward marketing management in organizations, the purpose of this book is to help you develop a marketing philosophy and to apply marketing principles in your practice, whatever your organizational or work environment may be. With the recent interest in entrepreneurial and intrapreneurial nursing activities and practices, marketing assumes new importance for both the profession and the individual nurse.

Examples of individual nurse managers and practitioners using marketing skills to manage their exchange relationships are plentiful. For instance, when nurses prepare résumés and tailor them to highlight past professional and educational experiences compatible with specifications for available positions, they are engaging in marketing activity. Individual salary negotiations between a head nurse and the employing hospital, or between a nurse consultant and a home health agency, are other examples of marketing. The case studies in Part 2 of this book are an eclectic assortment illustrating the many ways in which nurses are using marketing principles and strategies in their daily practices. These studies describe instances of the effective use of marketing by the larger health care organization, by the nursing organization as a whole (division), and as a subsystem (department or unit), as well as by the individual nurse.

Although the intended reader of this book is a professional nurse rather than a professional marketer, the functions of the two professionals can both be described as assessing, planning, implementing, and evaluating exchanges with others. The nursing process is familiar. Kotler and Clarke (1987) provide the professional marketer's description of the marketing process:

> Marketing is the analysis, planning, implementation, and control of carefully formulated programs designed to bring about voluntary exchanges of values with target markets for the purpose of achieving organizational objectives. It relies heavily on designing the organization's offering in terms of the target markets' needs and desires, and on using effective pricing, communication, and distribution to inform, motivate, and service the markets. (p. 5)

A point to note in this definition is that skillful marketing is not a series of unfocused or random actions, but rather a carefully formulated process designed to result in desired exchanges with one or more targeted groups. Marketing includes all the activities in the voluntary exchange of value for value by the involved parties. Since most of us specialize in our practices and have chosen specific populations as the foci of our services, targeting specific groups for special attention is an activity nurses have often performed without thinking of it as a marketing strategy. Throughout this book, the key concepts in this definition will be applied to nursing and nurses.

NEEDS, WANTS, AND DEMANDS

The essence of a marketing orientation is to assess the needs and wants of selected groups and to satisfy them through goods, services, or ideas, collectively called *products*. It must be stressed that, in a marketing approach to nursing management, the needs and wants of all parties must be considered—not only the patients', the nurses', the physicians', and the organization's, but *all* who are involved in the exchange. So often we do a less-than-complete assessment of the needs and wants of all parties affected by nursing service routines and procedures. For example, when patients' need for sleep is compromised for routine temperature readings at 6:00 a.m., whose best interests are served? It is consensus and balance among the needs and wants of the patient, other health care providers, the organization, and the goals and standards of the nursing profession that redefine high-quality care from a marketing perspective (Andreoli, Carollo, & Pottage, 1988).

Needs

Although a marketing approach implies activating and influencing wants, desires, preferences, and even demands, needs are not created by marketing efforts. All human beings have basic biological, psychological, and sociological *needs* (defined as a real or perceived deprivation). Nurses are familiar with Maslow's (1970) hierarchy of needs and their order of priority: physiological, safety, social, esteem, and self-actualization. The priority of needs changes as lower needs are satisfied, and according to the individuals' circumstances. Needs are influenced by what is valued at any particular time. There is also potential for conflict among various needs and how one chooses to meet them. It is very important for nurses to keep in mind that our perceptions of patients' needs may differ from the patients' perceptions of what they need and want.

Wants

Wants are satisfied by specific goods and services. Whereas water is a basic need, Perrier is a want. Health is a basic need; health care by a specific practitioner is often wanted, desired, or preferred. Needs are internal; wants, desires, and preferences are influenced by external cues that come to one's attention and stimulate interest in meeting a need in a specific way. We feel hungry—and then seeing an ice cream stand on the corner focuses our desire. After we are injured, we may ask to be taken to a specific practitioner for treatment.

When it comes to health care issues, people may not know exactly what they want from health care providers, and may have difficulty expressing their needs and wants. For example, surgical patients need safety during scheduled operative procedures. They may think they want a general anesthetic, but, after being informed of the risks, change their preferences to a local or regional block. Furthermore, patients may want certain health care services and amenities that are not closely allied with their basic needs for that care. Think of a patient, newly diagnosed as having diabetes, who wishes to live alone but does not want to be involved in self-care. Clearly self-care is a need for survival. Nurses are marketing when they point out to such patients that learning to inject insulin will help to satisfy their needs for a healthy existence, safety, and perhaps esteem.

Nurses must also consider the role of health care providers in patients' health care needs and wants. The patient has a need for restoration of well-being. Physicians may create the need for hospitalization by the mode of treatment selected for the patient. A patient's dependency brought on by surgical procedures and other forms of treatment creates a need for nursing care, but the patient perceives the need as restoration of health and independence. Danger lies in presuming to define well-being for patients and society. Because needs and wants are unique to each individual, it is important always to try to validate the meaning of well-being, through discussion and mutual setting of goals, in any marketing exchange with patients.

Demands

Wants become *demands* when parties to the exchange are able and willing to make a transfer of goods or services. Most people have many more wants than demands. Marketers try to influence which wants become demands by making the goods or services they provide more attractive, available, accessible, and affordable than those of competitors. The case studies in this book describe how nurse marketers analyzed needs and wants to turn them into demands for their nursing goods and services. We do this wherever we try to influence a patient to return to the hospital, clinic, nursing center, physician's or nurse practitioner's office, or wherever it is that we practice nursing. We turn wants into demands when we market nursing manuals or nursing and patient education programs. We also turn wants into demands when, as nurse managers, we recruit or retain staff nurses.

EXCHANGES

Exchange Theory

Exchange is another basic concept in the marketing definition. Marketing in all organizations, whether for-profit or nonprofit, occurs in a framework of voluntary exchange by all parties. Similarly, marketing by individuals, in this case by the professional nurse, is based on exchange. Social exchange theory describes all interactions among individuals as an exchange of resources (Beckman-Brindley & Tavormina, 1978). All parties to the exchange have power in proportion to the resources they control and the value of those resources to other parties. Something of value is offered by the organization or individual in exchange for resources needed to continue producing valued goods, services, or ideas.

Kotler and Clarke (1987) describe the three major theories used to predict exchange outcomes. The self-interest of individuals and organizations and utility maximization are basic concepts of the economic theory of exchange. Each party to the exchange identifies all expected benefits (money, health, self-esteem) and all expected costs (money, time, efforts, discomfort). Based on this analysis, the theory predicts one of three outcomes:

1. No exchange will take place if there is a net loss for both parties.
2. An exchange will take place if both parties anticipate a net gain (unless one party hopes for an even better offer in this exchange or another).

3. If one party will gain and the other lose, an exchange will not take place unless the offer is improved for one party, and the other is satisfied with less gain.

Fairness is the basic concept of the equity theory of exchange. It predicts that an exchange will take place when both sides consider the offer to be fair. The basic concept of the power theory is the use of power to achieve maximum gain in an exchange. As in economic theory, an exchange takes place when both parties would gain from it, but here the terms of the exchange depend on power and equity.

Exchange Elements

There are five elements in an exchange: (1) at least two parties; (2) each party has something that the other perceives to be valuable; (3) each party can communicate and deliver things of value; (4) each party has freedom to accept or reject the offer; and (5) each party believes it is appropriate to deal with the other (Kotler, 1988, p. 6). The voluntary exchange of value for value, and the communication process by which the exchange is effected, are central to marketing wherever it takes place. All parties must perceive that the exchange will be beneficial to them in order voluntarily to agree to be involved. Marketing concepts do not apply to an involuntary exchange in which goods or services are forced.

In an early article on use of the marketing process by nurses and nurse managers, Froebe (1982) indicted nursing leaders for ignoring the importance of voluntary exchange in interactions with nursing staff and patient markets. Although the nurse leaders' intentions were good, voluntary exchange was often missing in the decision-making and implementation stages of team and primary nursing systems. Participative management styles emphasize the voluntary exchange of values between nurse managers and staff nurses. Changing the time or location of patient services without surveying patients' preferences is an example of violating the voluntary exchange principle in patient transactions. We agree with Froebe that voluntary exchange is central to both the nursing process and the marketing process.

Consumers' Exchange Roles

Exchanges frequently involve multiple parties on at least one of the two sides of the exchange. In some of these exchanges, involving consumers in groups, there will be joint decisions, with group members sharing more or less equally in the decision. However, in many marketing exchanges with groups, different roles are assumed by members of the consumer group. Kotler and Andreasen (1987) describe five basic roles in the exchange process and the marketing management strategies to influence them. Each role calls for a specific strategy that is consistent, whether different individuals take on the roles or one consumer assumes all five roles. We added a nursing example for each exchange role strategy.

1. The *initiator* is the originator of the concept of a specific exchange.

Marketing strategy: Make initiators aware of consumer needs and preferences and of new market offers. For example, tell the benefits manager of the human resources department about your nurse-managed obesity clinic, so that it can be considered for inclusion in the benefits package.

2. The *influencer* is the person(s) offering heeded advice on the exchange decision.

Marketing strategy: Through implementation of a marketing plan, persuade influencers to recommend your product rather than a competitor's. If adding an employee weight-reduction clinic to the benefits package is suggested by the benefits manager, the influencer might be the staff member who researches obesity clinics in the area and who will recommend to hospital administration a provider of this service. This individual is a target of your marketing plan.

3. The *decider* is the person(s) who decides what action, if any, to take in the exchange, as well as how, when, and where the exchange will occur.

Marketing strategy: Through implementing a marketing plan, persuade deciders to choose your product. If the chief executive officer (CEO) of the hospital has been authorized by the board of trustees to make the decision, the CEO is targeted for a persuasive sales presentation by the director of the nurse-managed obesity clinic.

4. The *transactor* is the person(s) who makes the exchange transaction for the consumer group.

Marketing strategy: Facilitate the exchange by anticipating and removing any obstacles that might arise. Review the contract in advance with the director of the human resource department, who will be the transactor of the exchange, so that signing the contract is without impediment.

5. The *exchanger* is the end user (the consumer) of the offered product.

Marketing strategy: Initiate and maintain contact before, during, and after the exchange to ensure consumer satisfaction. Adhere to policies and procedures that support the marketing plan and to standards of nursing practice, from first contact with the client through follow-up and evaluation of care and outcomes. Client satisfaction with all aspects of the service would be monitored on a regular basis by interviews and questionnaires. The benefits manager should also be thought of as a party to the exchange and monitored for satisfaction with service overall.

Transactions

The exchanges between a nursing organization or an individual nurse and other parties are complex and vary in nature with individual *transactions,* the basic units of an exchange. In some transactions, the nurse manager represents the employing agency in exchanges with the nursing staff; in other transactions, the nurse manager is part of the nursing staff in exchanges with the employer. Similarly, staff nurses are involved in exchanges representing only themselves, and in group exchanges as part of the nursing staff. More than two parties are frequently involved in these transactions; for example, when a state nurses' association represents staff nurses in negotiating wages with an employer.

Values

Values, as defined in exchange theory, are the benefits received through the exchange, minus the costs or price paid in return. They are not defined in this context as operational beliefs. Many of the values exchanged in the marketing process can be classified as either goods or services. Both goods and services are referred to as *products* in marketing vernacular. *Goods* are objects that can be physically transferred from one person to another (for example, nursing supplies or money). *Services* are acts that one person performs for the benefit of another, such as nursing care.

Predicting what is of value in an exchange may be difficult, because of the unique cultural, psychological, social, and personal factors involved. Thus, it is imperative to validate perceptions of what values are being exchanged. Diagramming the perceived values in an actual or potential exchange helps in the validation process and fosters a marketing perspective. Diagrams of a few of the values exchanged between nurse and hospital and between nurse and patient appear in Figure 2-1. Diagrams must be tailored for individual transactions and updated frequently, because what is valued in any exchange process is subject to change.

MARKETING MANAGEMENT PROCESS

Through the use of marketing management techniques, nurses can identify and respond to the needs, wants, and demands of the groups and individuals with whom they exchange values. Consumer demands for goods and services must be managed so that the organization and nurse practitioners can also achieve their own objectives. Equalization of the supply of, and demand for, nursing services is essential to control costs, and exerts a powerful influence on the satisfaction of consumers and providers of health care. Nurse managers spend a great deal of their time matching demand for services with available resources through patient classification and staffing and scheduling activities. Shortages of human and material resources contribute to the frustration and burnout of all levels of professional nurses. (See Chapter 5 for more information on demand states of products.)

Marketing is a discipline that helps the nurse manager not only to identify management objectives, but also to obtain them. The marketing literature (Berkowitz & Flexner, 1978) describes a management process that can be adapted

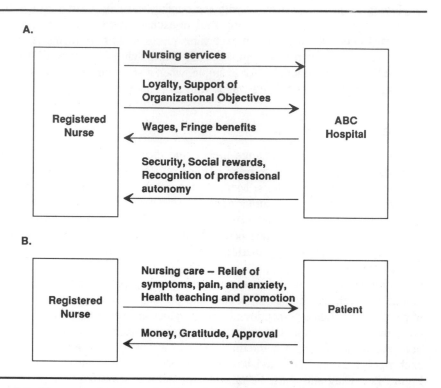

Figure 2-1. Diagrams of exchanged values. A. Registered nurse and hospital exchange. B. Registered nurse and patient exchange.

for use in any type of nursing organization, whether it is a hospital, nursing home, or community health agency, as well as for independent practice and professional nursing corporations.

The marketing management process begins with an analysis of the needs, preferences, and perceptions of current and potential consumers (users) and customers (buyers) in relation to the needs and capabilities of the organization and its personnel. Opportunities for exchange that are available to the organization or individual are explored. The marketing model then progresses to researching and selecting target markets, to planning marketing strategies and tactics, and to implementing the strategies. The process does not end after the evaluation phase, but begins again, in circular fashion. Emphasis on meeting the consumers' needs and preferences is the main difference between this model and many other nursing management models. It often requires research to determine these needs and preferences; too often, it is presumed that, by virtue of education or experience, the nurse already knows them. Other models that can be used to manage marketing activities are described by Galante in Case Study 7.

Marketing Philosophies

Marketing Orientation

Adding marketing functions to nurses' roles does not necessarily mean that they will manage their exchange relationships with a marketing perspective or orientation. Naming and using some aspects of a process does not necessarily mean that the entire process becomes part of one's orientation or philosophy. A *marketing orientation* implies that the energy of the organization or individual nurse is focused on identifying the needs and wants of its primary customers and on delivering the services that satisfy the customers. The assessed needs and wants are satisfied through designing, pricing, promoting, and delivering competitive goods, services, or ideas. These are the characteristics of excellent companies that Peters and Waterman (1984) describe as "staying close to the consumer" and "an obsession with service." Thus, a marketing orientation is also called a *customer orientation.*

Just as patient-centered nursing care is based on an assessment of patient needs, wants, perceptions, and preferences, a market-centered orientation for a nursing organization or individual nurse practitioner requires a similar assessment of all consumers and of one's own customer-focused behaviors. Qualitative and quantitative research and action based on the results are planned and implemented to better meet the customer's needs. In an organization, customer-centeredness is expressed by all employees in friendliness and a willingness to solve customer problems, and results in customer satisfaction.

As Shapiro (1988) points out, a market orientation is more than slogans and slick promotions. It comes from the philosophy and values deep within the organizational culture. He suggests that we answer the following five questions, which we have adapted for nurses, to evaluate whether we are committed to our customers.

1. Is it easy to do business with us?
     Are we accessible?
     Do we respond promptly to requests for information and other services?
     Do we provide information and services our customers need and want?

2. Are promises and contracts honored?
     Do we promise a higher level of nursing care than we have resources to deliver?
     Are we able to deliver services on a timely basis?
     Do we provide competent nursing staff?
     Do we provide well-oriented nursing staff?

3. Are standards met?
     Do nursing personnel know the standards of care?
     Are nursing standards reasonable for resources available?

4. How well do we respond to clients?
   Do we assess patients', physicians', employees', and organizational needs and wants?
   In our assessments and interventions, do we really listen to customers?
   Do we follow through on our actions?
   Do we have a *why not* rather then a *why* orientation?
   Do we treat customers as individuals by personalizing services?

5. Do we foster collegial relationships?
   Are we quick to share data, information, and sources?
   Do we share rewards as well as blame?
   Do we share in decision-making?
   Are we as concerned about the well-being of other workers and professionals as we are about our clients?

In addition to this customer/consumer philosophy, there are at least four other measurable attributes of the marketing orientation (Kotler & Clarke, 1987). All five are listed below. The answers to the questions following each attribute will give you an indication of the marketing philosophy of your organization.

1. Customer/consumer philosophy: Are consumer needs and preferences of primary importance in your nursing management goals, plans, and decisions?
2. Integrated marketing organization: Does the staff have marketing skills to carry out a marketing management process (including analysis, planning, implementation, and evaluation of marketing activities)?
3. Adequate marketing information: Do you and other nurses and managers in the organization receive the marketing research data that you need to be effective marketers?
4. Strategic orientation: Does top nursing management have an innovative strategic plan to achieve its long-term objectives?
5. Operational efficiency: Are your marketing activities cost-effective?

If you answer *yes* to these questions, a marketing orientation is part of your organizational culture. If you answer *no,* look for ways you can solicit top management support for a marketing orientation, as well as ways to initiate better hiring practices and reward market-oriented nurses. If there is no nursing strategic plan, or if it does not support this marketing orientation, your work will be more difficult.

Societal Marketing Orientation

Because of the nature of the health professions, the goal of nurses and other health care providers has been described as a *societal marketing orientation.* This means that the main focus of marketing efforts is to study and meet the needs, desires, interests, and preferences of the target markets so that the goods, services, or ideas exchanged benefit both the consumer and society. This marketing management philosophy differs from the marketing orientation described earlier by changing the emphasis to enhancing consumers' and society's well-being, while also satisfying their needs, wants, and interests.

A major concern of those who use the marketing process in health care is that the goals of marketing will overshadow or extinguish other justified and worthy goals, such as research and education. To meet marketing objectives, health care providers should not have to sacrifice professional and organizational values as identified in their mission statements, goals, and objectives. The societal marketing process helps to identify the interests of all parties to an exchange as well as those of society as a whole.

Conflict exists when what patients want is neither what patients need nor in their best interest. Examples of consumer conflicts of self-interest are smoking, substance abuse, speeding, drunk driving, and poor diet. Hospitals may provide a balanced diet when the patient wants a fast-food hamburger or a well-marbled steak and french fries. Patients have many wants, in the form of amenities, that are not associated with their health care needs: color televisions, cheerful rooms, and a choice in menu are among them. Generally, it is possible to meet some of the wants as well as the needs. However, not all of the wants are appropriate to satisfy, and others cannot be met because of the cost.

In a societal marketing orientation, society's best interests are assessed along with the individual's wants. Recent restrictions on smoking are a good example of the process. Marketers must take society's interests as well as consumer needs and wants into consideration and act responsibly.

Other Marketing Management Orientations

Three additional management orientations related to marketing may be prevalent within an organization. (Five are summarized in Table 2-1). A unit or department may emphasize one philosophy more than another, depending on the nursing unit manager or area director. You will recognize overtones of these philosophies from your nursing experiences in health care institutions. According to Kotler and Andreasen (1987), marketing evolved from a product orientation to production, sales, and eventually a customer orientation.

The *product orientation* is a particular danger in nursing and other health care organizations. It focuses on delivering services that the provider thinks are good for the consumer, regardless of the consumer's opinion. Since the provider (physician or nurse) values so highly the service being provided, there is resistance to changing it even when the service is not wanted. Some health care of the aging and dying suffers from this orientation, as do nursing procedures performed because "it is good for you." At times, these services are not in the patient's best interest, although the provider may think they are. In the nursing profession, this rigidity was most common during the heyday of functional nursing, with its

---

TABLE 2–1   Comparison of Five Orientations in Health Care Marketing

Orientation	Product	Production
Focus:	Delivering products the organization wants.	Efficiency in production and distribution.
Method:	Taking a paternalistic approach: "We know what is best for you."	Streamlining management and production; using high-tech/low touch; emphasizing productivity; losing patient in bureaucracy.
Outcomes:	Patient interests subjugated to interests of providers; customer dissatisfaction.	Patient interests subjugated to efficiency of system; customer dissatisfaction.
Examples:	Using technology to keep patients alive at all costs; keeping control of patient; nurse "Ratched"; team nursing.	Patients waiting long periods of time for diagnostic tests; functional nursing.

---

division of nursing labor by tasks. This philosophy is of particular concern during periods of nursing shortage.

A *production orientation* focuses on the efficient output and distribution of the product or service. It assumes that the health care consumer values most the affordability and availability of services. The human relations aspects of the work are viewed as less important than productivity. This orientation is frequently seen in large organizations and is also prevalent in health care. It is found in admissions departments, and in waiting rooms where patients may wait for a long time, enabling health care providers to make the most of their own time.

Unfortunately, this orientation is also present in nursing. Both functional and team nursing lend themselves to a production orientation. The patient frequently has to adapt to the process, regardless of condition, problem, wants, or needs. Often more attention is paid to satisfying the system than the patient. In nursing, this orientation is seen in the overly rigid enforcement of rules such as when treatments are done, temperatures taken, and the like. Not taking time to deal with patient anxieties before a surgical procedure, because the circulating nurse is opening supplies, is another example of a production orientation. Nursing shortages make it more difficult than ever to avoid the consequences of this

TABLE 2-1   Comparison of Five Orientations in Health Care Marketing

Sales	Marketing	Societal Marketing
Stimulating interest in existing products.	Identifying and satisfying wants and needs.	Satisfying and enhancing consumer's and society's well-being.
Increasing budget for public relations, advertising, outreach; emphasizing personal selling.	Systematically studying and changing needs and wants; acting on information to satisfy consumers.	Balancing profits, consumers' wants, and public interest; attending to items in mission statements not directly connected to patient wants, i.e., research and education in a teaching hospital.
Short-run increase in customers and revenues; questionable long-term results.	Increased consumer satisfaction; increased revenues short- and long-term.	Increased consumer and societal satisfaction; increased revenue short- and long-term.
Using public relations, ads, brochures, etc; recruitment of nurses without regard to retention; attraction of patients without attention to satisfaction.	Establishing after-hours pediatric clinic (Case Study 12); developing nurse retention program (Case Study 18); primary nursing.	Organ donation program (Case Study 4); Down Syndrome program (Case Study 6); recruitment to nursing programs (Case Study 15).

orientation, which are usually dissatisfied patients. What health care consumer cannot describe numerous instances in physicians' offices, hospital emergency departments, nursing units, and admission offices when efficiency was paramount?

The sales orientation has become a threat to health care organizations in the last 10 years with the great push to increase market share by "selling" rather than by changing services to meet consumers' needs and desires. The goal in a *sales orientation* to marketing is to stimulate interest in services presently offered by the organization through advertising, public relations, and sales calls. This is a short-term strategy, because the focus is not on developing products or services to attract a new segment of the population. An intensive sales campaign directed toward filling hospital beds is an example of a sales orientation. In his classic article about "marketing myopia," Levitt (1960) stresses the difference between selling and marketing:

> The difference between marketing and selling is more than semantic. Selling focuses on the needs of the seller, marketing on the needs of the buyer. Selling is preoccupied with the seller's need to convert his product to cash; marketing with the idea of satisfying the needs of the

customer by means of the product and the whole cluster of things associated with creating, delivering and finally consuming it. (p. 38)

The sales approach has often been used by nursing departments for recruiting staff. Recruiters are sent to job fairs and college career days. Ads are placed in newspapers and journals; slick brochures are produced. Other inducements, such as trips, bonuses, and cars, may be offered. Less thought and effort are put into retention. Short-term sales may go up, but long-term effects are open to question. If a marketing orientation is used instead of the sales orientation, a retention program would be developed. Nurses' job satisfaction would increase and turnover would decrease. Long-term benefits for the nursing division could be substantial.

A similar scenario often takes place in the bid for increased bed occupancy. Sales are emphasized, but nothing is done to increase patient satisfaction. Again, the method is short-sighted, and, in the final analysis, expensive.

Symptoms of having a product or sales orientation to marketing are suggested by Andreasen (1982) and adapted here for nurses. Some of these symptoms pervade nursing practice. Think of your consumers as all groups with whom you exchange anything of value (to consumers and you) as you evaluate whether there are elements of product or sales orientation in your practice.

1. *Perceiving the nursing service as inherently desirable.*

    Do you consider that your consumers, whether patients, employer, employees, or physicians, may not share your concept of the service you offer in the exchange?

2. *Thinking that the consumer is not knowledgeable and does not appreciate the value of your nursing services.*

    Do you really understand why the obese patient does not follow your diet instructions?

3. *Overemphasis on promotion.*

    Do you count exclusively on advertising to recruit nurses to your organization? What is it that really attracts staff nurses to the health care agency? Is it an ad, or hearing from a nurse colleague that your nursing organization is a great place to work?

4. *The secondary rule of consumer research.*

    Do you "know" what your patients, colleagues, and employer want from you, or do you use research to confirm your preconceived notions? Do you approach marketing research with an open mind to learn what you can from these studies?

5. *One best marketing strategy.*

    Do you stay close to patients, employees, and physicians so that you can plan marketing strategies that add value to your exchanges?

6. *Ignoring generic competition.*

    Do you evaluate *all* your competitors, some of whom are not as obvious as the hospital down the street or the nurse practitioners in the next office?

7. *A marketing staff selected for its knowledge of products.*

Are you on the marketing team because of your nursing knowledge, or because you understand marketing management and research as well as the customer market? (Andreasen's point here is that professional marketers need specialized education in marketing. We agree, but wouldn't it be helpful if the professional nursing staff had a marketing orientation as well?)

Unfortunately, nurses, like other health care professionals, sometimes project a "we know best" attitude and ignore consumers' (patients') preferences and desires in situations where options and choices are possible. In service professions, such as nursing and medicine, some consumers do not have all of the information they should have to make truly informed decisions about what treatments and services would be best. In most cases, though, they know what they need: a state of wellness.

Organizations

Most nursing and health care marketing activities take place in an organization of some type, whether it is a hospital, nursing home, community health agency, school, business, professional nursing corporation, or small consulting firm. Of the country's two million registered nurses, the Division of Nursing (1986) estimates that approximately 80% are employed in nursing. The breakdown of employment settings is found in Table 2-2. From these data it is apparent that only a very small percentage of nurses practice outside organizations; therefore, in this section, we consider the nursing organizational elements related to marketing management.

Structure

Organizing is one of the basic components of the management process. It involves establishing a structure through which the manager can coordinate resources to accomplish goals and objectives. The structure is the networks of communication, authority, and work flow that connect the workers in the organization (Stevens, 1985).

Three basic types of design or structure are used in organizations: (1) functional design, (2) product/project/program design, and (3) matrix design. Most health care organizations traditionally have had functional structures. In a *functional* structure, departments are organized by specialized knowledge, skills, and functions. Functional design is illustrated by the traditional nursing organization (Figure 2-2).

In the *product/project/program* structure, personnel representing a variety of functional specialities report to one manager for a specific service or program. Interdisciplinary ad hoc committees and task forces are short-term examples of

TABLE 2-2   Registered Nurses' Employment Settings in 1984 and 1988

Employment Setting	1984[a] Percent	1988[b] Percent
Hospitals	68.1	67.9
Nursing homes	7.7	6.6
Community health	6.8	6.8
Ambulatory care settings	6.6	7.7
Nursing education	2.7	1.8
Student health service	2.9	2.9
Occupational health	1.5	1.3
Private duty nursing	1.5	1.2
Self-employed	—	0.8
Other	1.4	2.7
Total	99.2	99.7

[a]*Source:* Division of Nursing. (1986). *The registered nurse population: Findings from the national sample survey of RNs, November 1984* (NTIS No. 0906938). Washington, DC: U.S. Government Printing Office.
[b]*Source:* Division of Nursing, Bureau of Health Professions, U.S. Department of Health and Human Services. (1988). National sample survey of registered nurses. Unpublished data.

this design, and are frequently found in health care organizations. As product line management became more popular in health care, this design was used increasingly for both long- and short-term projects. An example of the product/project/program design appears in Figure 2-3.

A *matrix* organization is created when the project team structure is superimposed on the functional structure (Figure 2-4). In this example, the nursing director in the home health project reports to both the vice president of nursing and the home health product manager. The financial officer of the project reports to the chief financial officer of the hospital as well as to the product manager. Another example from a nursing organization would be an oncology clinical nurse specialist who is accountable to both the oncology service director (product executive) and the vice president of nursing (functional executive). Although the product line executive oversees operations, finances, and marketing for the oncology line of services, the individuals who head the functional areas also bear some responsibility for outcomes of the service. (See Chapter 7 for more on this topic.)

Although form or structure usually follow function, as illustrated by the matrix structure examples, in some organizations executives may view the structure as inflexible. Thus, they inhibit creativity and changes suggested by nurse managers and staff who have developed a marketing perspective. It is important to assess the organizational structure and the climate for change in the organization before beginning marketing activities.

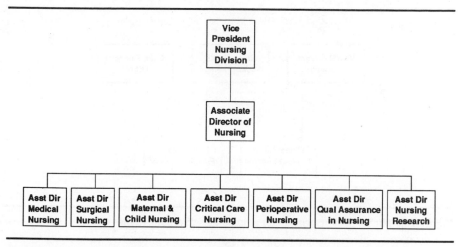

Figure 2-2. Functional design for a traditional nursing organization.

Culture

Another important organizational element to analyze before undertaking major marketing activities in a nursing organization is the corporate culture. *Organizational culture* is the implicit and explicit shared beliefs, values, and norms that shape the work environment. Schein (1985) describes three levels of organizational culture. First-level norms and values are observed in how the organization looks and feels, how staff members behave in their relationships and work activities. The second level is perceived when one learns the values and norms that

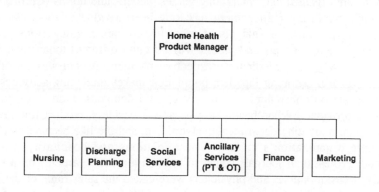

Figure 2-3. Product/project/program design for a home health organization..

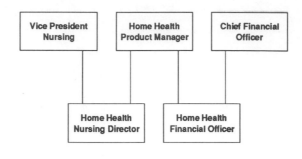

Figure 2-4. Matrix design (partial) for a home health organization.

leads to desired behaviors, whether or not the behaviors are practiced and can be observed. Underpinning assumptions that influence behaviors make up the third level of the culture, and are the hardest to discover.

To analyze a nursing organization's culture, begin by identifying the norms and values on all three levels. del Bueno (1987) provides a checklist that will help you in this assessment. It includes categories of image, deportment, status symbols and rewards, environment and ambiance, communication, meetings, rites, rituals, ceremonies, and sacred cows. Understanding whether the culture is compatible with projected marketing activities is important to marketing's success. The nurse manager's goal is to effect a match between the cultural values related to marketing activities and the activities themselves. In your organizational culture analysis, try to assess the degree to which individual staff nurses and nurse managers share the health care organization's marketing values, beliefs, and norms (Curtin, 1987).

Although marketing management has long been a value in for-profit multi-hospital corporations, an analysis of most health care organizations' culture related to marketing norms and values will be quite different today than it was before 1983, when the Medicare prospective payment system was introduced. Competition for a declining inpatient population makes marketing activities, with their emphasis on consumers' needs, wants, and demands, more acceptable to health care providers. When health care became a business, product line management, hospital marketing departments, advertising, and the like became part of the health care organization's culture. Guest relations and hospitality programs flourished. Professional journals began to publish marketing articles on a regular basis. On occasion, nurses and physicians were called the sales force of the hospital. Well over a billion dollars a year is now spent by the nation's hospitals for their marketing programs. For many hospital and community health nurses, marketing is now part of the organizational culture.

Resources

The third organizational element to consider when embarking on a marketing program in a nursing organization is *resources:* fiscal, material, and, particularly, human assets. Nursing and supporting personnel must be available for, and capable of, providing services. Capable means being both willing and able to meet the needs of the population to be served. In an era of nursing shortage, the nurse manager faces the challenge of projecting whether the necessary staff can be recruited and retained to initiate new programs and maintain existing ones. Maintaining adequate staffing consumes an inordinate amount of the nurse manager's time.

When nurses work without the staffing necessary for the workload, they often become frustrated and angry. A marketing perspective of meeting patients' needs, wants, and demands may then be difficult to cultivate. Patients interpret the nurses' behavior as lacking care and compassion, and this influences their choice of hospitalization in the future. A survey (Inguanzo & Harju, 1985) of 1,000 households, randomly selected throughout the country, identified that 79.5% have a preferred hospital for nonemergency care. The perception of receiving personalized and "good" care was the main reason given by 47.7% for their choice of hospital. Their doctor's recommendation was the main reason for only 8.3% of the participants.

Although a marketing perspective can be developed without investing a great deal of money, sophisticated marketing programs require a major commitment of fiscal resources. For example, for a nursing marketing project that began in 1988, an $800,000 grant from the Pew Charitable Trusts to the Tri-Council for Nursing is being administered by the National League for Nursing. This is a national, multimedia effort designed to inform the public about the role contemporary nursing plays in the delivery of high-quality, cost-effective health care services. The New Jersey Hospital Association's Nursing Resource Center is engaged in a $900,000, three-year marketing campaign to boost the nursing profession's image (Droste, 1988). Marketing, research, and promotional activities, including public relations and advertising, are costly, whether they are carried out by nursing personnel or professional marketers. In the last few years, the percentage of the average hospital's budget spent on marketing activities has spiraled.

Nursing Markets

Markets

A *market* is the group with whom values are exchanged. In marketing literature, market refers to a set of potential or actual buyers and users of goods and services. Buyers are usually referred to as *customers;* ultimate or end users are called *consumers.* Consumers are always customers even though they may buy indirectly (Drucker, 1973). Frequently the buyer is the user, but not always. Marketing efforts can be directed at both groups.

The buying concept is not straightforward in health care, because third-party payers, such as insurance companies and federal, state, and local governments, pay over two-thirds of the health care bills in this country. Of course, ultimately the user of health care services pays much of that amount through private health insurance premiums, fringe benefit payments from employers, and taxes. This third-party payment system places an intermediary between the health care provider and the ultimate user and buyer of the service, making the marketing process more complex.

To develop a marketing approach, the nurse must identify the markets with whom values are exchanged and those who have the potential for exchange. Primary internal markets for a nursing organization are the patient population, as consumers of nursing care, and the health care organization itself, as represented by the administrative staff. In a hospital, additional internal markets are the medical staff, other employees, volunteers, and trustees. Gillem (1988, p. 71) points out that "inside hospitals, each department or work area is an internal customer receiving some work product produced elsewhere in the institution, and in turn, each is a supplier to other departments or areas." External nursing markets include patients' families, visitors, the community, vendors, regulators, donors and supporters, professional associations, and nurse colleagues employed elsewhere.

In addition to defining markets as internal and external to the organization, they can also be categorized as potential, available, qualified available, served, and penetrated markets (Kotler & Andreasen, 1987):

1. The *potential market* is the set of consumers who profess some level of interest in a defined market offer.

2. The *available market* is the set of consumers who have interest, ability to transact, and access to a particular market offer.

3. The *qualified available* market is the set of consumers who have interest, ability to transact, access, and qualifications for the particular market offer. (The consumer meets qualifications determined by the seller.)

4. The *served market* is the part of the qualified market that the organization attempts to attract and serve.

5. The *penetrated market* is the set of qualified available consumers who are actually consuming the product. (pp. 237-239)

In designing marketing plans, a portion or segment of the potential market is targeted for special focus. Most organizations and individuals realize that they cannot serve everyone or meet all health care needs. The reason for targeting a particular subset of all potential customers and consumers can be based upon mission, philosophy, social need, resources, profitability, abilities of the provider, or many other possible considerations. As an example, when a new specialty nursing journal is published, the publishers send announcements to the target market of nurses known to have an interest in the subject of the journal, rather than to all registered nurses in the country. Thus, there is a higher probability of selling subscriptions. A gerontological nurse practitioner would likewise purchase senior citizen mailing lists instead of sending promotional brochures to the general public. In Chapter 3, segmenting and targeting markets are discussed at greater length.

The word *market* can also refer to the place where the exchange of goods and services is negotiated. In this latter sense, a nurse manager goes to the labor market to recruit nursing employees; a hospital controller goes to the financial market to sell bonds to provide capital to build a new wing. Hospitals or nursing homes are also markets where the patient comes to trade dollars for nursing, medical, and other health care technologies and service.

Publics

Publics are groups that have a potential or an actual interest in, or an effect on, an organization. An exchange of values is not the only basis for relationships between a health care organization and its publics. Kotler and Clarke (1987, p. 61) differentiate between a public and a market this way: "Once the organization starts thinking in terms of trading values with that public, it is viewing the public as a market."

Clearly, a nursing organization has many more publics than markets. A partial list of a nursing organization's publics might include the following:

- Local community
- Donors/foundations
- Suppliers/vendors
- General public
- Mass media
- Volunteers
- Competitors
- Regulatory agencies (JCAHO, HCFA, OSHA, ERISA, state health departments)
- Referring services (emergency medical services, nursing homes, community health agencies)
- Third-party payers (insurance companies, Medicare, Medicaid).

The groups with whom nurses exchange values most frequently are not listed here: patients, physicians, hospital administrators, and employees. Notice the overlap in the lists of publics and external nursing markets. Many of the groups listed as publics can and do become markets for nursing organizations and engage in exchanging values.

Kotler and Andreasen (1987) suggest several ways that an organization's publics can be classified. The relationships between an organization and all of its publics are not equally positive or reciprocal. If the organization appreciates the support of a public, it is a *welcome public*. An *unwelcome public* is one that has a negative relationship with an organization, usually because of controls and constraints the public imposes. A negative or indifferent public being courted by an organization is a *sought public*.

Publics are also divided into active and passive groups. *Active publics* help carry out the mission of the organization, directly or indirectly, by paid or volunteer work, selling supplies, or donating money to the organization, for example. *Passive publics* provide the tolerance and goodwill necessary for the organization to function, as exemplified by a community board or the immediate neighbors of a health care organization.

Using a systems approach, publics can be classified a third way, by their functional relationship to the health care provider or organization. Donors, regulatory agencies, third-party payers, and suppliers are then categorized as *input publics*, because they supply resources and exert constraints on a provider organization. *Internal publics* are responsible for converting these resources into desirable products. They include the board of directors, management, staff, and volunteers of the organization. *Intermediary publics* assist in the distribution and promotion of the organization's products to the ultimate consumer. These middlemen are less prominent in health care organizations than in consumer goods companies, but marketing research and consulting firms are examples of intermediary publics of increasing importance in the health field. *Consuming publics* are the customers of the health organization. They include the groups we call patients or clients, as well as families, communities, consumer and employer groups, the general public, competitive, and media publics. All these groups consume the output of the health care provider or organization, and, in turn, affect the organization's and practitioners' ability to achieve their goals.

SOCIAL MARKETING

Much of the marketing activity of nurses comes under the definition of social marketing. Kotler and Zaltman introduced the term *social marketing* in 1971. They used it to describe the use of marketing principles and strategies to further a social cause, idea, or behavior. The term now means a marketing management process that uses planning, implementation, and control strategies to increase the acceptability of an idea or behavior in one or more targeted groups (Kotler & Roberto, 1989). Fox and Kotler (1980) state that the terms "social cause marketing," "social idea marketing," and "public use marketing" are synonymous with "social marketing." Market segmentation, consumer research, product concept development and testing, directed communication, facilitation, incentives, and exchange theory are used to achieve the desired response.

The goal of social marketing is to effect change that is in the best interests of the individual or society. Social marketing uses traditional elements of social change theory with marketing and communications theory, in an integrated way. Social marketing generally encourages people to take some action that is beneficial to others as well as themselves. In Case Study 6, Frost shows how social marketing helped children with Down Syndrome and their parents while at the same time contributing to a positive image of nursing.

Social marketing can be, and has been, applied to a wide variety of social situations, including health care problems and practices. It is especially useful when information needs to be given to many people to encourage new behaviors. A recent example is the dissemination of information to control the spread of AIDS. Other areas in which social marketing has been used by nurses and other health care professionals are cancer detection and treatment, smoking cessation, diet, exercise, high blood pressure treatment, and immunization against childhood diseases.

Another use of social marketing has been to counteract the marketing of products that are undesirable or potentially hazardous to health, such as cigarettes, alcohol, foods that contribute to liver, heart, and lung diseases and obesity, and other problems that may cause accidental injury and death. The manufacturers of these products usually have large promotional budgets. Social marketing is now seen by many public interest groups, health care workers, and government agencies as an effective way to present the other side of the story and to encourage people to engage in more healthful behaviors.

A third important use of social marketing is to move people from wanting or intending to do something to actually doing it. It is one thing for people to know that they should quit smoking, have a mammogram, or change their diet. It is quite another to stimulate them to action. Social marketing can provide approaches that facilitate action. See Case Study 4 for a discussion of the use of social marketing to promote organ donation.

CONCLUSION

In this chapter, we presented the basic marketing concepts that you will need to understand as you progress through this book. These include the meaning of marketing and of a marketing perspective. Because marketing takes place within a framework of voluntary exchange, the theory, elements, and roles of exchange must be considered. Through the marketing management process, nurses can identify and respond to the needs, wants, and demands of individuals and groups with whom they exchange values. Much of Part 1 deals with this process.

REFERENCES

Andreasen, A.R. (1982). Nonprofits: Check your attention to customers. *Harvard Business Review, 60*(3), 105–110.

Andreoli, K.G., Carollo, J.R., & Pottage, M.W. (1988). Marketing strategies: Projecting an image of nursing that reflects achievement. *Nursing Administration Quarterly, 12*(4), 5–14.

Beckman-Brindley, S., & Tavormina, J. (1978). Power relationships in families: A social exchange perspective. *Family Process, 17,* 423–434.

Berkowitz, E.N., & Flexner, W.A. (1978). The marketing audit: A tool for health service organizations. *Health Care Management Review, 3*(4), 51–57.

Curtin, L. (1987). Healing the hospital. *Nursing Management, 18*(12), 9–10.

del Bueno, D.J. (1987). An organizational checklist. *Journal of Nursing Administration, 17*(5), 30–33.

Division of Nursing. (1986). *The registered nurse population: Findings from the national sample survey of RNs, November 1984* (NTIS No. 0906938). Washington, DC: U.S. Government Printing Office.

Droste, T. (1988). Tackling the nursing shortage through marketing. *Hospitals, 62*(12), 34–35.

Drucker, P.F. (1973). *Management: Tasks, responsibilities, practices.* New York: Harper & Row.

Fox, K.A., & Kotler, P. (1980). The marketing of social causes: The first 10 years. *Journal of Marketing, 44*(4), 24–33.

Froebe, D.J. (1982). The marketing process. In A. Marriner (Ed.), *Contemporary nursing management* (pp. 47–55). St. Louis, MO: C.V. Mosby.

Gillem, T.R. (1988). Deming's 14 points and hospital quality: Responding to the consumer's demand for the best value health care. *Journal of Nursing Quality Assurance, 2*(3), 70–78.

Inguanzo, J., & Harju, M. (1985). What makes consumers select a hospital? *Hospitals, 59*(6), 90, 92, 94.

Kotler, P. (1988). *Marketing management: Analysis, planning, implementation, and control* (6th ed.). Englewood Cliffs, NJ: Prentice-Hall.

Kotler, P., & Andreasen, A.R. (1987). *Strategic marketing for nonprofit organizations* (3rd ed.). Englewood Cliffs, NJ: Prentice-Hall.

Kotler, P., & Clarke, R.N. (1987). *Marketing for health care organizations.* Englewood Cliffs, NJ: Prentice-Hall.

Kotler, P., & Roberto, E.L. (1989). *Social marketing: Strategies for changing public behavior.* New York: Free Press.

Kotler, P., & Zaltman, G. (1971). Social marketing: An approach to planned social change. *Journal of Marketing, 35*(3), 3–12.

Levitt, T. (1960). Marketing myopia. *Harvard Business Review, 38*(4), 45–56.

Maslow, A. (1970). *Motivation and personality.* New York: Harper & Row.

Peters, T., & Waterman, R. (1984). *In search of excellence.* New York: Harper & Row.

Schein, E.G. (1985). *Organizational culture and leadership*. San Francisco, CA: Jossy-Bass.
Shapiro, B.P. (1988). What the hell is 'market oriented'? *Harvard Business Review, 66*(6), 119–125.
Stevens, B.J. (1985). *The nurse as executive* (3rd ed.). Rockville, MD: Aspen.

CHAPTER 3

Nursing Markets

MARKETS

All organizations, as well as individuals in a profession or business, have markets with whom they exchange values. However, all organizations do not engage in marketing, previously defined as the process of managing these relationships. *Markets* are sets of potential and actual buyers (customers) and users (consumers) of goods, services, and ideas. The identity of an organization's or an individual practitioner's markets may not always be clear. According to Drucker (1973, p. 81), there are two important questions to ask: "Who is our customer and who should he be?"

For most nurses, those engaged in clinical practice, patients are the primary market. (We use the terms *patients* and *clients* throughout the book; one definition of *client* is a customer). The employing agency should also be considered a primary market because of the volume and importance of exchanges that take place between nurse and employer. Since a hospital organization is the employer for approximately two-thirds of the country's registered nurses, it must, therefore, be part of any discussion of nursing's markets. Depending on the work environment and the degree of autonomy in the nurse's practice, physicians must be considered a primary market for many nurses.

Readers must evaluate who are their primary markets and who are secondary markets. The answer depends to a large degree on the nature of the nurse's practice and area of specialization. Nurse midwives might well include fathers in their primary markets. Whether families or significant others are included in primary or secondary market categories depends on the frequency and nature of exchanges. Occasionally, what is considered a secondary market might be targeted for a marketing campaign to convert group members from secondary to primary users.

In this chapter, we discuss patients, employees, and physicians as nursing markets. This is followed by a section on the nurse manager's primary market, the managed nurse group. Because the majority of nurses work in hospitals, the groups that are primary markets for hospital organizations are considered from that perspective.

PATIENTS AS A NURSING MARKET

As length of stay and occupancy rates declined, in most parts of the country, after introduction of the Medicare prospective payment system in 1983, competing for patients became a conscious effort on the part of hospital administrators. Some tried to instill a marketing perspective in physicians, nurses, and other staff members. The number of marketing articles in nursing and health care literature multiplied rapidly. Almost all nursing management textbooks now include a chapter on marketing. Graduate schools introduced marketing courses into health care administration and nursing administration curricula.

For the overwhelming majority of registered nurses working in hospitals and nursing homes, the patient market has been delivered to nursing units for nursing care without direct negotiation for that privilege on the part of nursing staff. Unfortunately, too few nurses and nurse managers realize how vital their role is in marketing nursing services to patients. Not enough thought goes into analyzing the values exchanged with patients. There has been a tendency to emphasize the nurses' side of the exchange: what they deliver, and at what professional and personal costs. To make us aware of how well we are meeting patients' expectations, needs, and wants, we have begun to think of quality assurance programs, patient satisfaction questionnaires, and complaints received from patients, significant others, and physicians as vital to the marketing management process.

Although the unique needs and wants of each patient are generally recognized, many research studies have investigated what patients value in the exchange with nurses and other health care personnel. Over a decade ago, Flexner and Berkowitz (1979) reported that patients most valued the technical quality of their health care, followed by cleanliness, supportive and friendly attitudes, and physical comfort. Eriksen's (1987) later research found that, in a sample of 136 hospitalized patients, for the most part there was an inverse relationship between patient satisfaction and the quality of nursing care as defined and measured by nurses. When nurses provided high-quality physical care, actively taught patients to deal with their illnesses, and emphasized adherence to procedures and policies, correlations with patient satisfaction were negative, although not all were statistically significant. However, moderate positive correlations (nonsignificant) were obtained when patient satisfaction was correlated with social courtesy and orientation to surroundings. This points to the value of these nursing behaviors for a sample of patients. The researcher concluded that professional nursing values and nursing administrative concerns can be in opposition to the values of patients.

What the patient considers to be high-quality nursing care may vary according to age, socioeconomic class, acuity of illness, place, time when service is rendered, and when satisfaction is measured. Patients make assessments of the quality of their nursing care before, during, and after a nursing service is rendered. At each time, they may define quality of care differently.

Each nursing unit should consider patient satisfaction issues as part of its unit-based quality assurance program. All nurses must evaluate their practice using patient satisfaction criteria as well as professional standards. As pointed out by Petersen (1988, p. 25), "evaluating the quality of care without determining if the client is satisfied is only half a measurement." We can no longer presume that we know our patients' definition of high-quality nursing care and what they value in the exchange with nurses. We must continually ask them. How much we adapt our care to patients' needs, wants, demands, and expectations is the measure of our marketing perspective.

MacStravic (1986, p. 61) advocates therapeutic pampering of patients to improve both the process and the outcome of their care. He describes therapeutic pampering as "the marketing equivalent to therapeutic touch. It transcends formal medical and nursing protocols to focus on the therapeutic value of personal interactions and specific organizational policies whose sole or chief purpose is to satisfy patient wishes." Responding to patients' wishes also results in long-term benefits for both patients and health care providers, such as continuity of care, compliance with the plan of care, and improved quality of life.

THE EMPLOYER AS A NURSING MARKET

The employing organization is not an end user of nursing services, but it is actively involved in exchanging tangible and intangible values with its nursing staff; thus, it meets the criteria for a nursing market. Just as patients differ in what they value, so do employers of nurses. Generally, they ask for the nurses' effort, time, knowledge, skill, loyalty, and support of organizational mission and objectives. In return, nurses receive salary or wages, fringe benefits, social rewards, and varying degrees of job security, recognition, responsibility, and professional autonomy. Notice that some of what the nurse receives in the exchange is influenced by the working environment, but is not completely controlled by the employer. While wages and fringe benefits are negotiated by the agency's governing body and executive officers, feelings of recognition, achievement, and professional growth are more intrinsically derived. What gives one nurse a sense of accomplishment may not have the same effect on her colleagues in the same nursing unit.

As discussed in Chapter 2, parties in an exchange have power in proportion to the value of the resources they control (Beckman-Brindley & Tavormina, 1978). When hospitals in some parts of the country laid off nurses in 1983 and 1984, nurses found themselves in a buyer's market. They were less valued by hospitals with empty beds. Three years later, although one-third of the nation's hospital beds were empty, the aggregate demand had increased, and the nursing supply was not increasing fast enough to meet demand (Prescott, 1987). This was followed by a period in which salaries and benefits once again increased significantly. Compression of wages for experienced nurses is now being addressed by some employers. Nurses have a seller's market.

The focus in this section is on nurses meeting the needs and desires of the employing agency; later, nurses are considered as a hospital market. If nurses cannot meet the employer's needs for revenue by keeping beds open, expect employers to look for other ways to bring health care services to patients. This may mean hospital administrators will support physicians in their ill-conceived attempt to bring registered care technologists (RCT) or other ancillary workers to the bedside. Long ago, many physicians substituted licensed practical nurses and unlicensed personnel for registered nurses in their offices. Nurses must work with the employer to redesign the staff nurses' work so that tasks not in the nursing domain are reassigned. The employer's survival and economic health are as clearly in the best interest of the nurse as are patients' well-being and health.

PHYSICIANS AS A NURSING MARKET

Physicians have a complex market relationship with nurses, particularly in the hospital arena. With the entire hospital organization, physicians exchange patient referrals in return for a fully equipped workplace, direct service, continuing education, and a number of other conveniences. Nursing services are part of this exchange. Although hospital administrators generally see their medical staff as a primary market, nurses prefer to think of physicians as colleagues and not as customers. However, the definition of marketing as exchange of valued goods, services, and ideas helps us to understand why physicians are an important nursing market.

The nurse wants to provide collegial service to support the physician's medical practice in the office, hospital, nursing home, and community. According to Berkowitz, as reported by Klann (1984), the physician wants efficiency and high-quality patient care. Luciano and Darling (1985) also point out some of the expectations of physicians in the exchange with nurses and ways nurses can more effectively meet the needs and preferences of physicians (see Exhibit 3-1).

In addition to physician-prescribed patient care and independent nursing functions, nurses provide direct services to physicians, including reporting and assistance with treatments and procedures. Although the patient is the recipient of both dependent and independent nursing services, it is the physician who often requests and charges the patient for them.

What values the nurse receives in the exchange with physicians, in addition to the very important patient referrals for nursing service, is not easy to define, varies greatly with individual nurse-physician relationships, and is much debated in nursing circles. Unfortunately, physicians and nurses as organized groups lack a marketing perspective toward each other. Rather than working with the nursing profession and the hospital industry to increase the values exchanged with nurses, in 1988 the American Medical Association unilaterally developed a plan to solve the nursing shortage by means of the RCT. Because the terms of an exchange are influenced by power, nurses need to solicit the aid of the end user of all health care services—the patient, client, consumer—in this and similar conflicts among health care providers. Neither physician nor nurse groups can afford to have adversarial relationships with each other.

In support of collaborative practice, Cerne (1988) reports on four demonstration projects that were beneficial to patients, nurses, physicians, and hospitals. Patients felt that the quality of care had improved. With more trust and respect for each other, physicians and nurses had more effective communication and higher levels of job satisfaction. In addition, one of the hospitals reported decreased costs and greater staff efficiency. All parties in the exchanges benefited. (See Case Study 9.)

THE NURSE MANAGER'S MARKETS

A primary market for a nurse manager is the group of nurses who are managed. In some exchanges, nurse administrators and managers represent the employing health care organization. It is the responsibility of nurse administrators to clarify performance standards and policies and to help the staff nurse understand the organizational culture, nursing philosophy, and objectives. Other terms of the exchange that should be explained before hiring, as well as during orientation, include the compensation package, professional development and promotional opportunities, and career ladders (Fine, 1985). As a representative of the employing organization, the nurse manager is frequently charged with describing the employer's terms in the offer.

At other times, the nurse administrator represents the nursing staff in exchanges with hospital administrators. When professional and employee values conflict with organizational values, nurse managers are in an uncomfortable situation that they must resolve on the basis of personal values. What are their ultimate benefits after deducting the price or costs they must pay in this conflict? For example, nurses rank support from nurse administrators very high in their list of employment wants (Huey & Hartley, 1988). Unfortunately, nurse executives and nurse managers' decisions in these conflicts are often perceived by the staff as favoring management at the staff's expense. Perhaps the reason for this perception is that the managers' benefits derived from supporting the employer meet lower order needs (physiological and safety) than do benefits from professional association with staff (social and self-esteem). Another factor contributing to this perception is that nurse managers do not always share the information that staff nurses need in order to understand all the variables in the conflict. For example, if budgeting and hospital financial conditions are not shared with the nursing staff, the nurses cannot be

EXHIBIT 3-1   Strategies for Effective Physician/Consumer Relations

1. The guiding objectives of the nursing department should include a statement about physician/customer relations.

2. The interpersonal behavior of the top nursing administrator will set the pace for departmental nurse-physician relations. The nurse executive must verbally reinforce and portray a posture of positive attitudes about physicians as customers. This can be accomplished by
   - Active listening and responsiveness to physician compliments and complaints;
   - Collaborative, nondefensive participation as a member of medical staff committees;
   - Congenial greeting in corridors, nursing units, and parking lots.

3. The nursing administrator or an appropriate nursing manager should meet with each new physician customer to
   - Find out the needs of the new customer (the service requirements);
   - Describe services available and ways they can be most efficiently used to meet customer needs;
   - Negotiate a mutually satisfactory service agreement. This is not a legal contract, but a verbal service agreement based on what the physician wants in relation to what the organization can give.

4. Nursing managers should develop a ''physician preference card'' about each member of the medical staff. This should
   - List all desired protocols, such as special dressings, management of drainage tubes, and progressive activity;
   - Be used for all new employee orientation, floating staff reference, and student nurse rotations;
   - Be kept current.

5. The nursing services department should have a strong, well-documented quality-assurance program.
   - Nursing activities to be surveyed should include problem areas that physicians find aggravating. These could include accuracies of intake and output totals, patient fall prevention, and expediency of discharge planning.
   - Quality-assurance data should be shared with a standing committee of the medical staff.

6. The management of physician complaints (valid or invalid) by the nursing administrator should include

- A recognition that a physician complaint is a customer complaint;
- An investigation that equals the reviews done for patient complaints or depositions;
- Assurance that delegated follow-up of physician complaints is managed with thoroughness and a commitment to resolving any identified deficiencies;
- Avoidance of memo wars (i.e., written communications that are sent up and down medical or nursing hierarchies and copied to directors of services). This practice escalates the problems rather than solving them;
- Problems brought directly to the attention of the nursing administrator should be followed up by a written or verbal response within 5 working days about the investigation and the corrective action taken.

7. Physicians should be asked to evaluate the services they receive in the nursing department. This rating can be done by
   - Informal questioning of physicians by members of the nursing administration team;
   - Formal, written questionnaires distributed annually or on an alternate-year basis;
   - The development of a joint practice committee with membership equally balanced between nurses and physicians.

8. Physicians must be involved in nursing services program development.
   - Physicians are often one of the groups affected by changes in nursing services (e.g., nursing station remodelling). Their input should be solicited.
   - Nursing managers need to learn from physicians how a proposed change will affect the medical staff (e.g., changes in a unit's assignment method for care delivery).

Source: From "The Physician as a Nursing Service Customer" by K. Luciano and L.A.W. Darling, 1985, *Journal of Nursing Administration, 15,*(6), pp. 19-20. Copyright 1985 by J.B. Lippincott. Reprinted with permission.

---

expected to understand when staffing or use of nursing supplies must be reduced to remain solvent. A marketing perspective will help the nurse manager recognize and meet the staff nurses' needs, wants, and demands in situations such as these.

Although many nurse managers above the head nurse or first-line manager level have limited contact with the patient market, their relationships with patients are very important. The nurse manager is responsible for assuring that *at least* a safe level of nursing care is delivered, at the right time, to the right patient, by the right nurse. When this cannot be assured, the responsible nurse manager must suggest to hospital administrators and medical staff that nursing units and departments be closed. Denying health care access to the patient market often has dire consequences for patients and providers. Therefore, nurse managers spend an increasing proportion of their working day marketing the profession and the employing organization in recruiting and retention activities. Some of these marketing activities are described in Case Studies 13 and 18.

One final point about the influence of the nurse manager on patient and nurse markets comes from a research study reported by Weisman and Nathanson (1985). They investigated the relationship of patient outcomes and the job satisfaction level of nursing staff in 77 family planning clinics. Findings suggested that, by providing working conditions conducive to nurses' satisfaction, nurse managers can improve patient outcomes. Job satisfaction was higher when nurses perceived that conflict among the staff was low and when they had high levels of control over clinic policies and procedures. Nurses' job satisfaction was the strongest determinant of patient satisfaction. That, in turn, predicted better patient outcome (as measured by contraceptive compliance, in this instance).

THE HOSPITAL'S MARKETS

For the hospital organization, patients, physicians, and employees are primary markets. Physicians are often identified as the most important target market for a hospital (Koger & Perry, 1985), but employees are not always included in either the primary or secondary hospital markets (Hisrich & Peters, 1985). Perhaps it takes shortage conditions to make hospitals realize the importance of their employee markets.

Patients

Although physicians are largely viewed by hospitals as the key to admissions, the greatest share (53%) of the average hospital marketing budget is spent on advertising and public relations aimed at potential patients (Droste, 1989), compared to 20.7% targeted at physicians. Advertisements for health care organizations are seen in newspapers, on buses, on billboards, and on television. Some surveys show that patients are exercising more control over the choice of hospital, often choosing a physician by hospital affiliation rather than vice versa. When 1,000 consumers were asked how they chose a hospital, courteous personnel, a wide range of specialists, and the latest hospital technology and equipment ranked higher in importance than a physician's influence (Droste, 1987). However, in another annual survey, the physician's influence over elective hospital selection increased from 36.9% reliance in 1984 to 48.9% in 1987 (Droste, 1988c). People more likely to perceive the physician as dominant in hospital selection lived in the East, were 35 to 44 or 55 to 64 years of age, had some college or vocational training, had one child under 18, and had annual incomes over $30,000. Single people under the age of 35, living in the West, with incomes under $15,000 or between $20,000 and $25,000, and without regular physicians were most likely to rely on themselves or their families for hospital selection.

To respond to patient satisfaction questionnaires and to the rise in consumerism, guest relations and guest hospitality training is given to hospital employees in all departments, as years earlier it was given to hotel employees. The purpose of these programs is to develop a spirit of responsiveness to guests, i.e., patients or clients. Kotler and Clarke (1987) define a responsive health care organization as one that tries to perceive and satisfy the needs and preferences of its markets while maintaining clinical standards and budgetary controls.

Although not meeting the strict definition of terms (see Chapter 5), nursing staff members have been called the "sales force" at a Florida hospital that sees them as the consistent link between hospital organization and patient population (Powills, 1985). This hospital wisely planned a marketing program with three components: marketing to the nursing staff, to patients, and to physicians. The nurses developed a post-discharge communication program of telephone calls, letters, and birthday cards as part of their marketing plan for patients.

Physicians

The hospital industry regards the physicians as a primary market because they are the gatekeepers to hospital admission. Emergency and ambulatory care departments are the only services to which the patient has some degree of direct access. Some oral surgeons have admitting privileges and, in a very few cases, nurse midwives and practitioners have obtained the right and privilege to admit to hospitals, usually under the auspices of a physician.

Once patients are admitted, nurses play a considerable role in deciding what and how much care patients receive, but this fact is not generally known or acknowledged in the hospital marketing literature. Nurses' role in "selling" hospital services may be little known outside hospital walls, and even by the patient market, because hospitals do not generally charge separately for nursing services. (A few hospitals do bill for nursing services. See Sovie and Smith [1986] for an example.) Additionally, nurses exert considerable influence on what services, drugs, and treatments physicians order for patients.

Since 1983 and the introduction of the Medicare prospective payment system, the federal government, through congressional legislation and regulation by the Health Care Financing Administration of the Department for Health and Human Services, has had an increasing role in determining what health care services will be delivered to the segment of the population over 65 years of age and where services will be delivered. While hospital occupancy rates have dropped to less than two-thirds of licensed bed capacity, ambulatory services have increased significantly. Pressure is exerted on physicians to order fewer tests and procedures and to discharge patients as quickly as possible.

Regardless of outside influences, physicians continue to play a large role in determining who will be admitted to a particular hospital and what charges will be billed. If the hospital wants the physician to admit patients, values must be offered in the exchange. As pointed out earlier, the hospital is an important work-site for physicians; therefore, they want from the hospital support services and instruments to carry out their work efficiently, whether that work is patient care, education, or research. The quality of the nursing and medical staffs is very important to physicians (Droste, 1988a). Koger and Perry (1985) point out that physicians, in their role as patient advocates, frequently complain about hospital services to patients.

Physician marketing strategies used by hospitals to increase revenues include: establishing an office of physician relations, recruiting physicians known to be heavy admitters, encouraging referrals from suburban and rural areas, providing office space, personnel, and equipment, joint business ventures, educational programs, and more. Hospitals have also been spending an increasing amount of their marketing budgets on the physician segment. This portion of the marketing budget was predicted to increase by 83% in 1988 (Droste, 1988b), but an average hospital in the United States spent less than 10% of its $236,600 (plus marketers' salaries) marketing budget on physician marketing in 1987 (Droste, 1987). The proportion of marketing staff time spent on physician relations increased from 12% in 1985 to 19% in 1987, second only to time spent on advertising functions (Neiman & Reczynski, 1988).

Nurses

Nurses are the largest segment of the hospital industry's employees. Because nursing employees, as a group and individually, are vital to a hospital's ability to achieve its basic financial goals through patient services delivered, they should be considered a most important hospital market. No other group of employees has as much patient and physician contact. Thus, nurses are enormously important to patient and physician satisfaction. The hospital's dependence on its nurses is not reflected in some of the benefit packages offered by hospitals to nurse employees.

Periods of nursing shortage emphasize the dependence of hospitals on an adequate supply of registered nurses. From 1953 through 1980, the vacancy rate in the country's general duty nurse market ranged from a high of 23.2% in 1961 to a low of 9.3% in 1971 (Feldstein, 1983). In a normal employment market, wages increase to meet demand, but this has not always been true for nurses employed in hospitals. According to Feldstein, hospitals have great market power over nurses because they employ over two-thirds of working nurses, and they practice collusion in setting nurses' wages. Sixty percent of hospitals compete with fewer than six hospitals for their registered nurses. Therefore, hospitals are largely oligopsonists, having to compete with few other employers for their labor markets. After the introduction of Medicare and Medicaid in 1965, nursing costs were retrospectively reimbursed by third-party payers, and nurses' wages increased more rapidly than did comparable professionals' wages. Several factors in the last five years have produced another shortage of nurses. Simply put, demand has increased and the supply is threatened as enrollments in basic nursing programs fall. Potential nursing students are attracted to fields offering better working conditions, higher salaries, and higher potential for income over the career span.

The current nursing shortage has made hospital organizations very aware of their need for this portion of their labor market. (In Case Studies 13 and 18, Mershon and Trofino discuss marketing strategies to recruit and retain nurses.) Without nurses, units close and quality of care suffers, resulting not only in patient and physician complaints but also in increasing negligence and malpractice litigation. Once again, hospitals are surveying the nurse market to see what is most attractive to nurses in the exchange with the employer, what will recruit, and what will retain nurses. Although there was not universal agreement among five surveys reported by Wilkinson (1987), top-ranked nursing wants were special pay for difficult shifts, better working hours, adequate nurse-patient ratios, and good pay. In a survey of *American Journal of Nursing* (*AJN*) readers (Huey & Hartley, 1988), the four factors most important to nurses who planned to leave their present employment were a competent RN staff, being allowed to exercise nursing judgment for patient care, an adequate RN-patient ratio, and support from nurse administrators. Joiner and Hafer (1985) point out that a marketing orientation on the part of hospital administrators would emphasize research to determine the extrinsic rewards (salary, fringe benefits, working conditions) and intrinsic rewards (recognition, accomplishment, esteem) that are expected and preferred by registered nurses.

SEGMENTATION

The entire market with whom nurses exchange values is too large, diverse, and geographically scattered to be considered for a collective marketing effort. The process of dividing a market into groups that share certain characteristics is called *segmentation*. Parties in any exchange may differ from one another in basic ways: needs, wants, preferences, perceptions, attitudes, behaviors, location, age, socioeconomic resources, personality, and values. These variables can have important effects on goods, services, and ideas developed for market segments, as well as on the marketing strategies the nurse marketer uses. In a segment of the market, each member should be enough like the rest of the group that they may be considered together when planning marketing strategies. However, the members of a segment should be enough different from other segments that they require separate marketing strategies (MacStravic, 1977). Products are often designed for small market segments, also called *niches,* when they are found to have a particular, often unfilled, need that provides a market opportunity for the developer of the idea.

Nurses' primary market segments have been identified earlier as patients and the employing organization. The basis for this macrosegmentation is the nature and frequency of exchanges between the nurse and each of these groups. Nurses provide professional and technical nursing services to patients to meet their health care needs, and work services to the employer that help ensure fiscal survival. Most of this section is devoted to a discussion of the microsegmentation of nurses' patient market, because there are so many variables to consider. Later in the chapter, segmentation of other nursing markets is covered. The process is similar, although the differentiating variables are not.

There are two major steps in segmenting the nursing market. The first is to identify the criteria that best differentiate the market segments. The second step is to compile the differentiating characteristics of each segment into a profile. Unfortunately, there is no easy way to decide on the best variables to use for segmentation; usually, various combinations must be tried before a meaningful profile can be developed. It is important to remember that the segmenting variables must be relevant to what is being offered in the exchange.

Although nurses try to personalize their services for each patient, broad groupings are commonly made to identify patients who require similar nursing services. Hospitals and other health care facilities reflect this segmentation, as do the areas of nursing specialization. Traditional health care segmentation has been based on sex, age (pediatrics, geriatrics), nursing or medical diagnoses (nutrition clinic, diabetic clinic, burn unit), acuity of illness (intensive care unit, long-term care unit), admission status and location of service (inpatient, outpatient), or even by payment scheme (private pavilion, HMO, health fair).

When a new opportunity for marketing nursing service is offered, take a creative look at segmentation, rather than using the traditional methods and criteria. Using a grid illustrates that segmentation can be based on a combination of factors and helps identify new possibilities and unmet needs. If a nutrition clinic were being developed, market segmentation might consider potential consumers by age and by previous usage of the agency's other clinics, as depicted in Figure 3-1.

Segmenting by Preference

Because the marketing process attempts to provide what the consumer wants and desires in an exchange, it is important to consider preference in segmentation. Kotler (1988) describes segmenting a market by consumer preference and the three patterns that can emerge in this type of segmentation. If you are deciding the hours a pediatric outpatient clinic should be open (see Case Study 12), and market research shows that all possible types of users prefer similar hours, the preference is *homogeneous.* Preference is *diffuse* if there is no agreement on clinic hours and the choices range over the 24-hour spectrum. If, however, the physician market prefers a clinic open from 5:00 p.m. to 11:00 p.m., and the potential patient market wants 24-hour service, this is a *clustered* preference pattern.

Behavioral Segmentation

Behavioral variables may be the best starting point for beginning to segment a market. One of the behavioral variables to consider is *occasions of use*. The question to ask is, "On what occasions would a patient use this service?" For example, a nutrition class might be sought by a patient after a coronary artery bypass procedure.

Benefit segmentation classifies consumers by the benefits or results they want from the product, such as the benefit of cardiovascular health from a fitness clinic, or the ability to cope with activities of daily living after treatment in a rehabilitation unit. The segmenting questions to ask are:

- What are the major benefits of this nursing service?
- What types of people look for each major benefit?
- Which major competitors offer similar benefits?

Kotler and Clarke (1987, p. 244) describe four core benefit segments in the health care market: (1) quality buyers who seek the best service without regard to cost; (2) service buyers who want the best nursing and personal service, while assuming that all health care is of acceptable quality; (3) value buyers who expect the price to reflect the level of service; and (4) economy buyers who emphasize low cost over quality, service, or value. Nursing research is needed to evaluate how nursing's consumers fit into this type of segmentation.

Other behavioral variables to consider in nursing markets are *user status* (user and nonuser) and *user rate* (volume). Are there groups of nonusers of the nursing service, first-time users, frequent users, or ex-users who could benefit from special marketing approaches? Sample user rate questions include: How often will the consumer use the nursing service offered? Can the potential market be segmented into heavy, medium, and low user segments? If it can, do heavy users share similar characteristics that can be included in their profile?

Segmentation can also be based on *loyalty*. How can you categorize potential users by their degree of loyalty to your service? Is the loyalty due to your quality of service, to habit, to price, or because no one else offers the nursing service in the geographic area?

Psychological and Psychographic Segmentation

Psychological variables to consider in segmentation include personality characteristics, attitudes, and buyer readiness stage. Are assertive feminists more likely to be interested in the women's health service you wish to offer than more passive and dependent women? Five readiness stages that help segment the consumer

**Markets by
Previous Use of Outpatient Clinics**

		No Previous Use	Infrequent Use	Occasional Use	Frequent Use
Markets by Age	**Babies** (to 1 year)				
	Children (2 to 17 yrs)				
	Adult (18 to 64 yrs)				
	Seniors (over 65 yrs)				

Figure 3-1. Segmentation grid using variables of age and previous use of outpatient clinics.

market are: aware, informed, interested, desirous, and intending to make the exchange. Assessing the percentage of the potential market in each of these readiness stages is very important in designing marketing strategies (see Chapter 4). Consumer attitudes toward a nursing service can be hostile, negative, indifferent, positive, or enthusiastic (Kotler, 1988). Each of these patient segments requires a different approach, as any practicing nurse can attest.

Lifestyle and values are segmenting variables categorized as *psychographics* (Green, Tull, & Albaum, 1988). Nurses planning wellness services would also segment potential consumers according to lifestyle factors (eating and exercise habits, degree of stress at work) as well as by values (fitness, health). Nursing services for women may use lifestyle as one of the segmenting variables (see Case Study 17). Commonly used terms such as *yuppies* and *empty-nesters* are lifestyle designations used by marketers.

Sociological Segmentation

Social class is a variable that is related to some types of health care problems and thus can be the basis for segmentation by health care providers. As an example, in marketing prenatal services, segmentation could consider the known relationships of low birth weight to lower socioeconomic class.

Demographic Segmentation

Closely related to psychographic and sociological segmentation is the use of demographic variables to divide the potential nursing market on the basis of scx, age, occupation, income, and payment source. Many nursing organizations' philosophy statements include a disclaimer regarding denial of services on the basis of race, religion, or income. The philosophy may acknowledge that there are social, cultural, racial, educational, age, and sex differences that affect health care needs and preferences. These differences have long been used to segment health care segments, whether consciously or not. By definition, gynecological nursing service markets serve women. Occupational nursing is often segmented on the basis of specific health care needs of groups of workers. A nurse practitioner who chooses to specialize in the chronic care of patients with sickle cell anemia will segment by race as one of the differentiating variables of this market.

Although philosophically there may be opposition to health care segmentation based on ability to pay and the quality of service to be rendered, these are normal segmentation criteria for most consumer markets, and also exist de facto in health care. The amenities offered in conjunction with health care, such as private rooms and private duty nursing care, are usually based on the patient's ability to pay for them. Income and payment source often determine where patients will be served and by whom. Nurse midwifery in the United States was developed by the Frontier Nursing Service because of the need for childbirth care for poor women in rural Kentucky (Kalisch & Kalisch, 1978). Most health care providers prefer a paying patient to one who is indigent, as the latter must be subsidized by other consumers such as governmental agencies and donors. Suffice it to say, it complicates the exchange of values between health care provider and patient when terms of the exchange are not met.

There are other examples of using payment source as a segmenting variable in health care. A nursing home or home health agency that is not certified for Medicare payment would ignore the segment of the health care market that relies on this federal program to meet health care expenses. Whether a patient is admitted to a private rehabilitation hospital or to a county rehabilitation unit often depends on the patient's insurance coverage. Payment contracts function as segmentation variables in health care.

Geographic Segmentation

The last of the types of segmenting variables to be considered as the basis for nursing service market segmentation are geographic factors. Most health care organizations, including nursing organizations, offer their services to a limited geographic area. However, the number of multihospital corporations (see Case Study 13), nursing home chains, and community health agencies with multiple sites (see Case Study 11) is growing steadily and is predicted to continue to increase. Hospital literature frequently reports regional differences in patient and physician markets. Nurses should consider geographic variables of region, city, and county size, as well as the density of population, when segmenting their markets. For example, after studying the profile of suburban and rural segments, a home health agency may choose, for a variety of reasons, not to serve the rural areas surrounding the city where it is situated, but include several suburban segments.

Segmentation of Organizational Markets

As more nurse entrepreneurs develop community- and hospital-based nursing businesses, there will be more opportunities for these entrepreneurs to market their services to organizations and individual patients. Clark and Quinn (1988) describe nurse entrepreneurs marketing their services to retirement communities (admission screening program), to hospitals (maternity fitness program), and business corporations (stress management workshops). Case studies in this book also discuss nurse entrepreneurs who marketed nursing products to other nursing, health care, and community organizations. Other case studies show how nurse intrapreneurs successfully effected exchanges within their own organizations as well.

Organizations can be segmented by some of the same variables used for the patient market. Consider the following factors suggested by Kotler and Clarke (1987):

1. *Size*. Can you provide services for a very large organization? Will it be profitable to serve a very small company?

2. *Geographic location*. Do you have the staffing to provide services out of the city, county, state, or region?

3. *Degree of interest*. Do you have the staffing and finances to pursue business with an organization that is unaware of or indifferent to your service?

4. *Resources*. Provided there is sufficient interest, can the organization afford your service? Does it have the ability to implement your program?

5. *Organizational culture*. What values does the organization stress in its personnel and benefit decisions? Are these values congruent with the nursing services you are offering?

6. *Red tape in the exchange process*. Will the documentation required and bureaucratic delays in decision making be compatible with your *modus operandi*?

Nurse Market Segmentation

Recruitment of nurses, especially in periods of shortage, requires segmentation of the potential nurse market. An example of market segmentation, with which all nurses can identify, is separating recruitment efforts for experienced registered nurses from those directed at recent graduates.

The recent graduate market can be segmented further into segments of nurses who had clinical educational experiences at the recruiting hospital and those who did not. Because beginning practitioners value internship and preceptor programs as well as longer orientation periods, the nurse recruiter and staff development department would develop different marketing plans based on the needs expressed by each segment. Student nurses are often targeted for recruiting efforts and offered summer work programs so that they begin the orientation and socialization process before graduation.

Experienced nurses are more likely than new graduates to be interested in opportunities for advancement through clinical and career ladders. Autonomy of practice, participative management, and decentralized structures may be valued more by this group. Efforts to remedy the compression of wages that plagues the profession are important for the experienced nurse market. Targeting experienced nurses for a marketing effort requires the nursing organization to review its benefit package, in regard to choice of benefits and retirement. For example, the segment of the nurse population with small children has been shown repeatedly to value child care as an employment benefit. More employers are addressing this need as one of their recruitment and retention strategies. The experienced nurse market can also be segmented by educational level, years of experience, past positions, and professional interests, if these variables make a difference in the marketing plan.

Some needs and preferences may be common to all segments of a market. An example might be the availability of alternate work schedules for both new graduates and experienced nurses; in this case, flexible schedules would be part of the profile for both segments. Segments need not vary in all factors, but only to the extent that they require a different marketing approach or a different form to the values exchanged.

Physician Market Segmentation

As discussed earlier, physicians, as a group and individually, exchange values with nurses. These relationships benefit from a marketing management approach. Segmenting the physician market by specialty group, geography, or some other variable depends on whether the segments require different services or different marketing strategies (see Case Study 14). Operating room nurse managers may decide to segment the surgeons by specialty when the managers plan a marketing program to improve room utilization.

After discussing the segmentation of nurse, patient, organization, and physician markets, it is important to reemphasize the multivariate nature of segmentation. Build segment profiles that describe the factors most crucial to the successful marketing of your product or service line. Market segments should be measurable, accessible, substantial, and serviceable given your resources and abilities (Kotler, 1988).

TARGETING

Segmenting nursing markets can be summarized as profiling the differentiating needs, wants, demands, perceptions, and other important characteristics of the various groups with whom nurses exchange values. Segmentation is a means of identifying opportunities for exchange. *Targeting* is the process of selecting one or more market segments for a directed marketing effort. The basis for selection is the probability of success in effecting the desired exchange. The choice is based on the best match of the product with the consumer in order to meet the provider's objective. In *target marketing,* segments are selected; a competitive positioning strategy is developed to communicate the difference between what you and your competitors offer to the same target markets; and a mix of strategies is planned to meet the exchange objectives. Positioning and other marketing strategies are presented in Chapter 5. We confine the discussion in this chapter to targeting in nursing's markets.

After the profiles of the market segments have been compiled, a decision must be made about the targeting strategy to pursue. There are three general directions to consider:

1. *Mass marketing.* No segment is targeted for special effort. An undifferentiated marketing strategy will be followed to exchange the same package of products to all possible consumers, focusing on needs and other characteristics common to all.
2. *Differentiated marketing.* At least two segments are targeted for a marketing campaign. A package of products is promoted for each segment, focusing on the unique needs and characteristics of that segment.
3. *Concentrated marketing.* One segment is targeted for major effort, with the product and marketing strategies focused on this particular segment.

Undifferentiated Marketing

Each targeting strategy has advantages and disadvantages. In undifferentiated marketing, offering one package of products to meet common needs of the broad market allows for economies of scale in production, service, research, training, and promotion. What is missing is the consumer satisfaction that comes from meeting individual needs and preferences. However, if the offered product meets the approval of the undifferentiated market, this can be a successful market strategy. In Case Study 3, Crawford and Fisher describe how they marketed their Joint Commission on Accreditation of Healthcare Organizations (JCAHO) checklist to all nurse executives of accredited hospitals. The nursing professional has always had a philosophy of trying to meet individual patient needs, but actual practice has been less differentiated than many nurses would like, due to the constraints of scarce resources. Reality shock, frustration, and leaving the profession can result from this disparity between philosophy and practice.

Differentiated Marketing

Competition in the health care industry in the 1980s, fueled by declining hospital occupancy rates and the resulting increase in ambulatory and home health services, led the industry to greater differentiation of products. In Case Study 13, Mershon describes how Humana created Centers of Excellence that target the markets for specific clinical specialties. The corporate nursing division also targeted nursing educators and student nurse groups to increase awareness of the organization and thus help recruit staff nurses. Products offered and marketing strategies were differentiated for the targeted market segments.

While differentiated marketing can lead to more exchanges (increased business) than undifferentiated marketing, it usually has higher associated costs for product development, research, communication, and promotion materials. Therefore, it is important that cost-benefit analyses be part of the evaluation process for differentiated marketing.

Concentrated Marketing

When nursing organizations or nurse entrepreneurs decide to target most of their resources on serving well one segment of the potential market, they are engaging in concentrated marketing. The targeted segment is usually the one thought to have the greatest need, volume, and potential for marketing success. Case Studies 12 and 17 describe how nurse managers targeted their services and marketing efforts on particular market segments (pediatric outpatients and women staff members) and identified needs of those segments that they were qualified to meet. Market research may be crucial in evaluating the needs of the targeted segment and the competing products already on the market.

This very focused marketing process facilitates efficient use of specialized resources. However, because the financial well-being of the effort depends on one group and a limited product line, there are risks as well. Frequently, an organization will expand its product line after a successful entry, as described in Case Study 3.

CONCLUSION

Having either a marketing or a societal marketing orientation requires that nurses broaden their perception of who nursing's customers are. We have tended to think only of patients as clients or consumers. If we are going to manage our exchanges with employees, physicians, and the general public, we must add these groups to our marketing management plans as targeted segments of the markets with whom we exchange something of value to both parties.

By segmenting potential markets according to their differentiating characteristics and wants, we can identify opportunities to exchange nursing products for economic and personal benefits to nurses. The targeted markets are those selected for a direct marketing effort, because they appear to have the best fit between consumer needs and preferences and nursing service capabilities and expertise.

REFERENCES

Beckman-Brindley, S., & Tavormina, J. (1978). Power relationships in families: A social exchange perspective. *Family Process, 17,* 423–434.

Cerne, F. (1988). Collaborative practice benefits nurses, patients. *Hospitals, 62*(3), 78.

Clark, L., & Quinn, J. (1988). The new entrepreneurs. *Nursing & Health Care, 9*(1), 7–15.

Droste, T. (1987). 1987: Physician marketing continues to grow. *Hospitals, 61*(24), 28–29.

Droste, T. (1988a). Nursing, medical staffs critical to admitting doctors. *Hospitals, 62*(14), 45–46.

Droste, T. (1988b). Physician marketing budgets to grow in '88. *Hospitals, 62*(2), 32, 34.

Droste, T. (1988c). The physician is still the main gatekeeper. *Hospitals, 62*(9), 38.

Droste, T. (1989). Marketers' survey: Advertising decline continues. *Hospitals, 63*(5), 52.

Drucker, P.F. (1973). *Management: Tasks, responsibilities, practices.* New York: Harper & Row.

Eriksen, L.R. (1987). Patient satisfaction: An indicator of nursing care quality? *Nursing Management, 18*(7), 31–35.

Feldstein, P.J. (1983). *Health care economics* (2nd ed.). New York: John Wiley.

Fine, R.B. (1985). Exchange behavior in administrative nursing marketing interactions. *Nursing Administration Quarterly, 10*(1), 53–55.

Flexner, W.A., & Berkowitz, E.N. (1979). Marketing research in health services planning: A model. *Public Health Reports, 94,* 503–513.

Green, P.E., Tull, D.S., & Albaum, G. (1988). *Research for marketing decisions* (5th ed.). Englewood Cliffs, NJ: Prentice-Hall.

Hisrich, R.D., & Peters, M.J. (1985). Comparison of perceived hospital affiliations and selection criteria by primary market segments. In P.D. Cooper (Ed.), *Health care marketing: Issues and trends* (2nd ed.) (pp. 82–90). Rockville, MD: Aspen.

Huey, F., & Hartley, S. (1988). What keeps nurses in nursing. *American Journal of Nursing, 88,* 181–188.

Joiner, C., & Hafer, J. (1985). Reward preferences of nurses: A marketing concept viewpoint. In P.D. Cooper (Ed.), *Health care marketing: Issues and trends* (2nd ed.) (pp. 99–108). Rockville, MD: Aspen

Kalisch, P.A., & Kalisch, B.J. (1978). *The advance of American nursing.* Boston: Little, Brown.

Klann, S. (1984). Good news and bad news in the marketing age. *AORN Journal, 40,* 790–792.

Koger, D.A., & Perry, F.L. (1985). Physician-centered marketing: A practical step to hospital survival. In P.D. Cooper (Ed.), *Health care marketing: Issues and trends* (2nd ed.) (pp. 91–98). Rockville, MD: Aspen.

Kotler, P. (1988). *Marketing management: Analysis, planning, and control* (6th ed.). Englewood Cliffs, NJ: Prentice-Hall.

Kotler, P., & Clarke, R.N. (1987). *Marketing for health care organizations.* Englewood Cliffs, NJ: Prentice-Hall.

Luciano, K., & Darling, L.W. (1985). The physician as a nursing service customer. *Journal of Nursing Administration, 15*(6), 17–20.

MacStravic, R.E. (1977). *Marketing health care.* Germantown, MD: Aspen.

MacStravic, R.S. (1986). Therapeutic pampering. *Hospital & Health Services Administration, 31*(3), 59–69.

Neiman, J., & Reczynski, D. (1988). Marketing function increases in health care. *Hospitals, 62*(13), FB24.

Petersen, M.B.H. (1988). Measuring patient satisfaction: Collecting useful data. *Journal of Nursing Quality Assurance, 2*(3), 25–35.

Powills, S. (1985). FL hospital nursing staff to market services to community. *Hospitals, 59*(11), 46.

Prescott, P.A. (1987). Another round of nurse shortage. *Image, 19,* 204–209.

Sovie, M.D., & Smith, T.C. (1986). Pricing the nursing product: Charging for nursing care. *Nursing Economic$ 4,* 216–226.

Weisman, C.S., & Nathanson, C.A. (1985). Professional satisfaction and client outcomes. *Medical Care, 23,* 1179–1192.

Wilkinson, R. (1987). Nursing shortages: Just the tip of the iceberg. *Hospitals, 61*(22), 68.

CHAPTER 4

Nursing Marketing Information and Research

PURPOSES OF MARKETING RESEARCH

The primary purpose of including a chapter on marketing research in a book for nurse managers and other nursing practitioners is to help you make better decisions about services that will meet the needs and preferences of your consumers in the variety of markets with whom you exchange values. These needs, wants, attitudes, and perceptions must be monitored in some systematic way so that you can develop strategies to satisfy your consumers. It is by means of various types of research and feedback systems that decisional information is collected, processed, and analyzed. *Decisional research,* commonly called *applied research,* uses existing knowledge to help solve immediate problems (Green, Tull, & Albaum, 1988). Marketing research is usually decisional in nature, rather than fundamental or basic research that develops theory and extends knowledge for its own sake.

Marketing research is a systematic process of designing the study of a specific marketing problem, collecting and analyzing the data, and reporting findings. The marketing research process is similar to any other research process:

1. Define the marketing problem and translate it into a research question.
2. Define the research objectives.
3. Collect data from both secondary and primary sources.
4. Analyze and interpret the data.
5. Communicate the results.

The purpose of marketing research is to provide information that will assist you in recognizing, assessing, and responding to marketing opportunities, challenges, and problems in your own career and in your employing agencies. After you have identified the users and potential users of a particular type of nursing or professional service, you can develop plans to meet the consumers' needs and to predict demand for these services. Market research can also provide opportunities to evaluate several alternative solutions to a marketing problem without the expense of implementing them (Burst, 1985). When conditions are changing rapidly, as they are in today's health care arena, market information is a very valuable resource for the nursing organization. It is often less expensive to obtain it through market tests and research than by making operational mistakes.

Differences Between Research for Goods and Service Products

Until recently, most market research was focused on goods rather than on services. Pope (1986) hypothesizes that this was because service businesses were usually small, personalized, and locally based and operated; therefore, they thought they knew what their customers wanted. As service organizations became large and began to merge into multicorporate, national businesses, they began to use market research methods regularly to keep in touch with their customers.

In general, research methods are similar for marketing goods and services, but the time at which research is done differs considerably for these different types of products. Product development research is difficult for services because prototype products cannot be developed for field testing. Simulation and pretesting of services is usually not practical; offering a new service is its own market test. Research of product acceptance can be conducted after a service is launched, but withdrawing a service usually leads to some dissatisfaction among customers and expense for the organization.

The need to test finished products, because they cannot be tested during development, has led service industries to shift their market research strategies significantly from those of the consumer goods industries (Pope, 1986). Service industries, including health care and nursing, specifically concentrate on overall studies of the market, its segments, and targeting opportunities. Service organizations can also study new service concepts, the need for additional services in the marketplace, and the attractiveness of the services to potential consumers. An example of a service concept research study is discussed by Hoffman and Aadalen in Case Study 8. They used the nominal group process to develop a national educational institute for public health nurse leaders.

USES IN SERVICE ORGANIZATIONS

Marketing research can be used to monitor and change present marketing strategies, to plan future strategies, and to evaluate new market opportunities. More specific uses for research in service organizations are suggested by Wilensky (1985). Characteristics of customers and their needs and wants can be identified, as well as customers' perceptions of benefits received from the services and their satisfaction with services. Research also is used to better understand who the competitors are and customers' perceptions of the competitors' services. The organization's image in regard to specific services and to competitors can be measured. Another area of research is the customers' assessment of price versus value received. Reactions to new services or barriers to trying new services can be studied. Finally, potential and actual customers' attitudes related to services can be measured over time.

In the health care industry, the most important uses for information obtained through marketing research are: monitoring patient satisfaction, identifying physician needs, gauging employee opinions and needs, soliciting local business employers' needs, assessing agency image in the community, developing new and innovative products, determining market share and market demand, and measuring the effectiveness of promotional activities (Keckley, 1988). Many nurse managers are involved in these activities to some degree, whether or not the activities are recognized as marketing functions. Whenever you are involved in planning new services or changing existing ones, in operating or evaluating nursing services, market research can help you make decisions with a greater probability for success. The greater the degree of risk in the marketing decision, the more you need marketing research to guide the decision. The motivation for new or continuing nursing services should not be emotional enthusiasm, but marketing information that objectively helps to identify potential markets and their needs and wants, as well as the financial feasibility of the services.

MARKETING INFORMATION SYSTEM

Many health care organizations now have an information system to manage the marketing process. Kotler and Clarke (1987) use the term *marketing information system* (MIS) to describe the system of collecting, analyzing, and disseminating information that facilitates decision-making regarding marketing plans, strategies, and evaluation. In this system, marketing information is collected from the nursing organization's publics, distribution channels, competitors, macro-environment, and particularly from its target markets, by means of various research methods.

The four MIS subsystems that provide the marketing information are: (1) internal reports, (2) marketing intelligence, (3) marketing research, and (4) analytical marketing techniques. Examples of internal records that provide valuable nursing marketing information include patient records, quality assurance reports, patient and physician satisfaction surveys, and exit interviews with nursing staff. The marketing intelligence system supplies the nurse manager with information on what is happening in the external marketing environment. Sources of this data are nursing periodicals, newspapers, television, hospitals' nursing newsletters, and nursing networks such as professional associations. Kotler and Clarke (1987) differentiate common types of marketing research from analytical marketing systems that require advanced statistical techniques and modeling procedures. The latter are not discussed in this chapter, but you can consult marketing research textbooks (such as Green, Tull, & Albaum, 1988) for further reading on these sophisticated research techniques.

In this chapter, we concentrate on ways that you can use existing internal reports, marketing intelligence, and marketing research to help make decisions that meet your marketing objectives. With the exception of survey and focus group methods, research methods are not described in great detail. With the information provided in this chapter, you will be able to decide when to hire marketing research consultants and when you have the time and research expertise to undertake your own investigation of consumer needs and preferences.

USING CONSULTANTS

Health care agencies use consultants for many reasons. Stevens (1978) outlines seven (see Exhibit 4-1), but here we discuss the hiring of a consultant to do tasks requiring skills that members of the employing agency do not have. There are consultants who are expert in communications, marketing management, and marketing research. The consultant is often hired as a project participant or manager, and actually carries out a project to completion. The use of a communications consultant is discussed in Chapter 5.

EXHIBIT 4-1   Uses for Consultants

1. To define or resolve problems.
2. To gain expert advice on a specific subject
3. To serve as a change agent or catalyst.
4. To educate staff.
5. To mediate or arbitrate conflicts.
6. To improve communication with the organization.
7. To do tasks requiring specialized skills.

Source: Stevens, B.J. (1978). The use of consultants in nursing service. *Journal of Nursing Administration,* 8(8), 7-15.

Marketing Research Consultants

An important issue related to the actual conduct of the proposed research is whether you should conduct the research yourself. If planning and carrying out a marketing research study is not feasible, a second issue is finding a consultant to do the study.

Three potential advantages to in-house research are: (1) decreased cost, (2) decreased time needed for the study, and (3) increased applicability of the study. In-house research is generally less expensive than that conducted by consultants because of the mark-up consultants must add in order to make a profit. This is true even when fully allocated costs for in-house studies are considered; the organization will have the cost of salaries and overhead but not the profit mark-up.

When an organization does its own research, provided that at least the person in charge has some research experience, less start-up time is needed. Insiders already know about the organization. They do not have to take as much time getting to know the needs and wants of the organization in order to carry out and interpret the research.

Of course, there are also disadvantages to in-house research. All the pros and cons must be evaluated carefully. Some of the disadvantages have to do with decreased objectivity and reliability. Both can be very costly to an organization. Decreased objectivity often occurs because the insider has opinions about the project and a vested interest in the study. Furthermore, even if the person managing the research is extremely objective, that person and the organization can be accused of bias. Always consider carefully whether in-house staff can be objective, and if it is important to enhance the appearance of objectivity through the use of an outside agency.

The inexperience of the staff may decrease reliability. Avoid assigning the project to someone with few skills in the area. Consider what work activities will not be done while staff are conducting the research. Remember that you need reliable results and a sophisticated level of data analysis. Make the decision about who does the research on the basis of: (1) attaining a useful, reliable outcome versus the ultimate cost of poor results due to inexperienced market researchers, and (2) the cost of using consultants. Unreliable results can be very costly to an organization. The best reason to use consultants is to avoid mistakes.

To help you decide who should do the research, consider each project individually. For example, you may be able to conduct focus groups or do a relatively small mail survey, but you could be overwhelmed by a phone survey involving hundreds of calls over several weeks. Some of the things that can go wrong are listed in Exhibit 4-2.

There are several sources to investigate when you need help with a market research study. First, look for assistance within the organization. Nurses on staff who have masters and doctoral degrees may be able to help you design a simple study. Those with MBAs will have more marketing knowledge, but perhaps less research expertise, than a nurse who completed a dissertation or thesis in an advanced nursing program. If you are working in a hospital or in a community agency such as the Visiting Nurse Service (see Case Study 11), the marketing department may have staff with research expertise. There is no point in seeking an outside research consultant unless you have a budget to pay for this service, or at least the possibility of securing payment. Before you seek outside help, find out if

EXHIBIT 4-2   Things That Can Go Wrong in Marketing Research

1. The wrong questions were asked.
2. The questions were worded incorrectly.
3. The questions were ordered incorrectly, resulting in a questionnaire that was leading and biased.
4. The sample was poorly selected.
5. The sample selected was not the appropriate target for study.
6. The research method was incorrect.
7. The results were inadequately or improperly analyzed or interpreted.

your study will be funded and if the marketing research consultant will provide a bid for services without initial cost to you. An idea suggested by Burst (1985) is to hire a marketing research consultant to evaluate each research project, including whether it can be done in-house. The cost of this consultation will generally be offset by doing the research well the first time around. Nursing research experience cannot be equated with market research. The tricks of the trade involve more than just research methodology.

Because the health care industry as a whole has become interested in market research only during the last decade, it may be difficult in some regions of the country to find a marketing research consultant with experience in health care. Sources for obtaining the names of consultants are a literature search, word of mouth, and "The Green Book." (This book, *The International Directory of Marketing Research Companies,* may be obtained by writing to the American Marketing Association, 310 Madison Avenue, New York, NY 10017, or by calling 212-687-3280. In 1990 the cost was $50.) Use of all these sources may be the best approach. Unfortunately, there is little evidence in the nursing literature that these outside marketing research consultants are made available to nurses in health care organizations, because of the investment required.

When selecting a market research consultant, Clarke and Shyavitz (1982) suggest looking for the following skills and attributes:

- Knowledge and understanding of the purpose and application of qualitative and quantitative market research.
- Expertise in a variety of research methods.
- Substantial experience in the use of qualitative research.
- Substantial experience in designing market research projects, including data collection and instrument design.

- Substantial experience in managing data collection.
- Substantial experience in managing data processing and data analysis.
- Strong statistical skills.
- Substantial experience in health care market research; if not possible, substantial experience in a variety of industries.

Marketing Management Consultants

Hiring a marketing management consultant is probably fraught with less difficulty than hiring research and communications consultants. If you are a nurse manager, you already are an expert in part of your consultant's job: management. You are looking for someone to bring marketing skills to your organization. Understand first that you will probably have to interview several consultants or firms (Carithers, 1977). Carithers also warns against using cost as the only guideline for hiring.

There is some important information to obtain when hiring any consultant. The person who meets with you to negotiate the contract should be the person who does the consulting. You need to get to know the person with whom you will be working. How comfortable you are with one another is an important criterion for hiring. Interviewing a salesperson does not provide this information. What the consultant proposes should make good business sense; be wary of the consultant who promises too much during the first meeting. Talk with the consultant at length. Try to see the consultant in action. Read work written by the consultant. Ask to see a finished report. Assess how information is conveyed.

Find out for whom the consultant has worked and what was done. You need to ascertain if the experience will bring something to your situation. It is helpful to call on references. Ask what the consultant did, if the project was completed on time, what were the consultant's style, strengths, and weaknesses, how long they worked with the consultant, and whether they would hire the consultant again.

To avoid misunderstanding during the project, understand the consultant's fee system and schedule of interim billing. The consultant may ask for a retainer to cover initial costs. When the full project is proposed, a detailed estimate of the costs should be included. Costs should parallel discrete parts of the project so that you can make cuts if necessary. Ask for a cost-benefit estimate for any component of the proposal.

Working with the Consultant

Consultants, as outsiders, are often perceived as intruders. Staff can be disturbed, resentful, and obstructive. You must do some groundwork in order to facilitate the consultant's work. It is important to inform all personnel about what is being done. The consultant's job and purpose must be understood by all. This will stop rumors and gossip and can help to ensure cooperation.

The consultant's work should be monitored. You should receive progress reports at regular intervals. Progress reports should be shared with personnel, as they serve to build interest in and commitment to the project. Staff may also be able to offer some useful insights.

According to Carithers (1977), one of the most frequent consultant recommendations to hospitals was to institute a comprehensive financial and reporting system. Although much progress has been made in hospital management information systems, nurse managers still have deficits in this area. Many nursing organizations lack control because they do not have easy access to essential information. The nurses association in Case Study 1 is a prime example. A marketing information system is necessary to recognize and take advantage of trends and opportunities.

Once you have the recommendations, it is important to implement them. While it is not necessary that you use all the suggested solutions, some of them may be useful and appropriate. In fact, there generally is not one solution but several alternate solutions or approaches to any problem. You should choose the one that is most cost-effective. It is often helpful to have the consultant assist in the implementation of the selected solution.

Evaluating Results

No project is ever complete until it has been evaluated. To assess whether it was a good investment, you will need to do a cost-benefit analysis. You need to know the outcome of the project and its costs, if the recommendations were implemented with minimal organizational upheaval, and if they are working. Other organizational changes may also have been brought out by the consultant's presence, and these should be assessed.

TYPES OF MARKET INFORMATION AND RESEARCH

Sources of Data

Marketing data and research are commonly categorized in several ways. One of these is based on whether the source of the data is primary or secondary. *Secondary data* were collected for a purpose other than the present study, while *primary research* generates original data that are collected through observation, interviewing, or questionnaires. Sources for secondary research are general publications, such as journals, books, and newspapers. The data gained from them can form a context for your problem. You can also obtain information from public, hospital, and university libraries, government reports, and fact sheets accompanying news releases. Throughout the case studies in Part 2, information from secondary research was relied on frequently.

The government, on the local, state, and national levels, publishes an enormous amount of data on a wide range of topics. This information is available at libraries, in brochures, or for purchase. Generally, the problem is ascertaining if the information you seek is available. There are three ways to facilitate finding the data you need: (1) ask the staff of elected officials such as senators and representatives to help; (2) consult librarians, particularly those who specialize; and (3) check for references to major studies and special reports in the popular press, such as *The New York Times*.

Important secondary data are probably available to you in patient records, staff exit interviews, patient complaints, quality assurance, and other records routinely used in your organization. Access to this information is easier if it was planned for in development of the format. For example, if patient demographic characteristics, patient complaints, and nurse exit interviews are coded and saved in the information system when received, access to the data will be easy. The trick is to make it readily available in a usable form.

Many studies are done each year by private groups and corporations, trade associations, and special interest groups. The cost of some of these reports is minimal, while others are expensive. You can find out about these studies from libraries, publications, experts in the field, and so forth. Case Study 11 refers to two studies done by private groups.

Secondary data must be assessed for relevance, impartiality, validity, and reliability. Even when data meet these criteria, you may find that you need to do primary research because you still have unanswered questions.

Qualitative or Quantitative Research

Market research is also commonly described as either qualitative or quantitative, depending on whether the results can be analyzed in a numerical framework. *Quantitative research* uses numbers to measure variables. The features that are measured in quantitative research must be valid aspects of the variables under study. Numerical scores must be reliable, objective, precise, and unbiased. Statistical analyses are applied to quantitative data to compare, differentiate, and make inferences. Quantitative research gives valuable information about the workings of the marketplace. When it is true experimental research, relationships among variables are identified, causality may be explained, and accurate predictions may be made.

Qualitative research is in-depth, subjective analysis of the characteristics and significance of human experience. Qualitative market research delves into why a number (often small) of consumers like or dislike a product, explores the depth of these feelings, and investigates what would change their perceptions and feelings.

The emotional content of responses is the focus of interest, rather than the number of yes-and-no responses. While qualitative research is considered "soft" research, because it does not generate the objective data of quantitative studies and does not use conventional scientific method, qualitative research is scientifically adequate. Properly conducted qualitative research meets tests of rigor. In business, and in marketing particularly, qualitative research has been useful for a long time. It is generally used when little is known about an area, as a base on which to build a quantitative study.

Both qualitative and quantitative methods are important in market research. They share four important requirements:

1. Rigor is essential.

2. The method is chosen to suit the specific problem.

3. Theory forms the base for the marketing research.

4. Cost-benefit analysis shows that the findings warrant the expenditures.

The choice between these methods is based on what you need to know. Each method has advantages and limitations. Creative, innovative answers are outcomes of the best marketing research. Table 4-1 summarizes some of the features of qualitative and quantitative research used in marketing.

TABLE 4-1   Choosing among Qualitative and Quantitative Methods

Approach	Use When You Want To Know	Advantages	Limitations
Qualitative Small-group study	A lot about a little: Early research Generate hypotheses	Natural Unobtrusive High validity In-depth	Unique Impressionistic Uncontrolled Low quantification
Quantitative Survey	A timely generalization: Test hypotheses Subgroup differences	Generality Quantitative Timely Replicable	Superficial Obtrusive Structured Self-reporting
Experiment	Causes and effects: Changes Time order	Control Powerful conclusions Across time Highest quantification	Costly Time-consuming Vulnerable Sensitizing

---

Adapted with permission of Macmillan Publishing Company from *Survey Research*, 2nd ed., by Charles H. Backstrom and Gerald Hursh-César, p. 16. New York: Wiley & Sons, 1981. Copyright © 1981 by Macmillan Publishing Company; Gerald Hursh-César, *The Research Information Workshop: Using Research for Public Policy Decision-Making*, Exhibit 11.3, Berkeley: Office of the Academic Vice President, University of California, 1977.

QUALITATIVE METHODS

Qualitative research is rooted in the 19th and early 20th centuries. The social problems of cities were exacerbated by urbanization and huge increases in population brought about by mass immigration. Journalists such as Lincoln Steffens and Ida Tarbell exposed many problems, and these exposés demanded responses. One response was the social survey. While social surveys presented large quantities of statistics on all sorts of issues, ranging from income to kinds and locations of toilets, the reports contained many detailed descriptions, interviews, sketches, and photographs. Also, while quantification was an important value at the time as a symbol of the scientific method, qualitative accounts were often more useful than the statistics. At the same time, anthropology also contributed to the development of qualitative research.

From the 1930s to the 1950s, development and growth of qualitative research was quiescent. Lazarfeld and Merton applied the group interview to a marketing question in 1942 (Merton, 1987). They developed the technique to promote the war effort through radio messages. For many diverse reasons, relatively little else was done to expand the use of qualitative research during this period. The 1960s, a period of great social change, brought renewed interest in qualitative research. Businesses began to use it for marketing studies by the late 1950s. The field of education came to accept qualitative research during the 1970s. The publication by *Nursing Research* in 1982 of Oiler's research report was seen by some as a turning point in nursing's slow acceptance of the method.

Observational Research

A qualitative research method that can be undertaken by most nurses is *observational research*. Nurses use personal observation daily in making patient care decisions, staffing decisions, and personnel evaluations. Personal observation can be done in a systematic way. An example would be observing every half-hour the number of patients waiting to be treated in the emergency department, when you are considering if staffing should be changed or the number of treatment rooms expanded.

Focus Groups

Focus group interviews are the qualitative research method used most frequently to discover consumers' needs, wants, preferences, and perceptions. They also allow observation of the product decision process. According to Bartos (1987), focus group interviewing techniques are based on psychoanalytical theory. The psychological approach to marketing research was advocated by the American Marketing Association as early as the 1930s. By the 1950s, the interviewing techniques were applied to motivation research and to discovering consumer responses to goods and services. As the use of marketing management has increased in the health care field, focus group interviewing has become common for groups of patients, physicians, and nurses.

Focus groups are small groups, selected from a target market, who are usually paid to share their feelings, opinions, and attitudes on a marketing topic. The topic can be a product, service, organization, idea, or any value that is exchanged in a marketplace (see Case Studies 9 and 20). The discussion lasts from one to three hours (average of one and a half to two hours) and is guided by a moderator. This research method is called a focus group interview because the moderator keeps the participants focused on the research questions. The *nominal group process,* described by Hoffman and Aadalen in Case Study 8, is another type of group discussion used to collect qualitative marketing research data. While the nominal group technique is used to reach consensus on issues and specific group decisions, focus groups are valued for their range and depth of opinions on the research questions.

The interviews are ideally held in a comfortable room with two-way mirrors, videotaping, and audiotaping facilities. The moderator and participants sit around a table so that they can see each other and be seen by observers, who often include the marketing client. Refreshments are usually served to create a relaxed, informal atmosphere.

Group composition

Focus group participants or respondents are brought together because they share certain characteristics and common interests that relate to the product that will be discussed. Usually participants are in the actual or potential market for that product. Group interaction is expected, and it is the moderator's duty to stimulate this interaction, so that new ideas or insights about the research topic will be generated.

Group members should be enough alike that rapport can be established and discussion not be inhibited by differences among members. Hisrich and Peters (1982) point out the advantages and disadvantages of heterogeneous and homogeneous groups. Diverse information can be generated in a heterogeneous group. If both sides of an issue are presented, commitment on problem resolution is enhanced. Alternatively, more information can be obtained from a homogeneous group. If the target market is precisely defined, focus group participants can be selected to fit its profile. This in turn increases the probability of gathering relevant information (Nasser, 1988). To avoid individual interviews within the group setting, focus group members should share the characteristics and experiences that allow full participation in the discussion. Burst (1985) recommends that focus group interviews be done in pairs, with duplicate groups of similar market subjects. This negates the influence of strong personalities and forceful opinions that may skew the results of a single focus group. In Case Study 9, Johnston conducted four physician and six nurse group interviews to obtain information for her marketing plan.

Several focus groups of dissimilar members may be interviewed to obtain the opinions of present users of a product, potential users, and providers of a service like nursing. For example, four types of focus groups to discuss establishing a nurse practitioner chronic care clinic might include a group of clients whose care is being managed by a nurse, a group of chronic care patients now managed by a physician, a group of nurse practitioners, and a group of physicians in the referral area. The number of focus groups of each type will depend not only on the scope of the research question, but also on the funding available to pay participants, moderators, and consulting market research firms.

If lists of target market members are available, such as lists of customers or potential customers for a product, selecting focus group members at random is recommended. Telephone calls are made at least two weeks in advance to invite participation and to screen out those who do not fit the specific profile characteristics. For groups of busy professionals, more advance scheduling may be required. Nasser recommends eliminating competitors' employees, members of news media organizations, and anyone who participated in a focus group within the last year, to avoid respondents more interested in payment than in the topic at hand.

Group Size

Focus group size ranges from 4 to 15, but usually is 10 to 12. Tull and Hawkins (1987) call groups of four or five *mini groups,* and recommend their use when a topic needs deeper probing than can be done in the larger focus group. The ideal size of a focus group depends on the topic, age, profession, and other demographic characteristics of the group. As an example, 15 senior citizens might participate in a focus group because group discussion is less familiar to the elderly, and they tend not to speak as freely as younger respondents would. In contrast, a smaller group of six to eight physicians might be ideal because, in general, they eagerly give their opinions, unless protecting a vested interest (Droste, 1988b). Two or three extra participants are usually recruited to ensure the desired group size. The extras should be thanked, paid, and dismissed if everyone shows up for the group interview.

Uses

The primary reason for focus group interviews is to learn directly the needs, wants, expectations, perceptions, and degree of satisfaction with goods or services prior to or after their introduction to the marketplace. Specific uses for the data obtained from focus groups are to:

1. Generate hypotheses that can be further tested quantitatively.
2. Generate information used to design structured survey questionnaires.
3. Provide background information on a product or service category.

4. Provide comparative perceptions on existing providers and their products or services.

5. Get impressions on new concepts, services, products, and/or procedures for which little information is available.

6. Stimulate new ideas to improve market position and penetration. (Hisrich & Peters, 1982, p. 13)

These uses point out that focus group interviews are exploratory and descriptive in nature. In general, they should not be used to arrive at marketing conclusions. Focus groups are better used to evaluate new ideas or products than those already available in the marketplace. In Case Study 20, Berg and O'Riordan used focus group research to explore the potential market for a nurse executive magazine. Focus groups should not be used to predict the level of utilization of a new service, but rather to explore what the service should offer (Droste, 1988b). Data obtained through focus groups should not be generalized.

In the nursing profession, focus group interviews are useful to assess nurses' attitudes about the employing agency, new services, nursing products, nursing organizations, and methods of operation, such as recruitment and retention strategies. Advertising concepts for nurse recruitment can be tested by groups of nurses before they are used. The issues raised in focus groups can be the basis for a quantitative survey of the entire nursing staff or a random sample thereof. Focus groups have been used recently to study the nursing shortage, and also by nursing schools competing for a shrinking student pool. See Exhibit 4-3 for a brief synopsis of focus group research on the nursing shortage conducted by the American Hospital Association.

Moderator

Successfully obtaining useful data from a focus group depends largely on the skill of the moderator, provided that the group has been chosen well to represent the target markets. A most basic requirement for the moderator is knowledge of group dynamics and consumer behavior. Rapport must be developed and participation encouraged from each group member. Without taking a substantive part in the discussion or influencing what is said, the moderator must be able to guide the discussion. Biases are introduced if the moderator verbally or nonverbally encourages or discourages responses, shifts topics before all opinions are expressed, misses cues, or influences results in other ways (Tull & Hawkins, 1987).

One of the most difficult requirements for some professional focus group leaders is to be familiar with a variety of marketing topics and the industries represented. Unless the moderator specializes in a particular field, extensive background reading and briefing may be necessary. The moderator should develop a discussion guide based on the objectives and suggestions of the client who is paying for the focus group interviews. However, the moderator should not depend on a questionnaire to guide the interview. *Serial questioning* that follows a precise

EXHIBIT 4-3   Focus Group Research on the Nursing Shortage

Objectives

1. Identify perceptions and causes of the nursing shortage from viewpoints of three groups: (a) practicing registered nurses, (b) student nurses, and (c) nurse executives and hospital administrators. 2. Compare the perceptions of the three groups. 3. Provide data to compare with views published earlier.

Groups

Three focus groups, each with 9 or 10 respondents, were drawn from the Chicago area. There were different criteria of age, experience, agency affiliation, etc. for each group. Criteria common to all three groups were: no other focus group participation in the past year and no involvement by self or family in news media, advertising, or public relations firms.

Procedure

The interviews lasted about two hours. They were all audiotaped. Only the hospital and nurse administrators were videotaped. The discussion questions and topics for the three groups had some similarities. For example, student nurses discussed when and why they decided to enter nursing, education and entry into practice issues, expectations of the profession and their role, and perceptions of their future in nursing. Practicing nurses also discussed when and why they selected a nursing career and their plans for the future. Hospital and nurse administrators answered questions about the changing needs for nurses, advantages and disadvantages of a nursing career, and the problems facing nurses today. Only the latter group discussed solutions to these problems.

Source: American Hospital Association. (1987). *The nursing shortage: Facts, figures, and feelings* (pp. 1–24). Chicago, IL: Author.

order, without regard to the discussion, such as adhering to the order of a questionnaire, eliminates the group interaction that is one of the major benefits of focus group interviewing. This type of questioning should be avoided (Hisrich & Peters, 1982).

Durgee (1986) describes three depth-interviewing techniques the moderator can use: laddering, hidden-issue questioning, and symbolic analysis. In the *laddering technique,* the interviewer moves from questions on tangible product features and basic needs to desired end values such as self-esteem, self-actualization, or health. Using this technique, a focus group of patients discussing nursing care might be asked first about nurses answering their calls, and then move to questions about being respected and encouraged to assume more of their own care. *Hidden-issue questioning* moves from hidden personal issues to sensitive life themes that are widely shared. By delving into private fantasies, the moderator is looking for emotional connections with the product, idea, or organization being discussed. A moderator using this technique in a staff nurse focus group might ask questions about the proudest moment in the nurses' career, work goals, or leisure interests, and use this data to help a marketing firm create effective advertisements for staff nurses. *Symbolic analysis techniques* solicit data on how the opposites of the topic are perceived by the consumer group, in order to learn more about the idea, product, or organization of interest. One way to study the opposite of a service is to explore how members of the focus group feel about not using the service, or what they might substitute. Another way is to have the group discuss opposite types of service. A third symbolic analysis technique is to solicit attributes of an imaginary non-service as opposed to a real service. For instance, the focus group might be asked to describe a hospital stay without nursing care. Using these techniques to explore the feasibility of opening a nurse practitioner clinic, the moderator might ask focus group members who are potential clients where they would go for primary care if they came to the clinic and found it permanently closed. Alternatively, they might be asked to describe someone who would never use this service.

Analysis of Data

Regardless of the technique used to guide discussion, the contents of the interview must be available for careful examination after the discussion is finished. If videotaping, or at least audiotaping, is not possible, notes must be taken, preferably by an observer and not the moderator. Fedder (1986) recommends that notes be taken not in chronological order, but according to the topics outlined in the discussion guide. This helps the moderator target the major issues without getting sidetracked, as well as facilitating content analysis of data.

After the focus group interviews are concluded, the moderator or another marketing researcher prepares a report for the client, summarizing the predominant issues and analyzing the reactions and emotional content of the responses. Excerpts from the typed audiotape or videotape transcripts are used to establish categories of themes elicited on each topic area. A quantitative aspect of content analysis involves counting the number of themes in each topic area and the number of individual responses on each theme (Hisrich & Peters, 1982). Expectations of the client for the depth of analysis should be discussed when contracting for focus group interviews.

Advantages

When skillfully handled by the moderator, focus group interviews offer several advantages over other types of market research methods. The group interview is usually more stimulating and interesting for the respondent than an individual interview, completing a questionnaire, or participating in a telephone survey. The multidirectional flow of communications among group members is a prime advantage over individual interviewing techniques. More candor and spontaneity may result. Another advantage is that the respondents' reactions to each other are observed and analyzed to gain understanding of the selecting and purchasing decision-making processes (Goldman, 1962). The dynamics of attitudes, opinions, and product decision-making are made more apparent, as participants respond to new information and to one another, during the course of the session. These interviews can be used for illiterate adults and for children. Executives of the client manufacturing firm or service company whose products or ideas are being researched can observe focus groups from behind two-way mirrors or on videotape to see firsthand the consumer reactions.

Disadvantages

The main disadvantage of focus group interviewing is that the participants are not likely to be representative of the entire target market, because of the way they are selected, the small sample size, and the possibility of obtaining incomplete, less-than-candid responses. One dominant personality can skew the results by unduly influencing the rest of the group. Another disadvantage is that results largely depend on the skill of the moderator, and not all focus groups are led by experts. In the nursing field, many focus groups are moderated by amateurs, and the results are not always discounted accordingly. Even when conducted by expert moderators, generalizations cannot be made to the population without supportive quantitative research.

Costs

Although less expensive than individual depth interviews, the focus group method of marketing research is relatively expensive, on a per subject basis, when compared to telephone and mail surveys. Professional marketing researchers charge substantial fees to moderate groups, as we learned when we investigated for our professional association marketing research. In 1987, when we obtained bids on a focus interview contract, charges ranged from a low of $1,500 for six groups to a high of $4,000 per group. There were additional charges of $250 to $350 per group if focus interviews were conducted in facilities designed for this purpose. Participants are customarily paid fees ranging from $25 to $200 each. Recent payment for participants in a food product focus group in New York City was $35 each. Estimated total costs for a hospital employee or a physician group range from $1,200 to $3,000 (Droste, 1988b). The difference depends on how difficult it is to recruit the group members. According to Keckley (1988), the typical fee to a physician for a one-hour focus group is $100 to $150. A nurse manager or nurse practitioner might expect $100 for a one and a half- to two-hour group interview, and a staff nurse considerably less, because the pool is larger and pay is lower.

As in all marketing research, it is essential that the cost of focus group studies be in proportion to the importance of the topic. When recruiting a registered nurse is projected to cost between $5,000 and $20,000, focus groups that provide data valuable to retaining staff nurses can be extremely cost-effective. On the other hand, it may not make sense to spend $10,000 on market research to help develop a nursing manual that might produce a profit of $500 each year, even after factoring in the intangible gains such as reputation enhancement.

Individual Depth Interviews

The *individual depth interview*, also called a *one-on-one*, is another of the methods used in marketing research to obtain qualitative data. In a 30- to 60-minute session, the interviewer has freedom to explore the research question in depth. The basic rule is to avoid influencing the respondent's answers. Information flow is unidirectional from respondent to interviewer.

Individual depth interviews require a greater investment of the researcher's time, and thus cost considerably more than group interviews of the same number of respondents. Tull and Hawkins (1987) report that interviewing 35 respondents individually takes about four times as long as the same 35 respondents in four group interviews. The participant may be given a gift or payment similar to a focus group respondent. The complete cost for 30 individual physician interviews may be up to $7,500, when preparation and analysis are included, and take from 4 to 12 weeks to complete (Droste, 1988c). If the interviews are taped, the transcription and content analysis costs are greater than for focus groups. However, the quality of ideas offered by each individual has been found to be higher than in focus groups (Fern, 1982). This is because the interviewer can pursue relevant and interesting responses without worrying about neglecting other participants.

There are circumstances when individual depth interviews are the most appropriate method to use. Some topics may be too personal, sensitive, confidential, threatening, or embarrassing to discuss comfortably in a group of one's peers. A nurse may prefer a private discussion of salary, financial investments, agency administrators, or even the quality of nursing care delivered on a hospital unit. Potential consumers might not wish to discuss in a group whether they would use an AIDS screening clinic or a detoxification service if one were to be established in the local hospital. Individual interviewing is also recommended when strong social norms and mores exist related to the marketing problem. For probing complex behaviors, attitudes, preferences, and decisions, the individual depth interview may facilitate obtaining the data needed to answer the market research question. Investigating high turnover rates in a nursing organization, including the process of deciding to quit, is an example of a complex issue best studied by individual depth interviews.

QUANTITATIVE METHODS

Until the mid-1980s, quantitative studies were the accepted means of conducting nursing research. Going back to Florence Nightingale, nursing has a long tradition of systematically quantifying aspects of the world in order to improve our lives. Nightingale was a pioneer in the uses of social statistics and their graphic representation (Cohen, 1984). At Scutare, she systematized chaotic recordkeeping and collected a large amount of data. When she returned to England, she saw the potential of using the statistics she had gathered for improving health care in hospitals. Because of her collection and analysis of quantitative data and how she presented it, major reforms in sanitation and hospital care were effected. The use of quantitative studies for marketing purposes has been evolving since the turn of the century.

Research Instruments

The two main categories of quantitative research instruments used by market researchers are questionnaires and mechanical instruments. Of the two, mechanical devices are used relatively infrequently. They include galvanometers, tachistoscopes, and audiometers (Kotler, 1988). We do not discuss them here because of their lack of applicability to marketing nursing services.

Questionnaires are by far the most common instrument with which to collect primary data for marketing. A broad definition of *questionnaire* is a set of questions given to respondents for answers. It is frequently self-administered. There are many ways to write questions. Therefore, they must be developed with great care and validated before they are administered on a large scale. Casually prepared questionnaires often yield inaccurate, unusable, meaningless information. The questions and their form, wording, and sequence must be chosen carefully and tested for reliability and validity. (For more information, see a research text such as Polit and Hungler (1978).)

Experimental Research

Experimental research is considered by many to be the most scientifically valid approach. It is the most rigorous form of quantitative study, and its goal is to find cause-and-effect relationships. This method calls for carefully selecting random or matched groups of subjects, treating them differently, controlling variables, and evaluating response differences for statistical significance. A true experiment must have three characteristics: (1) manipulation, (2) control, and (3) randomization.

While experimental research is important to the development and validation of marketing theory, its limitations (see Table 4-1) militate against its widespread use in marketing research. Additionally, random, controlled study conditions are difficult to attain in marketing research situations. We do not discuss experimental research any further, but urge interested readers who think an experiment might be appropriate for a marketing research project to consult marketing and nursing research texts.

Survey Research

Surveys are the most well-known and most frequently used form of market research. Polit and Hungler (1978) define *survey research* as:

> that branch of research that examines the characteristics, behaviors, attitudes, and intentions of a group of people by asking individuals belonging to that group (typically only a subset) to answer a series of questions. Survey research is an extremely flexible research approach and, therefore, is quite diversified with respect to populations studied, scope, content, and purpose. Surveys can serve a descriptive, explanatory, predictive, or exploratory function, and some research projects concentrate on more than one of these objectives. (p. 206)

The steps of the survey research method are found in Exhibit 4-4.

A *survey* is a formal procedure to obtain current information. Because of the rapidity with which the world changes, studies quickly become outdated. Basing marketing decisions on outdated information can be very costly. We therefore constantly need to test for current information.

There are eight important characteristics of survey research. Survey research is systematic, impartial, representative, theory-based, quantitative, self-monitoring, contemporary, and replicable (Backstrom & Hursh-César, 1981). It is systematic, in that it follows a set of rules and progresses in a logical, orderly fashion. Impartiality is demonstrated in the selection of the sample without prejudice or preference. While the personal values of the researcher influence the questions posed and the method used, surveys can be reasonably free of the researcher's personal biases. The information produced is more reliable than personal judgments and guesses.

Representativeness is achieved by the inclusion of all aspects of the problem under study and the population affected. Relevant principles of human behavior, laws of probability, and statistics guide the survey, making it theory-based. The survey assigns numerical values to nonnumerical characteristics of human behavior in ways that quantify and permit uniform interpretation of these characteristics. Surveys can be self-monitoring, in that their procedures can be designed to reveal any unplanned and unwanted biases that do occur. They are contemporary, in that they give current facts. Other people using the same methods in the same ways can replicate survey research to increase the generalizability of the findings or raise questions about the initial results.

Survey research is best suited for description. Surveys tell us about what people know, their beliefs, perceptions, attitudes, preferences, satisfaction, and so on.

EXHIBIT 4-4   Steps of the Survey Research Method

1. Define the problem to be studied.
2. Search the literature for information on the problem.
3. Develop the hypothesis; specify relationships.
4. Design the study; choose principles and procedures.
5. Organize resources; staff, funds, materials.
6. Choose the people to interview.
7. Develop the questions.
8. Construct the questionnaire.
9. Pretest the instrument; does it give the desired data?
10. Teach interviewers good data-gathering techniques.
11. Interview; obtain data from respondents.
12. Code; assign numerical value to responses.
13. Assure that all data is usable.
14. Program computer to handle data.
15. Organize data into tables.
16. Analyze data.
17. Apply measures of statistical significance.
18. Present findings and conclusions.
19. Apply findings and conclusions.

They measure the incidence of these aspects in the population. In Case Study 10, for instance, Kelly measured the kinds of continuing education programs nurses preferred. Through a survey, we found (in Case Study 1) that nurses were generally not aware of their district professional association. McAnnally describes the survey used to compare the quality of care expected and perceived by parents of children treated in a private clinic (Case Study 12). Cohen and Lowell (1989) used survey research to develop a nurse recruitment program.

Personal Interviewing

There are three contact modes of interviewing. Information can be obtained in person, by telephone, and by mail. (See Table 4-2 for characteristics of the interviewing modes.) Survey research for marketing gained credibility through personal interviews. Of the three contact methods, this is the most versatile. Personal interviews can be conducted in offices, shopping malls, the street, hospitals, or homes. They can be done wherever there are people who meet the target population description. It is often possible to ask more questions than by telephone or mail. For studies requiring lengthy interviews lasting an hour or more, this is the contact method of choice.

More administrative planning and supervision are required for personal interviews, which contribute to high costs. Personal interviewing is the most expensive contact method, but it enables us to acquire or verify certain data that we could not get with any other method. For example, we may get more reliable data if we directly observe a respondent's race than by asking for this information on the telephone. This is also the case if we want to ascertain the medications used by the respondent, verify weight, and so on.

While personal interviewing has many advantages, it is no longer the dominant survey method. Commercial surveys now generally use the telephone or direct mail to obtain needed information.

Interviewing by Telephone

Telephone interviewing is the best method for gathering information quickly. Telephones have an almost unlimited geographic reach. More than 90% of all United States homes now have telephones, making it possible to sample general populations thoroughly. Although only people with telephones can be interviewed, weighting techniques can be used to balance the sample for people less likely to have phones. Telephone surveys are most appropriate when studying general issues and populations that can be located through a directory, such as association members, officials, college students, physicians, and the like.

Studies show that the quality of data gathered by telephone and personal interviewing is comparable (Groves & Kahn, 1979). If questions are broken down into simple parts, it is possible to get information on complex topics. Good questions are understandable regardless of the method of contact.

Mail Surveys

Many articles in the marketing research literature deal with methodological issues involving mail surveys. These articles focus on timing or technique. The following issues have been studied in an attempt to improve response rates:

1. Notifying in advance by letter or telephone that a questionnaire is being sent.
2. Calling potential respondents requesting permission to send questionnaire.
3. Using white, off-white, or colored stationery.
4. Using a specific kind of postage such as commemorative stamps, metered mail, or specific denominations of stamps.
5. Including stamped or franked return envelopes.

6. Shortening or lengthening the questionnaire.

7. Evaluating various categories of sponsorship.

8. Identifying sponsorship of survey.

9. Making the questionnaire attractive.

10. Adding title under sender's name.

11. Personalizing the correspondence.

12. Assessing differences in titles of senders.

13. Assuring anonymity and confidentiality.

14. Composing the cover letter: permissive versus firm, a plea for help, a request for a favor, stressing social usefulness of study, importance of respondent to the success of the study.

15. Enclosing an incentive such as money or a small gift (pencils, trading stamps, etc.).

16. Promising a small gift for completing and returning the questionnaire.

17. Giving a deadline for return of the questionnaire.

18. Following up with reminders by mail or telephone.

19. Timing of the follow-up.

The results of these studies have been, to say the least, inconsistent. For example, personalizing the correspondence has increased the response rate in some cases, decreased it in others, and had no effect in still other cases. The same kind of results have been found with the use of different kinds of postage, composition of the cover letter, and other techniques. Reviews of the literature by Kanuk and Berenson in 1975 and Yu and Cooper in 1983 have not clarified whether these techniques actually work. That many of these efforts have been inconclusive is clearly stated by Kanuk and Berenson (1975, p. 451): "Despite the large number of research studies reporting techniques designed to improve response rates, there is no strong empirical evidence favoring any techniques other than the *follow-up* and the use of *monetary incentives* [italics added]."

Erdos (1974) maintains that incentives are necessary whenever the topic of the survey is not interesting enough or the sender's prestige is not impressive enough to induce a high return rate. The use of monetary incentives significantly increases the number of questionnaires returned, often by 50% or more. This was the case in our nursing association mail survey, when a dollar bill was enclosed as an incentive to return the questionnaire (Camuñas, Alward, & Vecchione, in press).

Advantages and Limitations

The greatest advantage of survey research is the flexibility and broadness of scope the method provides. Surveys can be adapted for many populations, they can gather information on a wide range of topics, and the information generated

TABLE 4-2   Choosing among Interviewing Modes

Interview Mode	When to Use	Advantages	Disadvantages
Personal	When timely generalization is desired	Complicated topics	Interviewer biases
	When combined with observation	Probing	Respondent availability
	When visual stimuli are used	Better rapport	Interviewer-respondent perceptions
	When rare groups are defined by geography	Better control of respondent	Expensive
Telephone	For immediate results	Anonymous	Disruptive
	For general issues, general audiences	Fast, cheap	Uncomplicated topics
	For simultaneous national/regional interviewing	Geographically flexible	Less control of respondent
	To verify survey data	More than 90% of homes have phones	Underrepresents minorities and low-income groups
		Free of perceptual biases	Imprecise local areas
		Monitors interviewer biases	
Mail questionnaire	For nose-counting sample enumeration	Cheapest	Low response rate
	For specialized, well-defined populations	Capable of census	No control of respondent
	For low-risk populations	Free of perceptual bias	Junk mail irritation
	For diary keeping	Pictorial, technical content	Slow returns
	To verify personal interviews		Requires literate respondents

Adapted with permission of Macmillan Publishing Company from *Survey Research*, 2nd ed., by Charles H. Backstrom and Gerald Hursh-César, p. 18. New York: Wiley & Sons, 1981. Copyright © 1981 by Macmillan Publishing Co; Gerald Hursh-César *The Research Information Workshop: Using Research for Public Policy Decision-Making*, Exhibit 11.4, Berkeley: Office of the Academic Vice President, University of California, 1977.

can be put to many uses. While they can be more expensive than experiments, they generate a large amount of information and can therefore be cost-effective.

There are also many limitations to survey research. In order for findings to be generalizable to large populations, the survey must be conducted according to strict procedures regarding sample size and selection. The sample must be large enough so that statistical analysis leads to reasonably valid conclusions. Respondents must have the same characteristics as found in the larger population. For instance, characteristics such as race, sex, religion, and political affiliation may be important. Achieving a sufficient sample size and mix of characteristics can make survey research expensive.

The data obtained in most surveys are generally superficial. Because of the time constraints and artificial circumstances under which surveys are conducted, probing very deeply into complex human behavior and feelings is not possible. This is not necessarily a weakness. Survey methods are better suited to extensive rather than intensive analysis.

Because the process of survey research is one of researchers communicating with respondents, often through interviewers, there is a lot of room for human error. Surveys are intrusive: that is, they are unnatural occurrences in respondents' daily lives. Respondents are very aware that they are being studied. Often they respond differently than they would if they did not know they were being studied. An added, related factor is the artificiality of the survey exchange. Surveys are structured situations. Each participant has a well-defined, almost mutually exclusive role. Interviewers ask the questions; respondents answer them. Questions and acceptable answers are determined by the researcher in advance. The questions and issues may be irrelevant or outside the respondent's experience; they may have no meaning relative to assessing the respondent's opinions.

Another limitation is that respondents self-report. Respondents do not always give the unvarnished truth. Nonresponse is also a limitation. When people do not respond, there is a risk of distortion in the representativeness of the sample.

PRESENTING RESEARCH FINDINGS

In addition to tabular results, a complete market research study includes one or more management reports, with or without charts or graphs. The major findings that are relevant to the marketing decisions facing management are presented. They should be written in a clear, straightforward way. Management must be able to understand the reports in order to make use of them.

It is often helpful to have a meeting to review the findings with the people for whom the study was done. A meeting gives them an opportunity to gain a better understanding of what was done and what the results mean. Presentation meetings often add to the value of the study.

Written reports should be tailored to meet the needs of the people using the information. Some people want very brief reports, while others want very detailed ones. Charts and graphs are important for still others. The format to use is the one that best conveys the study results. Generally, a study report includes the following:

1. Statement of purpose and objectives.
2. Short review of how the study was done.
3. Results of the study, with conclusions.
4. Recommendations based on results.
5. Detailed study findings on which conclusions and recommendations were based.
6. Appendix containing other, less important information.

JUSTIFICATION OF RESEARCH COSTS

Marketing Myths

Over a billion dollars is spent each year for marketing research in the United States (Tull & Hawkins, 1987). The hospital industry spends approximately $40 million to $50 million a year on marketing research, with a typical hospital spending $14,000 to $29,000 in 1987 (Droste, 1988a). According to Droste's report, the Steiber Research Group found that 50% of hospitals' marketing research is devoted to patients, 23.5% to physicians, 12.1% to businesses, and 14.5% to other referral markets.

In nursing management, as in many small businesses and nonprofit organizations, there is a tendency to associate marketing research with high costs, advanced statistical procedures, time-consuming surveys, and expensive consultants. Andreasen (1983) describes the following pervasive myths about marketing research:

1. The *big decision myth* is that marketing research is only required for major decisions; it is not necessary or practical for daily decisions.
2. The *survey myopia myth* is that the only marketing research method is the field survey with its random samples, questionnaires, and computer analyses.
3. The *big bucks myth* is that only large corporations can afford marketing research.
4. The *sophisticated researcher myth* is that only experienced researchers are prepared to use the complex methods that are required.

5. The *most research is not read myth* is that much marketing research is a waste of time because it is poorly designed or is superfluous. (p. 74)

Andreasen refutes all these myths and offers several low-cost approaches to marketing research. He suggests that the decision of whether to use marketing research should be based on a cost-benefit analysis, regardless of the magnitude of the decision. Are the projected benefits worth the cost of the research project? In this analysis, consider not only the cost of research, but what the costs will be if you make a poor decision. If you are determined to go ahead with a test of a new service to a targeted market, regardless of research results, the test can be your research. There may be little point in expending additional funds for preliminary research. Frequently, though, research can be done quickly and inexpensively, leading to a better decision. It need not be a sophisticated design to be useful. One of the alternative methods to a large survey is focus group interviews. Others are systematic observation of consumers' reactions to services, and the use of internal management reports and secondary sources that describe similar services and their acceptance by consumers.

In refuting the myth that "most research is not read," Andreasen reminds us that the key to sound marketing research is good planning by the researcher and by the ultimate user, if they are not the same. Both must be clear about the relationships between alternate decisions and the required marketing information. Marketing research results must be clearly understood by nurse users if the results are to be useful in planning marketing strategies.

Budgeting for Market Research Costs

Keckley (1988) provides some practical guidelines for budgeting marketing research. As pointed out earlier, the cost-benefit ratio is an important consideration. The research budget should be scaled to the degree of financial risk inherent in the marketing strategy, and no research should be done if there is no risk in the marketing decision. Keckley's advice is that you should not spend in excess of 20% of the total marketing budget for research on any service or program.

Because outside consultants may charge higher fees to gather secondary data from the library and computer sources, you may be able to use your own resources to collect data within the organization. Use your nursing resources whenever you can. If the health care organization has a marketing department or a nursing research department, you may be able to reduce your market research budget by asking these departments for assistance. Graduate students affiliating at health care agencies are often looking for interesting projects and should be considered valuable resources for market research activities.

In competing for scarce fiscal resources in today's health care organizations, justification of budget proposals is crucial to approval by budget committees and ultimately by the governing board. Each institution has its own system for budgeting, but the following guidelines can assist you in the justification of market research expenses. When market research is undertaken by a nurse or nursing organization, a budget must be prepared that incorporates all the costs associated with the study. This is easier when you contract with a marketing research consultant who can give an all-inclusive price for the project, and more difficult when it is a shared project or one conducted entirely by the nursing organization. In addition to allocated salary expense, fringe benefits, overhead, and administrative costs must be included. Burst (1985) reminds us to factor in the expenses of "opportunity loss," based upon what the staff would be doing instead of this project. Supplies, computer expenses, statistical consultation, fees for focus group participants, postage, telephone, and office space must be included in direct and indirect expense categories. The projected budget for conducting the study internally can be compared to bids from outside consultants and to the costs of testing the market without research.

Compare the costs of internally and externally conducted research to the cost of making a mistake with a new product that you might have avoided through market research. In considering the cost of a possible marketing mistake, again add the hidden costs of opportunity loss, direct salary expense, overhead, and administrative expense involved in trying out optional programs and services without conducting market research. It may be difficult to calculate the indirect costs of management time and organization morale in making the wrong choice, but they are important considerations in making your research decisions.

CONCLUSION

Market research helps us to understand our world and solve our problems. In order to make effective nursing and health care decisions and policies, we have to understand the nature of the problems and of the proposed solutions. We must have a solid information base about conditions, behaviors, awareness, feelings, beliefs, attitudes, and values. The goal of obtaining the knowledge is not to enable us to manipulate people, but to satisfy needs and wants. A continuous, up-to-date flow of information helps us to make informed judgments about policy and to design strategies that satisfy nursing's many customers.

REFERENCES

Andreasen, A.R. (1983). Growing concerns: Cost-conscious marketing research. *Harvard Business Review, 61*(4), 74–77.

Backstrom, C.H., & Hursh-César, G. (1981). *Survey research* (2nd ed.). New York: John Wiley.

Bartos, R. (1987). Qualitative research: What it is and where it came from. *Journal of Advertising Research, 26*(3), RC3–RC6.

Burst, A. (1985). Market research in the nonprofit sector. In E.E. Bobrow & M.D. Bobrow (Eds.), *Marketing handbook: Volume I: Marketing practices* (pp. 252–266). Homewood, IL: Dow Jones-Irwin.

Camuñas, C., Alward, R.R., & Vecchione, E. (in press). Survey response rates to a professional association mail questionnaire. *Journal of the New York State Nurses Association.*

Carithers, R.W. (1977). What to expect from an outside consultant and how to get it. *Health Care Management Review, 2*(3), 43–46.

Clarke, R.N., & Shyavitz, L.J. (1982). Market research: when, why and how. *Health Care Management Review, 7*(1), 29–34.

Cohen, I.B. (1984). Florence Nightingale. *Scientific American, 250*(3), 128–137.

Cohen, J.B., & Lowell, L. (1989). Market research gives nurse administrators an edge. *Nursing Management, 20*(5), 44–46.

Droste, T. (1988a). Are marketers drowning in data? *Hospitals, 62*(15), 42–46.

Droste, T. (1988b). Focus groups provide insight into marketplace. *Hospitals, 62*(11), 45–46.

Droste, T. (1988c). Research: Matching the method to the project. *Hospitals, 62*(15), 45.

Durgee, J.F. (1986). Depth-interviewing techniques for creative advertising. *Journal of Advertising Research, 25*(6), 29–37.

Erdos, P.L. (1974). Data collection methods: Mail surveys. In R. Ferber (Ed.), *Handbook of marketing research* (pp. 2-90 to 2-104). New York: McGraw Hill.

Fedder, C.J. (1986). Listening to qualitative research. *Journal of Advertising Research, 25*(6), 57–59.

Fern, E.F. (1982). The use of focus groups for idea generation. *Journal of Marketing Research, 19*(1), 1–13.

Goldman, A.E. (1962). The group depth interview. *Journal of Marketing, 26*(4), 61–68.

Green, P.E., Tull, D.S., & Albaum, G. (1988). *Research for marketing decisions* (5th ed.). Englewood Cliffs, NJ: Prentice-Hall.

Groves, R.M., & Kahn, R.L. (1979). *Surveys by telephone: A national comparison with personal interviews.* New York: Academic.

Hisrich, R.D., & Peters, M.P. (1982). Focus groups: An innovative marketing research technique. *Hospital & Health Services Administration, 27*(4), 8–21.

Kanuk, L., & Berenson, C. (1975). Mail surveys and response rates: A literature review. *Journal of Marketing Research, 12*, 440–453.

Keckley, P.H. (1988). *Market research handbook for health care professionals.* Chicago: American Hospital Publishing.

Kotler, P. (1988). *Marketing management: Analysis, planning, implementation, and control* (6th ed.). Englewood Cliffs, NJ: Prentice-Hall.

Kotler, P., & Clarke, R.N. (1987). *Marketing for health care organizations.* Englewood Cliffs, NJ: Prentice-Hall.

Merton, R.K. (1987). The focused interview and focus groups: Continuities and discontinuities. *Public Opinion Quarterly, 51*, 550–566.

Nasser, D.L. (1988). How to run a focus group. *Public Relations Journal, 44*(3), 33–34.

Oiler, C. (1982). The phenomenological approach in nursing research. *Nursing Research, 31,* 178–181.

Polit, D.F., & Hungler, B.P. (1978). *Nursing research: Principles and methods.* New York: Lippincott.

Pope, J.L. (1986). Marketing research for service industries. In V.P. Buell (Ed.), *Handbook of modern marketing* (pp. 36:1 to 36:10). New York: McGraw-Hill.

Stevens, B.J. (1978). The use of consultants in nursing service. *Journal of Nursing Administration, 8*(8), 7–15.

Tull, D.S., & Hawkins, D.I. (1987). *Marketing research: Measurement and method* (4th ed.). New York: Macmillan.

Wilensky, S. (1985). Services marketing research. In E.E. Bobrow & M.D. Bobrow (Eds.), *Marketing handbook: Volume I: Marketing practices* (pp. 221–234). Homewood, IL: Dow Jones-Irwin.

Yu, J., & Cooper, H. (1983). A quantitative review of research design effects on response rates to questionnaires. *Journal of Marketing Research, 20,* 36–44.

CHAPTER 5

Marketing Strategies

STRATEGIC MARKET PLANNING

Chapter 4 discussed research as one of the two key elements of marketing. Without research to discover, verify, and monitor the needs and preferences of targeted markets, there cannot be a marketing orientation. The other major element of marketing is the strategy that evolves from mission or purpose, market research, and strategic planning. Ideally, the top-level administrators of the organization or the nurse entrepreneur will have formulated a strategic plan that includes the mission, goals, and objectives for the next few years. Strategic planning requires assessments of the external and internal environments, both present and projected. Strengths and weaknesses in all areas of the operation should be analyzed when long-range plans are made. Strategic market planning is an essential part of the whole process.

Kotler and Andreasen (1987, p. 159) define the strategic marketing planning process (SMPP) as the "managerial process of developing and maintaining a strategic fit between the organization's goals and resources and its changing market opportunities." They delineate 10 steps in the SMPP:

1. Setting out the mission, goals, and objectives to which the process must contribute.
2. Assessing external environmental challenges and threats.
3. Evaluating internal strengths in resources and skills, vis-à-vis the external challenges.
4. Determining the marketing mission, goals, and objectives for the planning period.
5. Formulating the marketing strategies (paths) for goal attainment.
6. Putting in place the marketing systems and structure necessary to implement the strategies.
7. Establishing tactics or programs that follow the strategies for the planning period, including a timetable and assignment of responsibilities.

8. Establishing criteria to measure achievements.

9. Implementing the plans.

10. Measuring performance and adjusting strategies and tactics as necessary.

Note that it is the nursing organization's external and internal environmental analyses (steps 2 and 3) that help determine the marketing mission, objectives, strategies, and tactics for achieving objectives. This assessment would include an analysis of the factors set out in Exhibit 5-1.

EXHIBIT 5-1   Environmental Analysis Factors

- Community served by the organization
- Reimbursement and regulatory climate
- Competitors
- Availability of nursing personnel
- Collective bargaining environment
- Competency of nursing personnel
- Current and projected use of services
- Patient case mix
- Patient acuity and dependency factors
- Medical staff requirements
- Physical plant conditions
- Strengths and weaknesses of the nursing division
- Strengths and weaknesses of the organization as a whole

Some of the questions that must be answered in developing a nursing marketing plan have been adapted by Alward (1988, p. 201) from those suggested by Shaffer (1984).

1. What special skills does this nursing organization (department, unit) bring to the health care arena?

2. Who are the important target groups with whom the organization exchanges values?

3. What image of the nursing organization is held by the target groups?

4. What are the primary and secondary services to be offered to each target group and in exchange for what value to the nursing organization?

5. How can the services be improved and more effectively promoted?

6. Which services are profitable and which are not? (Profit is conceptualized here as any gain when compared to the expenditures needed to produce the service.)

7. Are the services priced appropriately for each market segment and for the financial health of the organization?

8. Who and where is the competition? What action is expected from them?

9. What market data is readily accessible and what must be collected specifically for the marketing effort?

10. What are (or should be) the nursing organization's mission and objectives? Based on the answers to questions 1 through 9, what business is this nursing organization in (or what business should it be in)?

Product Portfolio Planning

Most modern health care organizations have many market opportunities from which to select their offerings. They usually offer to their consumers in multiple markets a portfolio of many types of services. Planning this product portfolio raises continual questions about where and when to increase, maintain, decrease, or withdraw resources in producing these services. New product opportunities must be evaluated. The Boston Consulting Group (BCG) and the McKinsey/General Electric approaches to product portfolio analysis and management are now widely used. Both of these methods first separate individual or similar goods and services into strategic business units (SBU). A *strategic business unit* contains products that can be planned for together because they essentially are marketed to the same customers, in a similar way, and have the same competitors (Kotler & Andreasen, 1987). Nursing services offered to young families during their childbearing years might form one SBU in a group nurse practitioner practice. The two approaches differ in how they assess the SBU's performance and the attractiveness of actual and potential markets.

The BCG approach uses a grid to rate each SBU on two dimensions: its annual rate of growth in the marketplace and its share of the market compared to the leading competitors (Figure 5-1). The grid identifies SBUs falling into the four quadrants as *stars* (high market growth, high relative market share), *cash cows* (slow market growth, high relative market share), *question marks* (high market growth, low relative market share), and *dogs* (slow market growth, low relative market share).

The McKinsey/General Electric method of portfolio evaluation uses the dimensions of market attractiveness and organizational strength in a strategic business planning grid (Figure 5-2). In general, markets are more attractive if they are large, have high growth and high profit potential, and if they offer economies of scale as the volume or usage increases. Markets are less attractive if they are cyclical, seasonal, and have many strong competitors. Organizational strength is evaluated by factors of marketing effectiveness and knowledge, program quality, and efficiency level. Market attractiveness and the strength of each SBU are plotted on the grid to help with strategic market planning.

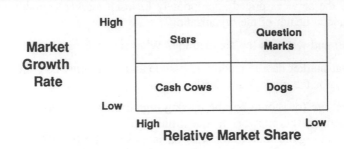

Figure 5-1. Boston Consulting Group portfolio planning grid.

Although product portfolio planning strategies are useful in marketing for both profit and nonprofit organizations, we must be mindful of the difference in emphasis on profitability when we deal with nonprofit agencies, and specifically with health care and nursing organizations. Profit is not the bottom line in all these decisions, as it most generally is in commercial, for-profit businesses. Hospitals and other health care providers often offer services that are not profitable because they are part of the mission of the provider. Alternatively, providers may be prevented from eliminating losing services by conditions in the internal and external political or regulatory environments (Solovy, 1989).

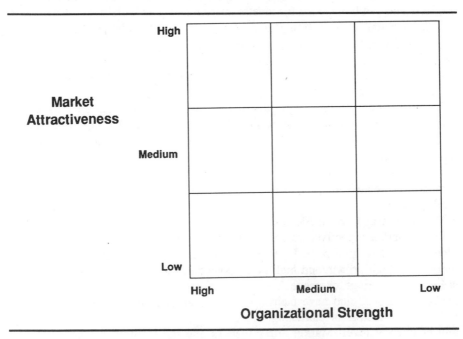

Figure 5-2. McKinsey/General Electric portfolio planning grid.

CORE MARKETING STRATEGIES

Three key components of the core marketing strategy to achieve marketing goals are selecting target markets, competitive positioning, and developing an effective marketing mix. We discussed segmenting and target marketing in Chapter 3. The focus of *competitive positioning* is to develop and communicate the attractive characteristics of your offer, stressing its significant differences from competing products. Positioning strategy often has to do with image and perceptions. The strategic question is, "How do you want to be perceived by consumers in comparison to other health care providers in the same market?" What is important is not what you think of your product, but whether it is perceived by the consumer as being better than, and different from, your competitors' products. To position yourself competitively, you must understand how consumers evaluate and choose among competing nursing services.

Bloom (1984) pointed out that it is much more difficult to distinguish among competing professional services than among consumer products such as cereals. He suggests (as we did in Chapter 4) using market research to discover what attributes patients perceive as making one health care service more attractive than, or different from, competitors' services. Market strategies can then be focused on developing and communicating a distinctive image, while delivering services that appeal to the target markets. Bloom describes three attributes that professional services, such as nursing, can use to distinguish themselves from other nursing care providers: more experience and specialization, more brain power in solving problems, and better procedures. We would add caring, compassion, and empathy as important differentiating nursing characteristics.

MARKETING MIX

Megamarketing

Marketing mix is the customized blend of marketing strategies used to achieve marketing goals and objectives. McCarthy (1981) originated the well-known classification of strategic components called the *four Ps* of the marketing mix: product, price, place, and promotion. When these strategic elements are used in health care marketing, Cooper suggests they be called service, consideration, access, and promotion (Keith, 1985), because these terms are more descriptive for the industry. Place components are frequently called *distribution,* and promotion is also known as *communications.*

More recently, Kotler (1986) recommended that two more components, power and public relations, be added to the marketing mix when strategic thinking is needed to attract markets to whom access is blocked or protected by third parties, as it so often is in the health care field. He calls the strategic process needed in protected markets *megamarketing*. Marketing and megamarketing are contrasted in Table 5-1. In the case of the protected health care market, gatekeeping third parties include physicians, insurance companies, governmental agencies, labor unions, employers, and public interest groups.

TABLE 5-1   Marketing and Megamarketing Contrasted

	Marketing	Megamarketing
Marketing objective	To satisfy consumer demand	To gain market access in order to satisfy consumer demand or to create or alter consumer demand
Parties involved	Consumers, distributors, dealers, suppliers, marketing firms, banks	Normal parties plus legislators, government agencies, labor unions, reform groups, general public
Marketing tools	Marketing research, product development, pricing, distribution, planning, promotion	Normal tools plus the use of power and public relations
Type of inducement	Positive and official inducements	Positive inducements (official and unofficial) and negative inducements (threats)
Time frame	Short	Much longer
Investment cost	Low	Much higher
Personnel involved	Marketers	Marketers plus company officers, lawyers, public relations and public affairs staff

Public relations, as a strategy to pull the nursing organization into the marketplace, is the topic of Chapter 6. Before turning to the traditional marketing mix components, we should discuss power as a push strategy. *Power* is the ability to influence others to do what otherwise they might not have done. Much has been written in the nursing literature on our need for political skills and strategies to keep and use power effectively in obtaining desired goals. Without understanding how to use power and politics in the work place, your influence will be limited. (For references on power and politics in nursing, see Chapter 1.) After identifying the gatekeepers to a target health care market, the nurse marketer must determine what strategies and incentives need to be negotiated to gain access to the ultimate user of the offered nursing service. In some cases, it may be power rather than value that wins over the gatekeeper. Thus, Kotler (1986, p. 121) states that "marketing is increasingly becoming the art of managing power."

When direct access to a market is blocked, the three broad strategies suggested by Kotler to overcome opposition are: (1) organize coalitions of allies, (2) make allies of neutral groups, and (3) compensate opponents for losses. Nurses must think of consumers, particularly of patients—the end users of nursing services—as allies and form coalitions with them, as well as with other health care workers. Although at times we are discouraged by our slow progress in forming coalitions that include physicians, we must persist, particularly in those markets where the product is interdisciplinary health service.

In health care, another important "p" component of the marketing mix is the people who deliver the service (Kotler & Clarke, 1987). An essential way to improve the quality of health care is to exert influence on the providers, who are often professional, self-regulating practitioners. Since many of these are not employees of the health care agency in which they practice, service incompetence is even harder to control than clinical incompetence. The latter is subject to peer review and various policies of the organization. However, if the organizational culture supports empathic care, over time this value has a positive effect on most of those practicing within that health care facility.

The Seven Cs of Health Care Marketing Mix

Before turning to the traditional four Ps of the marketing mix, there is a set of service benefits or attributes that Ireland (1985) has called the "seven Cs." They are important to the health care strategies mix. Nurses would do well to keep them in mind when planning marketing strategies for exchanging their services with patient markets.

Care—Technical capacity and competence in personnel, equipment, management systems, and plant.

Caring—Compassion, warmth, empathy of caregivers for patients.

Comfort—Room service amenities, including food service and selection, telephone, and interior design.

Convenience—Benefits that reduce aggravations for consumers: preadmission testing, admission, scheduling, parking, visiting, waiting rooms, hours of operation. (These are extremely important to patients in the United States.)

Curative—Service attributes that assist the patient to get well, ranging from those that are lifesaving to those less significant, but still valued, that increase levels of wellness.

Cope—Benefits exchanged to help patients adapt to illness, injury, loss of function, or self-image problems. For example, psychosocial nursing services, patient education, discharge planning.

Cost—Attributes that help control health care costs, such as those that contributed to the development of outpatient surgery, birthing centers, home care, and computer-assisted management systems.

PRODUCT

A *product* in its broadest sense is defined as whatever is offered to a market to satisfy a need, desire, or preference, and as a set of benefits "that can be offered to the market for attention, acquisition, or consumption" (MacStravic, 1986, p. 35). The common categories of products are goods or physical objects, services, and ideas. An organization's products can also include feelings of accomplishment, satisfaction, pride, self-esteem, and belonging. Products can include persons, places, programs, and organizations, because the value package or offering of these products can be thought of as services.

To develop products in any of these categories, you should distinguish the core, tangible, and augmented levels in the product concept. The *core product* is what the consumer is seeking in order to answer a basic need. In the case of nursing products for patients, the core product is improvement or maintenance of health. Nursing service per se is not our core product; it is a vehicle or means of restoring health and thus is a production function. Carmel's (1985) research indicates that the core product or outcome (improvement of health) is a more important predictor of the patient's satisfaction with nursing care and hospitalization than is the process (health provider's services). It is thus a useful exercise to identify the needs and wants at the core of each product you offer in a marketplace exchange, as well as its hoped-for result, so that the core product is clear and can be marketed by describing outcomes anticipated from the services. In the case of interdisciplinary health services, this is more complex, because of the number of health care practitioners involved in the production process who thereby affect the outcome.

The *tangible* level of a product is identified by five characteristics: features, styling, quality level, packaging, and brand name. Not every product has all these features, but most products that are goods have at least some of them. Nursing services might be identified by features (primary nursing), quality level, and even brand name (Visiting Nurse Service). In Case Study 3, some of the tangible features of nursing manuals are discussed.

The third level is the *augmented* level of a product, in which services and benefits are added to the tangible product. These added values are for the purpose of differentiating products from those of competitors or for meeting additional needs and wants. An example of this augmented level of a nursing product is the outpatient visits provided without additional cost after inpatient care, as described in Case Study 19.

Characteristics of Service

A *service* is an intangible activity or benefit that is offered to another party without that other party becoming owner of the product. Some services are connected to a physical product, others are not. An increasing segment of the labor force is employed in service industries such as health care, government, finance, education, insurance, entertainment, travel, trade, communications, food, lodging, social, and management services. These services account for about 75% of the nonagricultural jobs in the United States and about 70% of the national income. In the past three decades, most of the women and minorities entering the work force, in 44 million new positions, were absorbed by the service industries (Heskett, 1987).

Pope (1986, p. 36-2) defines a *service industry* as one that "controls the distribution of the product or service to the end user, as well as provides or produces the product or service." The differentiation for Pope is not whether the product is tangible or intangible, but the control over distribution to the end user. Thus McDonald's is a service business while Campbell's is not.

Many of the characteristics of services, including health care services, are similar to those of commercial products. Tyson (1977) points out six common features. Health care services and commercial products (1) are developed to meet customers' needs, (2) require investment of capital for research, development, and operation, (3) have special features that should be packaged to obtain consumer acceptance, (4) are exchanged with (sold to) select market segments, (5) bring revenues or goodwill to the producer/provider, and (6) are similar to other marketplace offers.

Other characteristics of services are not similar to those of goods. Kotler and Andreasen (1987) describe five differentiating characteristics of services that must be considered when planning marketing strategies. The important features of services are intangibility, inseparability, variability, perishability, and consumer involvement.

Intangibility

Services cannot be tested by the senses before they are exchanged with consumers, nor can they be returned for credit as one might return a uniform that does not fit properly. The service purchase decision is made on the basis of trust or confidence in the provider. For the patient, this may involve trust in an attending physician, nurse practitioner, or nurse midwife, as well as in an institution. Health care providers can use tangible devices and techniques to increase the patient's confidence, but all too frequently these are dismissed as unnecessary or time-consuming. Tangible aids include drawings and brochures to describe procedures, name tags with positions clearly identified, clean and neat personnel, attractive facilities, and quick response to call bells or telephone calls. Another strategy to increase consumer confidence is to identify the provider by a brand name. In Case Study 13, Mershon describes how Humana used the corporate name to communicate a positive image to the nursing community. Zeithaml, Para-suraman, and Berry (1985) also suggest that creating a strong organizational image, after-purchase communications, and cost accounting to help determine fair prices will enhance consumer trust. On the other hand, permission forms with a very long list of risks, although necessary for obtaining informed consent, can undermine confidence in health care providers, especially if that trust was weak in the first place. Unkempt, rude, or inconsiderate health care employees are tangible symbols of a poor service offer to clients.

Inseparability

A service cannot be separated from the providing source. It is consumed as it is produced and is often sold directly by the producer of the service. Unlike consumer goods, services cannot be produced, tested, and held in inventory until they are needed. Instead, the service producer must be physically present at the exchange. This characteristic of services has led to quality problems in the health care industry in general, and for the nursing and medical professions in particular. Human productivity is limited, while demand for health services can be very inconsistent and urgent. One of the strategies for dealing with this problem is to select, train, and supervise other service providers in whom patients can trust. The nursing profession is once again at this point, as the demand for registered nurses exceeds the supply. Maintaining the quality of nursing services, while delegating some of the tasks of nursing and nonnursing functions, is our challenge in this environment.

Variability

Another characteristic of services that has a substantial impact on quality is their variability from one service occasion to another, and from one provider to the next. We know that the level of service provided by a very competent or even expert nurse will vary depending on whether the practitioner is rested after three days off or fatigued after working a mandatory double shift, and whether the nurse is angry, depressed, harassed, or happy and satisfied with working conditions. We are also aware of the difference in the competence and caring of nurses with similar educational backgrounds and years of service. Orientation, quality assurance, and guest relations programs are attempts to control the variability of services to patients by providing a more consistent level of quality. Process and outcome standards define the level of nursing care that is acceptable in each nursing organization. Another approach to the variability aspect of services is to customize them to meet individual patient needs, as nurses have attempted to do through the nursing process and nursing diagnosis.

Perishability

Because services cannot be stored until they are needed, they must be con-sidered perishable. No revenue can be obtained from an unoccupied bed, although a nurse is on duty and assigned to care for any patient who might be admitted to that bed. If variable staffing, based on patient dependency and acuity measures, is practiced, the perishability of nursing services is not the huge problem it is when fixed staffing is based on unit capacity. The use of part-time and per diem nurses helps match the supply and demand and assists the nurse manager in preventing payment for unclaimed and thus perished services.

Consumer Involvement

Although consumer involvement is possible in producing goods through the use of kits and self-assembled products, the consumer plays a much larger role in the production and delivery of services. The quality and cost of nursing services vary not only according to the competency and productivity of caregivers, but also according to the cooperation, participation, interest, and abilities of the patient and family members. For example, when communication between nurse and patient is blocked by language or psychological problems, nursing services will be less effective and efficient than when there are open communication channels. In addition to an emphasis on self-care theories as a basis for nursing services, we are seeing more interest in consumer involvement from a cost-containment viewpoint. Cooperative care units, such as the model developed at New York University Medical Center (Gibson & Pulliam, 1987), have been shown to be successful in containing health care costs and improving the quality of care. MacStravic (1988) describes how patients involved in self-care can promote high quality of care, reduce the cost of care, and thus increase the provider's surplus or profit. Patients can also contribute information useful to marketing activities, buy additional services, and promote health care services to others. MacStravic encourages health care providers to make patients active participants in their own health care, rather than passive recipients of services.

Types of Services

The generic production processes that describe and unify manufacturers of commercial goods—such as assembly line, batch, or continuous flow—are not applicable to service industries. A service business often claims that it operates in a way that is unique or different from other types of service industries, but services can be classified by some common key elements: labor intensity, equipment or technology intensity, consumer involvement, purchase motive, and personalization. In fact, functional nursing might be compared to an assembly line, team or modular nursing to batch processing, and clinic nursing models to continuous flow product production.

Although we tend to think of the hospital industry as labor-intensive, Schmenner (1986) points out that a modern hospital has a relatively low labor intensity when it is measured by a ratio of labor to plant and equipment costs. Utilities, communications, banking, hotels, and hospitals have higher capital investments in plant and equipment than in personnel. In comparison, high labor intensity services include stock brokerages, insurance agencies, data processing, wholesale and retail sales, and personal service companies (laundries, beauty shops, mortuaries). When the health care industry is measured on consumer involvement in the service process and customization of service to satisfy individual needs, it rates higher than hotels or airlines.

Schmenner creates a grid with degree of labor intensity on one axis and degree of interaction and customization on the other axis. Hospitals fall into the *service shop* quadrant (low labor intensity and high interaction and customization). Independent nurse practitioners would fall into the *professional service* quadrant, along with physicians, lawyers, and architects (high labor intensity and high interaction and customization). The *service factory* quadrant includes airlines, trucking, hotels, and other services with low labor intensity and low interaction and customization. The fourth quadrant, called *mass service,* includes schools, retail banking, and stores with high labor intensity and low interaction and customization.

Personalizing a service can be programmed, such as in the guest relations approach, or it can be customized for each individual. While these two types of personalization focus on process, *option personalization* focuses on outcome by allowing the consumer to choose from alternative services (Surprenant & Solomon, 1987). Nurses use all three types of personalization in their practices.

Marketing Challenges for Services

Hospitals and Other Health Care Organizations

In the health care industry, marketing challenges arise from the necessity of dealing with proliferating technological advances and the high costs of professional and skilled personnel. As difficult as it is to manage the supply of health care workers during peaks and valleys of census and acuity, this challenge must be tackled, because the demand for health care is often not elective and controllable. In a quasi-regulated industry, such as health care, where over two-thirds of payments come from governmental sources, costs must be kept down, because they cannot be freely passed on to consumers. At the same time, services must be customized for patients who are involved and intervening in the services they receive. Quality must be maintained for humanitarian, professional, ethical, legal, and marketing reasons. To provide high quality-services that satisfy the consumer, employee loyalty and satisfaction must also be sought.

According to Schmenner (1986), control of hospital services is one of the greatest challenges the industry faces. Control is affected by the unpredictable nature of health care, the need to schedule use of expensive equipment, and the variety of health care workers involved in patient care, as well as the uncertainty involved with patients' satisfaction and their perception of the quality of care. For nurse entrepreneurs and nurse practitioners, control is a more individual problem, less constrained by equipment and other health care workers, unless there is a medical community acceptance problem.

Professional Services

Professionals are distinguished from generic service providers by expertise acquired through higher education, expert judgment, recognized group identity, and self-regulation (Hill & Neeley, 1988). Until recently, health care professionals have not had a marketing orientation. Increasingly in the last decade, they became aware of the challenges and opportunities to use marketing strategies that help their consumers' decision processes, while increasing their own market share of the potential clients.

Some marketing challenges are more prevalent for professionals than for industries that market goods and nonprofessional services. Bloom (1984) isolated seven of these challenges; we suggest applications for nursing professionals.

1. *Strict ethical and legal constraints.* Serving and pleasing nursing's consumers is governed by the ANA Code of Ethics, the Nursing Practice Act of each state, and other professional and regulatory bodies.

2. *Buyer uncertainty.* Buyers and users of nursing services often lack the technical knowledge and skill to assess the required nursing competencies.

3. *Need to be perceived as having experience.* No nursing consumer wants a service provided by an inexperienced nurse who has not performed a particular service previously.

4. *Limited differentiability.* It is often difficult to distinguish one nursing organization's services from another's; a distinctive positive image is difficult to project.

5. *Immeasurable benefits of advertising.* The results of advertising professional nursing services are difficult to measure. In addition, advertising is expensive, hard to target, and not yet completely accepted by the public or the profession.

6. *Converting "doers" into "sellers."* All nurses need to acquire a marketing orientation and realize how essential they are to patient satisfaction and repeat business.

7. *Allocating time for marketing.* Formal and informal marketing activities should be recognized as a nursing responsibility. Nurses should be rewarded for serving as educators and liaisons to the community and patient groups.

Hill and Neeley (1988) recommend that the differences between generic and professional services should form the basis for marketing strategies. Because there is often a threat to well-being involved in the exchange, the consumer of professional services has a higher level of perceived risk in choosing a health care provider than one who is merely choosing a soap. There is greater dependence on the health professional to diagnose and describe the problem. In the search for a provider, the health care consumer is willing to expend greater effort and often seeks recommendations from trusted friends. It is more difficult for health care consumers to compare and evaluate treatment alternatives, because many of the criteria are unknown. The impact of the choice of the health care service provider on the outcome is uncertain and often serious.

These known differences in the consumer decision processes for generic and professional services are the basis for the marketing strategies that Hill and Neeley suggest to professional service providers. We have adapted them for nursing professionals. The strategies and tactics will help you market nursing, consulting, educational, and other professional services.

Marketing Strategy 1: Provide more information to your potential and actual consumers and targeted markets.

Tactics:

1. Always carry a supply of business cards.
2. Provide nursing colleagues, other health care professionals, and potential clients with information about your credentials, qualifications, and specialties.
3. Increase your visibility through presentations, publications, and professional networking activities.
4. Develop brochures describing your professional services, highlighting how they are unique, superior, and cost-effective.
5. Prepare videotapes outlining specific services and expected outcomes.
6. Provide references and recommendations from previous customers.
7. Use interviews and initial appointments to provide specific, understandable information to potential clients.

Marketing Strategy 2: Help consumers control the decision process by increasing their involvement.

Tactics:

1. Involve clients in planning the service and in deciding the extent of services.
2. Involve clients in the implementation and delivery phases of the service.
3. Involve clients in follow-up activities and evaluation after service, emphasizing the importance of consumer satisfaction.

Marketing Strategy 3: Minimize risks.

Tactics:

1. Discuss all possible risks when obtaining informed consent from patients and research subjects, as well as with all other consumers. (Physicians are

responsible for discussing the risks of medical treatment and nurses for discussing risks of nursing services.)

2. Offer incentives that reduce risk, such as a free initial consultation and follow-up calls or visits.
3. Provide grievance or redress procedures for dissatisfied clients.
4. Maintain your professional expertise.
5. Refer clients to other experts as necessary.
6. Select and train support personnel very carefully to maintain good customer relations.

Conflicting Service Goals for Health Care Organizations and Professionals

Nurses are well aware of the conflicting goals of cost-containment, efficiency, and personalization that affect the design of nursing delivery systems. Good or excellent nursing service is usually described as meeting an individual's physical and psychosocial needs. As pointed out in Chapter 4, the profession has not always emphasized patient satisfaction, nor definitively studied the nursing actions that contribute to patient satisfaction and excellent outcomes. Hospital marketing departments are expected to study customer satisfaction more closely as resources become scarcer and competition for the health care dollar escalates. They will be tracking the effect of various types of services and improvements on both patient and nurse retention and on the bottom line (Droste, 1989).

Research by Surprenant and Solomon (1987) led them to reject the conventional wisdom that personalized services of whatever type are always better. Although not a study of health care services, we would do well to heed their warning that there are costs to the service organization and to customers from personalized services that may not be justified. The value added by personalization needs careful assessment. They found that some aspects of personalization are more pleasing than others. For example, consumer confidence in the provider's abilities and satisfaction with effectiveness were decreased by programmed personalization techniques. Computer-generated letters using the recipient's name throughout is an example of this technique. Because the perceived quality of nursing service is so important to the profession and nurses' employers, systematic investigation of these complex constructs is necessary. You could begin by studying the effects of your guest relations program on patient satisfaction. Are the techniques perceived as genuine or programmed?

Managing Demand for Services

Managing demand for goods and services so that organizations or practitioners can achieve their objectives is the essence of marketing management. Equalization of product supply and demand is essential to cost control, and influences satisfaction of consumers as well as providers. The desired demand for nursing services may be above, below, or consistent with the actual demand of any given market. Kotler and Andreasen (1987) describe eight common demand states and the marketing tasks for dealing with them. We have added a health care example of each demand state.

1. *Negative demand.* A large part of the potential market dislikes or fears the product and may actively avoid it.

   Examples: Surgery, chemotherapy, hepatitis vaccine.

   Marketing task: Analyze the reasons for avoidance and whether the market's attitudes and behaviors can be influenced through product, price, place, or promotion changes.

2. *No demand.* The potential market has no interest in the product.

   Example: A tuberculosis testing service adjacent to an AIDS clinic for drug addicts.

   Marketing task: Create demand by making the market aware of the advantages of the product.

3. *Latent demand.* There is a demand for a product not available.

   Example: Vaccine for HIV.

   Marketing task: Measure the size of the market and develop a product to satisfy the demand.

4. *Falling demand.* Previous levels of demand are declining.

   Example: A clinical nurse specialist's requests for consultation decline 25% because of reimbursement denial by an insurance carrier.

   Marketing task: Analyze causes of the decline and increase demand through creative marketing strategies.

5. *Irregular demand.* The demand is inconsistent and creates inefficiencies in staffing for production and distribution.

   Example: Wide swings in pediatric unit census.

   Marketing task: Analyze trends in demand (seasonal, monthly, daily, hourly) and find ways to alter demand through incentives of price, place, or promotion.

6. *Full demand.* The actual demand is congruent with the desired demand.

   Example: Nursing workload matches available staffing levels on a nursing unit.

   Marketing task: Maintain full demand as competition increases by measuring customer satisfaction and providing high-quality products to meet changing consumer wants.

7. *Overfull demand.* The actual demand is higher than the desired demand.

   Example: More emergency department patients than can be safely treated.

Marketing task: Reduce demand by demarketing techniques such as less advertising, increasing prices, or referring nonemergency patients to ambulatory clinics.

8. *Unwholesome demand.* The product is judged undesirable by a segment of society who may form an alliance to discourage demand. All consumers may not agree with this judgment.

    Example: The present campaign against smoking cigarettes in public places.

    Marketing task: Encourage consumers to give up cigarettes through advertising, public service announcements, personal selling, taxes, and so forth.

Marketing a New Service

Much of the earlier marketing literature discussed marketing goods rather than services. With the more recent application of these principles and strategies to marketing of services and ideas in nonprofit organizations, we are learning where the differences lie and how a new service can best be tailored to meet consumers' needs and preferences. Some consumer goods require more capital investment and take longer to develop than services. However, new hospital services may be subject to certificate of need regulations of individual states. The internal structure of health care organizations often hinders rapid development of new products. As we discussed earlier, it is difficult to understand all the factors that enter the service customer's decision process. Lost opportunities for future exchanges are difficult to evaluate for both goods and services.

New products often fail. The reasons for failure are usually found in planning deficiencies and sometimes in the execution of plans. Market research may be poorly designed, poorly done, or poorly interpreted. Even with good research, results may be ignored by managers. The product may not be designed to meet identified needs. Costs and time for developing the product may be greater than expected. Promotion strategies may not be sufficient, and may fail to show the uniqueness of the product or its benefits to the target market. Competitors may react quickly to the new product. The following steps will help you avoid some of these pitfalls in developing a new nursing product.

Steps in Development

Although many services are developed without following a formal development process, you should at least consider following the nine major steps outlined below (Kotler & Andreasen, 1987). They will increase the probability of success for the new offering. Hoffman and Aadalen applied some of these steps in developing a continuing education program for public health nurses (Case Study 8). We also discuss developing a new nursing product to deal with the nursing shortage in a typical hospital.

1. *Idea generation.* Commit to a systematic method for seeking creative new ideas for products that might be offered to each of your target markets. Responsibilities should be specifically assigned to an individual or group. Establish formal reporting mechanisms and due dates. Do not count on serendipity or chance. Try to avoid old approaches in reaching for new products. Formalize procedures to scan a variety of sources for new ideas: competing health care agencies, other nursing organizations, health care and nursing publications, newspapers, conferences, patients, families, visitors, physicians, vendors, consultants, and other employees. Use *brainstorming,* a technique for generating creative ideas without prejudging their worth, by asking heterogeneous, small groups (five to seven members) to suggest new products or solutions to problems.

For our example, we appoint a Nursing Shortage Task Force to generate creative ideas. Structure and procedures for the process are provided, including meeting schedule, techniques to be used, and the time frame for reporting ideas to the vice president of nursing.

2. *Idea screening.* From the array of ideas generated, select those that seem the most promising. A rigorous screening process will pay off. A screening committee, made up of experts in related areas, should use weighted criteria developed by top management to evaluate each idea. In our example, the hospital executive council determines the financial investment they are prepared to make, the targeted number of nursing employees needed (by educational level), a time frame acceptable for reducing vacancies from 20% to 5%, the role the human resources department will play, and so forth. Each criterion is then weighted according to its importance in the process.

A screening committee is formed, composed of the associate director of nursing operations, the assistant directors of medical-surgical and critical care nursing, a head nurse, an experienced staff nurse, and a new graduate. All ideas generated by the task force are evaluated according to the criteria, and receive a value rating and a certainty rating, the latter indicating how confident the raters are of each rating. The three ideas ranking highest are selected for further development.

3. *Concept development and testing.* Expand ideas that seem promising by breaking them down into alternative concepts of how the goal expressed in the idea might be reached. This is one of several stages in the product development process where cost-benefit analysis may be helpful. This technique helps you make choices among competing concepts, with high benefits at the lowest costs preferred, whether costs and benefits have a monetary component or not. Of course, the analysis is usually more difficult if you are dealing with unquantifiable costs and benefits.

If, in our example, one of the high-ranking ideas is to establish a retention program for new graduates employed in the hospital, there are several ways this could be done. One way is to have the preceptors used during orientation continue to follow the new graduate for the next year, providing encouragement and dealing with disillusionment or problems that may develop. An alternative concept would be to have staff development educators support new graduates through formal and informal social and educational gatherings.

In order to test these two concepts, we interview not only new graduates but also preceptors and staff educators who would be involved in this market exchange process. Again, a ranking process helps determine which of the two concepts has the highest market potential. In this case, new graduates preferred maintaining their relationships with preceptors over the staff educator relationship. The preceptors were excited about the added responsibility, while the staff development department had several vacancies and felt overworked and stressed. The preceptor alternative was selected for the retention program.

4. *Marketing strategy planning.* After a new service or program is selected, market strategies are planned to introduce the service to the marketplace. The plan contains the long-term goals and marketing mix strategies, a description of the target market, including size and anticipated response, as well as the revenue (if applicable) and expenses for the first year of operation.

For the new graduate retention program, the long-term goal (five years after implementation) is a 95% retention rate at the end of one year of employment. This goal was based on a study of voluntary separations during the past three years. Marketing mix strategy plans describe how the new product will be introduced and operated, where it will be housed, how it will be promoted, and the cost to operate the program.

5. *Business analysis.* At this stage in the new product development process, fiscal impact on the organization's budget must be examined by top management. This often includes an analysis of the break-even point.

In our example, the hospital chief executive officer (CEO), chief financial officer, and vice presidents of nursing and marketing estimate how many new graduates must be retained over the present survival rate in order to justify the costs of the new service.

6. *Offer development.* If a product concept is approved, plans can proceed for implementing the service. Brochures and ads should be tested in the target market during development.

For the nurse retention program, action plans include introducing staff educators to the program, so they in turn can orient preceptors to their expanded role. Procedures and policies are written. Preceptors' job descriptions and performance evaluations include the new responsibilities. The concept is featured in newly designed recruitment brochures and in ads for the local newspaper and a national nursing journal. The brochures and ads are tested on a group of new graduate nurses.

7. *Market testing.* After the implementation plan and its timetable are approved, the product offer and its marketing program are tested by the actual marketplace. Only through test marketing can actual reactions to a new product be evaluated.

As mentioned earlier, it is more difficult to test the market for a service than tangible goods, but a service can be piloted on a limited segment of the target market.

We test the new graduate nurse retention program on a medical-surgical nursing unit, a critical care unit, and in the operating room. We need to evaluate if the new graduate and the preceptor will invest time and energy in this relationship, since in this case there is not a direct exchange of money for the service. (The preceptors are to be paid a bonus by the hospital based on the retention rates of new graduates they assist.) Further testing might involve alternative marketing strategies among the three units, for example, by altering frequency of meetings between new graduate and preceptor, place of meeting, and format of meetings.

8. *Commercialization.* This is the term used for the set of steps taken to broaden the offer to its potential market after positive market test results. These plans are generated by decisions on when, where, and how to launch the service.

In the nurse retention program, one of the questions to answer in this phase of the development process is whether to begin the program in June, when many new graduates begin their first job, or wait until they have passed state board exams. Another alternative is to begin immediately with any newly hired nurse within 12 months of graduation. Determining how to launch the full-scale program includes assigning the responsibility for implementing and supervising the program to the director of the staff education program. Finally, a timetable is set up outlining the tasks to be accomplished, in sequence, with target dates for completion. Cost parameters may be set out with this schedule.

9. *Launch.* The nine steps in the development of a new service culminate in the launch of the program to its target market.

Business Plans

Another way to approach new product development is by writing a business plan. This written document describes in narrative and financial detail the nature and expectations of the new product. The business plan for a nursing product would contain answers to the questions found in Exhibit 5-2. Vestal (1988) describes the business plan as a guide to operation and a source of management information to facilitate decision-making and performance measurement. Business plans are tailored to organizational specifications, and vary in format, length, and depth according to their purposes and uses. The quality of the business plan for a new service is important in the approval process as well as to the product's ultimate success in the marketplace.

Following Vestal's outline (also see Johnson, 1988), the narrative section of the business plan begins with a *title sheet* that includes the name of the product, the author(s) of the business plan, and dates of the document and projected product implementation. A one- or two-page *executive summary* includes the purpose of the product and how it supports the organizational mission, its market position and plans, and a financial overview of the initial costs and expected return on investment, with time frames. This very important document is found at the beginning of the business plan, but is written last. After the *table of contents*, the product's purpose is described in relationship to the organization and its consumers (*description of product*). The *product value section* gives the rationale for this product at this time, at this price, in this place. A *market plan* summarizes the environmental analysis, potential consumer research, and marketing objectives and strategies to be followed. The last narrative section is a *description of operations*, outlining how the product will be produced and priced. In the case of a nursing service, it would summarize staffing, organizational structure, quality control, physical design, capital equipment, and compensation practices.

EXHIBIT 5-2   Development Questions for a New Nursing Product

- Does the product fit your mission (purpose), philosophy, goals and objectives?
- Is there a need for this product?
- How large is the need?
- Who else in your market area supplies this product?
- Do competitors produce a good product?
- Is there a broader need for the product (national and international)?
- Is the product a logical extension of your product line(s)?
- What benefits (profits) can you expect in the marketing exchange?
- What human, capital, material resources do you need to produce the product and what is their source?
- When can you begin to produce the product?

The financial section of the business plan begins with a *description of the investment* needed for the next few years. Projected revenues and expenses are summarized here. *Financing sources* describe where funds will be sought, and might include banks, bonds, donors, and foundations. The cost of borrowing funds would be described here. Nurse administrators would usually confer with the financial officers of an organization. In the case of a private venture, nurse entrepreneurs might consult with financial advisors. A forecast of the volume of usage or sales (patient days, clinic visits, nursing manuals) is found in the *key assumptions* section. Predicting demand for a new product is crucial to its success. These predictions should be based on market research and not on guessing. *Pro forma financial statements* for three to five years include balance sheets, income statements (also called earnings reports or profit and loss statements), and cash flow statements. The operating *budget* identifies projected revenues and expenses for the first year of operation. The capital budget describes major equipment required.

Supporting information might include résumés, staffing plans, and other detailed information.

Product Life Cycle and Management

The performance of a new product in the marketplace usually progresses through four distinct stages of growth and decline. Although it has been argued that all health services do not follow the predicted stages of economic growth and decline, Breindel (1988) reports that hospital patient days and HMO growth are predicted by this economic theory. The product life cycle predicts a typical S-shaped curve (see Figure 5-3) when the four stages are plotted against usage (sales) and time axes. The *introduction* phase is generally one of slow growth in revenue and market share. The new offering is in the *growth* phase when it shows rapidly increasing acceptance. The third stage of the life cycle is the *maturity* phase, during which the product attains its highest market share, and usage (or sales) level off and then begin to decline. In the last stage, the *decline* in usage and revenues continues, until eventually the product is taken off the market, changed, or redesigned.

Not all products follow this S-shaped pattern. If sales rise to the mature stage, level off, and then rise due to changes in the product, market, or uses, the life cycle shows a scalloped pattern. A cyclical pattern, such as we see in the registered nurse market, reflects alternating periods of higher and lower supply or demand. A third anomalous product life cycle pattern is the fad pattern, marked by an early peak and decline.

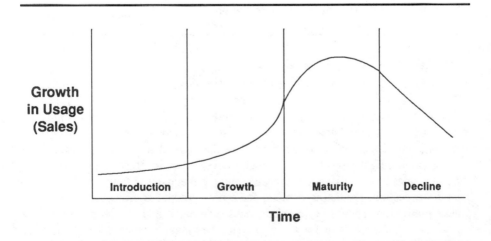

Figure 5-3. S-Shaped product life cycle curve.

Each stage in the more desirable S-shaped life cycle pattern has marketing strategies that traditionally are considered appropriate to that phase. Strategies during the introductory stage of a service are aimed at making potential users aware of the service and its advantages over competing or similar services. Persistent promotional strategies are very important at this stage, and should be aimed at reaching *early adopters,* who are the individuals most likely to respond to an innovative idea. They are important in spreading information and recommendations to other consumers.

In the growth phase, marketing efforts are directed toward maintaining or improving the quality of the product so that the early adopters who tried it will return for additional purchases, if and when that becomes necessary. New features may be added as consumer feedback becomes available. Other strategies are to search for new market segments and new ways to reach targeted markets. For growth to occur, consumers must use the product that they became aware of in the introductory phase. During the growth period, revenue may begin to exceed expenses, but the surplus is often reinvested in the search for new consumers.

The third stage of the product life cycle is the maturity stage. The rate of growth slows and stabilizes when most of the potential users have been made aware of and have accepted the product offer. This phase generally lasts longer than the introductory or growth stages, and demands a great deal of marketing management. Innovative strategies may be necessary to ward off competitors and maintain market share. For instance, during this stage a pediatric unit may recruit new pediatricians or encourage referrals through a continuing medical education program for community physicians. In Case Study 12, McAnnally describes how a pediatric clinic was improved to attract private patient admissions for a mature pediatric service.

The final stage of the product life cycle is decline, characterized by loss of market share as consumers, either abruptly or slowly, lose interest in use of the product. Although there is a continuing need for health care services, patients may choose other providers of that care, new technologies, new places, and even health care at better prices, as their consumer orientation increases and as the health care environment changes. As an example, we need only think of the shift from inpatient to outpatient cataract extraction surgery that resulted from advances in technology and Medicare prospective payment program regulations. Regardless of the lack of demand and decline in the life cycle of health care products, if you are the only provider of health care services in the area, it is a difficult decision to phase out weak products.

Demarketing

Before the introduction of prospective payment systems in the 1980s, the health care industry as a whole was in a cycle of growth. The focus was on expanding programs and facilities, as well as providing more highly qualified personnel. In hospitals, there was a trend toward hiring all registered nurse staffs and more baccalaureate-prepared nurses. Since 1983, alternative delivery systems are competing for patients, and employers are exercising more control over health care insurance costs. Hospital and health maintenance organization executives monitor physicians' use of services. To decrease hospital losses from unreimbursed services, health promotion and cost-effective methods of treatment are stressed. Health care managers are now challenged to reduce the growth of resource consumption. Cooper, Maxwell, and Kehoe (1985, p. 33) use the term *demarketing* to describe a "systematic marketing effort aimed at decreasing consumption of a given item or service." For instance, they suggest that the demand for physician services can be demarketed by promoting health education and self-care, as well as by convincing physicians that nurse practitioners and physician assistants can assume some primary care responsibilities. Demarketing techniques are used in Great Britain to discourage elective surgery under the National Health Service.

As defined by Breindel (1988), *nongrowth* marketing policies, procedures, strategies, and tactics are those that cause the volume of a market or service to be maintained at the present level, decreased, or deleted. In his nongrowth opportunity mix, Breindel describes several strategies for preventing growth in services, markets, or both. *Stabilization strategies* involve maintaining services to meet current levels of demand and prolonging the maturity stage of a service. Strategies to maintain occupancy rates at previous levels are examples. *Market retrenchment* refers to maintaining the services offered but decreasing the demand in targeted segments of the market. These strategies would be exemplified by nurse practitioners who attempt to decrease unreimbursed care without changing their services. Using *market divestiture strategies,* a segment of the market is no longer offered services, such as deleting adolescent admissions to a pediatric unit. *Service retrenchment* involves decreasing the size or scope of a service, usually because it is underutilized. Closing 12 ophthalmology service beds because of a shift to outpatient surgery is an example. *Shrinkage* is the strategy when both service and market scope are decreased. Fewer services are offered to consumers who demand less, perhaps because prices have escalated or the services are less convenient and accessible. *Service divestiture* means that a service is eliminated, but its market is retained by absorbing it into another service. Transferring clients from a dedicated Weight Watcher's clinic to a broader-based nutrition clinic is an example of this strategy. When a service is deleted and its market is lost to the health care organization, the strategy is called *liquidation.* The service and the market are lost when a hospital closes its home health department and refers clients to the Visiting Nurse Service. As nursing organizations evaluate the plethora of new services developed during the 1980s, and respond to economic forces in the health care industry, these strategies for decreasing their markets, services, or both will receive more attention.

PRICE

Simply defined, *price* is the sum or amount of money or its equivalent for which anything is bought, sold, or offered for sale. Defined more broadly, "price is the sum of the values consumers exchange for the benefits of having or using the product or service" (Kotler & Armstrong, 1987, p. 290). Price is of primary importance in marketing. It is the key to the profitability of a business and basic to economic theory. Pricing is the area that is most imprecise for practically all businesses.

Health care organizations have had persistent problems in applying pricing concepts to decisions. Price decisions in health care have often been vague, unclear, and underemphasized. (You will see this in the case studies we present in Part 2.) This has nothing to do with the fact that the authors are nurses or women; rather, it is because of the way health care is structured. Issues surrounding third-party reimbursement are the root cause. These issues include third-party payments, the constant threat of change in policies regarding money, regulated pricing structures, consumer price insensitivity, and lack of consumer price awareness (Kotler & Clarke, 1987). Setting pricing objectives for health care organizations is very complex because of these factors, but it must still be done.

Price describes the actual charge made by a health care organization to a patient. However, it is not the only cost to the patient. There are effort costs, psychic costs, and waiting costs as well as money costs. For example, getting women to have baseline and periodic mammograms involves the following costs: (1) the actual price of the test; (2) the time, cost, and trouble of getting to the test center; (3) the fear of hearing that one has a breast malignancy or other pathology; (4) the time waiting for the test to begin; and (5) the time having the test. Finding ways to reduce any of these costs may lead to more sales; that is, more women may have the test done if some of these costs are minimized.

Issues surrounding transportation are part of effort costs. The difficulty a patient has in getting to the health care organization is an example of a cost that brings no revenue to the institution. However, indirectly transportation benefits the organization. The organization provides care at one site; all the patients come there. This arrangement allows the organization to provide care to more patients. Lower costs for the organization may result.

Price is one of the marketing mix tools that an organization uses to achieve its marketing objectives. Health care organizations must coordinate their price decisions with product or service, place, and promotion decisions in order to develop a consistent and effective marketing program. Decisions made for one aspect of the marketing mix affect each of the other strategies. For example, the decision to establish private doctors' offices in an upper-class neighborhood means that higher fees will be charged in order to cover higher costs. Likewise, a cosmetic surgery organization choosing to promote its services with prime-time television ads must charge high fees to cover costs.

Costs are the expenses incurred in producing a product. They determine the base or minimum price that a health care provider must charge for its service if it is to break even or make a profit. Costs take two forms: fixed and variable. *Fixed costs,* also called *overhead,* are those costs that do not vary with the use of services. These are the bills the organization must pay each month, such as rent, heat, electricity, water, administrative salaries, and so forth. Fixed costs continue no matter what the bed occupancy or clinic use. *Variable costs,* such as nursing personnel and supply costs, fluctuate directly with the level of service provided. Providing care for patients with varying acuity results in changing costs, because patients require different levels of care. *Total costs* are the fixed and variable costs combined. The charged price should at least cover the total costs and an acceptable percentage of surplus. If it costs an organization more to provide a service than it costs competitors, the organization is at a disadvantage; either the organization must charge more or be satisfied to make less surplus or profit.

Internal costs set the base or floor for prices, and external factors of the market set the top or ceiling prices. Customers balance the price of a service against the benefits of having it. Generally, there is a relationship between price and demand. Buyer perceptions of price affect the pricing decision and the ultimate demand for the product. Price-demand relationship varies for different kinds of markets. In some markets, the seller has more freedom in setting the price. Economists identify four types of markets. These types are pure monopoly, pure competition, monopolistic competition, and oligopolistic competition. Each of these markets requires different pricing strategies.

A *pure monopoly* is made up of a single seller, and can be a government monopoly (United States Weather Bureau), a private regulated monopoly (New York Stock Exchange, utility companies), or a private nonregulated monopoly (diamond and coffee cartels). In each case, pricing decisions are different. A government monopoly can often set several pricing objectives. It could set a price below cost because it is important to distribute the product to consumers who cannot afford to pay full cost. Or the price could be set high to discourage use. In a regulated monopoly, the government allows the producer to set rates that allow a fair return. Nonregulated monopolies are free to set a price at what the market will bear. These companies do not always charge the highest price for several reasons: they fear government regulation, they do not want to attract competition, or they want to penetrate the market faster by setting a low price.

Pure competition markets are made up of buyers and sellers dealing in a uniform commodity such as wheat, soybeans, pork bellies, and financial securities. The individual buyer or seller has little effect on the going market rate. Sellers cannot charge more or less than the going price, because no one would buy the product at a higher rate, and because they can sell all they want at the market price. The role of marketing is small as long as the market is one of pure competition.

In contrast, in a *monopolistic competition,* the market is made up of many buyers and sellers who trade over a wide range of prices, instead of a single price as in pure competition. This is possible because the sellers differentiate their products. Buyers see differences in products and will therefore pay varying prices. Branding, advertising, and personal selling, as well as price, are used to make products stand out. Each company is affected less by the marketing strategies of competitors than it would be in an oligopolistic market.

The *oligopolistic competition* market is composed of a few sellers who are very sensitive to one another's pricing and marketing strategies. Steel, aluminum, and health care are examples of oligopolistic industries. There are few producers of steel and aluminum in the United States. In health care, there is a limited number of local hospitals. It is difficult for new sellers to enter the market because of plant costs and regulation. Each hospital carefully watches the competition. If hospital X raises nurses' salaries by 10% and hospital Y does not, nurses may quickly switch employers. To compete, hospital Y could raise salaries, increase benefits, or both. Organizations in an oliogopoly have to keep prices equal to those of their competition or risk losing customers.

Price decisions are influenced by many factors. These factors include those that are internal to the health care organization and those that are external. Internal factors include the organization's marketing objectives, marketing mix strategy, revenues, and expenses. External factors include the nature of the health care market, demand, competition, government policies, economic and other environmental forces.

Pricing for a health care organization is a complex issue. There are four stages in developing a pricing structure. The first stage is determining the pricing objective. Objectives include maximizing profit or surplus, usage, and other factors discussed below. The second stage is determining the pricing strategy. Included in this stage is the decision as to whether the price will be primarily cost-based, demand-based, or competition-based. Cost-based strategy means setting prices on the basis of costs. Demand-oriented marketers estimate the value customers place on the offering and set the price accordingly. Competitive-based strategy determines the price largely on what price the competition is charging. The third stage is considering pricing in terms of whether the market is reimbursed or paid directly by the consumer. The fourth stage is anticipation of changes in reimbursement policies and procedures and how to respond to the changes.

Setting Pricing Objectives

Even though health care is an extremely complex marketplace, because of variables in payment, such as self-pay, charges, costs, negotiated prices, no-pays, retroactive denials, DRGs, and the like, managers must still determine objectives for their organization. Because of this complexity, price is redefined in light of the specific situation. For example, in self-pay situations, price is the correct term to represent the amount of money consumers must pay out of pocket. Price is also the term used to refer to a charge based on costs or a negotiated charge based on competitive bids in other reimbursement situations. The following factors must be taken into account when setting pricing objectives in health care: surplus maximization, cost recovery, net patient service revenue maximization, usage maximization, public relations enhancement, cross-subsidization, and market disincentivization.

Surplus Maximization

Surplus or *profit* is the difference between net revenue and expenses. In the past, there was less emphasis in nonprofit health care organizations on making a profit or surplus than there is today. Then, as now, they often operated at a loss. External funding from donors, grants, and the like kept them in business. However, external funding to subsidize operating losses has dried up or shrunk significantly since the late 1970s. As a result, health care organizations must now look to making a profit in order to make capital improvements and to get the organization through financially tight times.

It should be pointed out that making a profit and maximizing profit are different objectives. In setting objectives to make a profit, the organization might seek only to make a surplus that will cover short-term operating and capital needs. In contrast, maximizing profit means that the largest possible surplus is sought. For-profit health care organizations experienced large earnings growth in the 1970s and early 1980s because of expansion, aggressive pricing and collection strategies, and operating efficiency based on economies of scale and effective management. An important objective was to maximize the profits returned to shareholders while remaining competitive with nonprofit health care facilities.

Cost Recovery

The cost recovery objective is to set a price per unit of service that allows for recovery of all, or a reasonable part, of costs. This pricing objective is common in health care. Cost-based reimbursement was developed to achieve this. Insurers such as Blue Cross have traditionally provided full cost recovery. Under cost-based reimbursement, though, there is little inducement for an organization to cut costs. Prospective payment based on DRGs was intended to eliminate traditional cost-based reimbursement. The payment for each DRG is based on average, nationwide resource consumption rather than an individual hospital's cost. In any third-party payment system, cash flow problems may result from retroactive denials and delayed payments.

Partial cost recovery is the pricing objective for some health care organizations. These organizations have external sources to make up for the unrecovered costs. Nursing schools and public hospitals are two examples of organizations seeking partial cost recovery from students and patients. Both could charge higher prices. However, by raising tuition to cover costs, nursing schools could price themselves out of business. Instead, they look to contributions, gifts, grants, bond issues, and various other sources to raise operating and capital funds. In the case of public hospitals, higher prices could mean denial of care to those patients for whom such hospitals were originally intended: the poor. These hospitals receive money from government to stay afloat.

Net Patient Revenue Maximization

The objective for health care organizations is to maximize net patient service revenue; that is, total revenues minus discounts, bad debts, contractual allowances, retroactive denials, and disallowed expenses. One way to do this is to increase the number of charge-based (usually commercially insured) patients serviced. These patients bring higher revenue and higher surplus per unit of service than do those reimbursed through the Medicare and Medicaid programs. Another way to do this is to increase ambulatory, rehabilitation, and other types of service still reimbursed on the basis of cost.

Marketing strategies can help maximize net patient revenue by attracting the largest possible number of targeted patients. Revenue is maximized by ensuring that as many of these patients as possible are commercially insured and are not a financial risk. However, this strategy has ethical implications. The poor and those patients without health insurance also need health care. Some compromises must be made to provide care to such patients. Other considerations are how financial and accounting decisions regarding allocation of costs affect net patient service revenue. High fixed costs are often allocated to those services that are used most by cost-reimbursed patients. This explains why health care finance and accounting managers are involved in pricing decisions. The interested reader may refer to the hospital financial and accounting literature for more information on this area.

Usage Maximization

This objective is based on a concept that has been almost universally accepted by economists and business people. It states that as price decreases, demand increases. Health care organizations may decide to maximize use if costs are low and relatively fixed, each user represents additional revenue, and increased volume can be handled without a proportionate increase in expenses. In addition, there should be no revenue caps. Health promotion programs often have usage maximization as a pricing objective, as do those organizations that believe users and society benefit from their services. The smoking cessation program in Case Study 2 and the women's health care program in Case Study 17 are good examples of this.

In many industries, low price does stimulate increased use, and may produce more revenues over time. The specific situation must be carefully evaluated before adopting a usage maximization objective. The incentive provided by a low price must be compared to the disadvantage of a low price indicating low or poor quality (Shapiro, 1968). In addition, usage maximization is often one of the strategies employed to achieve the objective of maximizing net patient service revenue.

Public Relations Enhancement

Prices can be set based on a public relations objective. Hospitals often set daily room rates as low as possible because of the attention these charges receive. To compensate, charges are raised on services and supplies that receive less publicity. "The Diabetes and You" patient education program in Case Study 2 is an example of pricing for public relations enhancement.

Cross-subsidization

Many health care organizations seek to balance surpluses and losses with cross-subsidization. This is the process of using funds from one product to compensate for losses from another. Hospitals have traditionally lost money on obstetrics and pediatrics, but it is usually important for the organization to continue to provide these services, for a variety of reasons. It may be the only provider in the area, or the losing service may have great public relations implications. The hospital thus must support the losing service with surpluses gained from profitable services, such as medical-surgical departments and operating rooms.

Cross-subsidization based on third-party payments also occurs. Medicare and Medicaid often reimburse at rates that do not cover full costs. Health care organizations then cross-subsidize these deficits with surpluses from private insurers such as Blue Cross. This is often called *cost shifting*.

Market Disincentivization

To achieve market disincentivization, prices are set to discourage as many people as possible from buying a product. This technique is another form of de-marketing. There are at least four reasons for market disincentives. They are used when (1) the product is bad for people, (2) the organization has reached its limits for production, (3) there is a shortage, and (4) the organization wants to discourage certain segments of a market.

The tax on cigarettes is an example of a market disincentive intended in part to reduce smoking because of the associated health risks. Substantial revenue is produced for the government by this tax. There is fear that raising the tax high enough to be a true disincentive would decrease needed revenue. However, because tobacco use is an addiction, cigarette taxes could, in fact, be raised much higher before this would happen. For example, although in Scandinavia cigarette taxes are significantly higher than in the United States, the Scandinavians' rate of smoking is considerably higher. Initially, United States cigarette companies were reluctant to raise their prices, but they did so after they saw that people would buy cigarettes despite taxes. While prices went up 42% between 1960 and 1970, sales still rose by 11% (Davis, 1989).

Higher prices are also set to discourage usage when the organization is working at full capacity and does not want additional business. An example of this is charging higher fees for inappropriate use of emergency services, walk-in visits to clinics, and broken appointments. Raising the price will discourage purchase of the products during a shortage. Several common situations in health care call for market disincentives. Hiring a private duty nurse has become too costly for many patients. The cost was raised in part because of the current nursing shortage. Fewer nurses are available for private duty, so prices are raised to decrease demand. As a result, fewer patients have private duty nurses, especially if their insurance does not reimburse them. Using price to discourage certain segments of a market is common in luxury goods and service markets. Hospitals use this technique when pricing their private pavilions and amenities programs. Third party payers usually do not cover the additional costs, so only patients who can afford to pay out-of-pocket use these services.

Pricing Nursing Services

Nurse managers must know what it costs to deliver nursing services if they are to justify nursing budgets and obtain sufficient funding. Cost information is also essential to evaluate the kind of care that can be provided for any given level of funding. Knowing the cost of services allows for the development of a sound marketing plan. Costing out of nursing services is the first step in developing realistic pricing strategies. In addition, costing allows more effective management of resources and productivity.

There are at least four methods for costing out nursing services. See Table 5-2 for a comparison of these methods. The first, employed by Wood (1982) at Massachusetts Eye and Ear Infirmary, uses a disease trajectory based on patient care classification and length of stay. Holbrook (1972), at Montana Deaconess, and many others use a second method, based on patient classification or acuity with associated average costs for each patient category. The third method uses a task-based technique. DRGs form the basis for the fourth system.

PLACE

Place refers to how products are made available and accessible to consumers. Traditionally, the term *distribution* is used by marketers to delineate this aspect of marketing. All providers of services must consider place in developing marketing mix strategies. Most of the marketing literature on distribution deals with tangible goods rather than services, and discusses channels of distribution, warehousing, inventory, retailing, wholesaling, and other areas. Because of the services provided by health care organizations, these aspects of distribution are for the most part not applicable to health care. However, there are exceptions. Medical suppliers and pharmaceutical companies distribute goods: cardiac monitors, dialysis machines, x-ray equipment, medications, and intravenous solutions. Additionally, health care

TABLE 5-2   Systems for Costing Out Nursing Services

	Massachusetts Eye and Ear (Wood)	Montana Deaconess (Holbrook)
Source of the new costs	Mathematical derivation from old costs	Mathematical derivation from old costs
Basic assumptions	Nursing is reflected in time	Nursing is reflected in time
Conversion system	1. PETO units cumulated into total nursing time per day in a trajectory for a given diagnosis 2. Patient charged by the "norm" of nursing units per the "day" of the trajectory in which he fits via his diagnosis and therapy	1. Four level patient classification system used twice daily 2. Average nursing time associated with each level 3. Costs determined by multiplying level times average hours per level, cumulating per hospitalization
Criterion	Medical diagosis and/or medical/ surgical therapy	Level of nursing care required, i.e., patient acuity
Relationship of criterion and conversion system	Daily nursing norms calculated for each medical/surgical entity based on average patient response trajectories	Nursing norms per patient classification calculated on a twice daily actual patient assessment

TABLE 5-2   Systems for Costing Out Nursing Services

	Task-Based Costing	*DRG-Based Costing*
Source of the new costs	Actual cost studies of nursing hours and equipment and supplies used	Differentation of nursing resource costs from other resource costs for statistically sound number of cases per each DRG.
Basic assumptions	Nursing is reflected in both time and level of personnel	Nursing resources can be differentiated from other resources of care.
Conversion system	1. Average time is calculated for each task 2. Costs are calculated by multiplying time by average salary of worker who normally does the task 3. Indirect costs are apportioned	1. Average nursing costs would be calculated (by whatever method) for most commonly seen types of patents in each DRG category. 2. An average nursing cost per DRG category would be extracted by calculating percentages of each type of "case" within the DRG category. 3. The cost norms would be assigned to future patients according to their DRG placement.
Criterion	Tasks done by nurses best reflect use of resources	Patient data grouped for another purpose can be statistically manipulated to produce at least normative nursing costs.
Relationship of criterion and conversion system	Cumulative billing per task, per day	Extracted norms per case would be statistically satisfactory but there would be little assurance that a projected cost had anything to do with a specific patient case. to do with a specific patient case.

Source: Reprinted from *The Nurse As Executive*, 3rd ed., by B.J. Stevens, p. 286, with permission of Aspen Publishers,

organizations and nurses can produce and distribute tangible products such as software packages and manuals. See Case Study 3 for one example.

There are three important distribution decisions for health care organizations to make. These are: (1) physical access, including channels, location, and facilities; (2) time access; and (3) information and promotional access, including referral. Although access is an old concept in health care, some of these decisions have received little attention. Among health care professionals, having access usually means financial access to care and having a regular source for clinical care. Marketers generally see these as consumer variables rather than as distribution variables.

In fact, much innovation in distribution has been severely criticized by the health care industry. Dental offices, medical clinics, and emergicenters are the recipients of much disparagement, when what they have done is make care more accessible in all aspects—physical, time, promotional, and referral. Often they are located in shopping malls, are open 7 days a week from 12 to 24 hours a day, and require no appointment. They offer the consumer convenient health care.

Physical Access

Channels

Kotler and Andreasen (1987, p. 473) define a *channel* as "a conduit for bringing together a marketer and a target customer at some place and time for the purpose of facilitating a transaction." A pregnant woman may have many options in choosing a channel for care, such as a solo or group nurse midwife practice, a solo or group obstetrical practice, a neighborhood health center, a hospital-based nonemergency ambulatory care unit, a hospital-based emergency room, a freestanding walk-in clinic, or an HMO. A similar assortment is available for well babies, and other health care clients.

Health promotion and disease detection channels have increased and expanded significantly. Channels that distribute good nutrition information have grown from mere posters in classrooms to community health fairs, cable television, videotapes, hospital closed-circuit television, computer-assisted instruction, and telephone hotlines. Just about every imaginable phase of illness and health is covered using one or more of these methods.

An important aspect in the use of unconventional channels is bringing health care to the consumer rather than making the consumer go to a central source. Mobile vans are a popular way to deliver health care, education, and screening. Telephone service brings care, in the form of diagnosis and advice, into the home.

Location

There is an old saying that the three most important things for a successful business are location, location, and location. Four of the most important factors to assess in choosing a location are competition, demographic characteristics of the area, accessibility to transportation, and the need to be near other medical facilities or a referral base. The importance of location for health care organizations is now recognized by most providers. Patients often segment themselves by proximity to a source for care. As with the purchase of other products, people tend to buy health care where it is most convenient. This is most obvious in an emergency. It is also true for routine, nonemergency care. Distance from the facility becomes less important as the urgency and risk of the health problem decreases, as the patient's level of education and income rises, and as the consultation or admission goes from unplanned to planned (Kotler & Clarke, 1987).

Many strategies have been used to reach different segments with problems related to transportation. Providing emergency care to the patient in the shortest possible time is an example of a situation in which transportation is critical. Community nurse service or home care is provided when it is better to go to the patient than to have the patient come to the institution. Use of storefront clinics, churches, and mobile units maximizes access to health care by decreasing transportation costs. Transportation to the health care provider may be paid for by government, through social services, when appropriate and necessary. For example, in New York and other cities, teams of mental health professionals and outreach workers move about assessing the homeless for care needs.

Some health care organizations located in rough neighborhoods have opened offices or satellites in wealthier parts of town in order to retain upscale patients who dislike and refuse to travel in bad parts of town, or who want to use a facility closer to their homes and offices. Health care organizations must look at transportation as part of the price they expect patients to pay, even though the organization does not receive the income. When selecting a site, ease of access must be a major consideration, as it has a significant effect on use and satisfaction (MacStravic, 1985). Transportation difficulties may require increasing service benefits to keep utilization at needed levels.

There is now a trend toward multihospital corporations, both nonprofit and for-profit. For their welfare and survival, health care organizations must now consider factors with which retail businesses have traditionally dealt: how many branches, of what size, where to locate, and what specialty services to include. The renowned Mayo Clinic in Rochester, Minnesota opened branches in Scottsdale, Arizona, and Jacksonville, Florida. The Presbyterian Hospital in the City of New York, a tertiary care institution, opened a community hospital nearby and a doctors' office building several miles away in a more prosperous section of the city.

Location has an impact on nurse recruitment. Health care organizations located in low-income areas often have difficulty attracting and retaining professional staff. Because of a lack of funds, lower salaries may be paid. Additionally, professionals may not want to live in the surrounding community. However, nurses who work at the hospital in a very wealthy neighborhood may not be able to afford to live in the community. The hospital may have to offer subsidized housing in order to attract and retain sufficient staff.

Facilities

The appearance of the facility is an important aspect of physical access. Inpatient and ambulatory care facilities must be designed with concern for their look and feel. Patient and staff satisfaction are affected by the atmosphere of a building. Disappearing are the long, narrow, poorly lit corridors, hospital-green walls, and cold, institutional furniture; hospitals are now designed and decorated to make them comfortable, hospitable, cheerful, and functional. (See Chapter 6 for further discussion of corporate identity.) Nursing stations are planned to bring nurses and patients closer together, to facilitate nursing activities, and support nursing functions. Nurses should be included in all stages of new hospital design. They can help the architect design patient care units that assist nurses rather than making their jobs more difficult. Nurses should also be included in all stages of facility renovation. Their knowledge of the work of patient care can contribute to an improved facility.

Many health care organizations cannot provide optimal facilities because of financial or regulatory constraints. They should, however, strive to make the facility as attractive as it can be. If a facility is run-down, patients and staff will deprecate both the facility and the care, because people often do not differentiate between the tangibles and intangibles of service.

Time Access

There are three issues concerned with time access. They are: (1) the hours a service is provided, (2) the time spent waiting in the health care facility for the service, and (3) the amount of time between getting an appointment and actually receiving the service. All three issues have important implications for service use and customer satisfaction. Until recently, little attention was paid to time access. Health care organizations provided care at their convenience. Generally, outpatient services were open weekdays between 8:00 a.m. and 5:00 p.m. People with jobs had to take time off from work for appointments. Hospitals also had limited hours. Diagnostic procedures and surgery were done only during the day, Monday through Friday. These time access barriers showed no consideration of the needs and wants of the consumer; they came about solely for the convenience of providers and staff who disliked working evenings and nights. By limiting time access to usual working hours, the health care organization saved money on shift differentials, staff salaries, and overhead expenses such as heat and electricity.

A greater number of health care providers are now beginning to develop channels to cope with time access problems. Case Study 12 describes an evening pediatric clinic, for example. All such programs are not new, however. The Boston Evening Medical Center (originally called the Boston Evening Dispensary) was established over 100 years ago (Kotler & Clarke, 1987). In many areas, physicians now make nighttime house calls.

The time spent waiting is a major source of patient dissatisfaction. This is true whether the wait is between the making of and the actual appointment or in the health provider's waiting room. No one wants to wait six weeks to see a neurologist or spend hours in the waiting or examining room of a gynecologist. Walk-in medical and dental clinics are a response to these time access problems.

Informational and Promotional Access

Health care organizations are dependent to a great extent upon referrals. Referral involves the use of intermediaries to distribute information on and promote the organization. Physicians are the most visible intermediaries in health care, and are the primary gatekeepers. Hospitals rely on physicians for admissions. Physicians were the targeted market in Case Studies 9, 11, and 14. All three of the involved organizations put much effort into courting and meeting the needs and wants of the gatekeeper physicians.

Organizations have the choice of using push or pull strategies. *Push strategies* rely on intermediaries to inform and promote (push) the organization to the consumer. In Case Study 13, Mershon describes how Humana used push strategies with nurse educators to recruit nurses. Kolatch used nurses to encourage physicians to refer their patients for visiting nurse services (Case Study 11). Personal selling is a basic push strategy. *Pull strategies* do not use intermediaries. They rely on advertising and other promotional activities to pull the consumer to the organization. Ware, in Case Study 19, used a pull strategy for an eating disorder service.

The push strategy has been the traditional form used by health care organizations to generate demand for their services. It is likely to remain the most important strategy, for two reasons. It is appropriate because the sensitive, personal nature of health problems makes advertising difficult, and because consumers generally must rely on gatekeepers or intermediaries to diagnose the health problem and prescribe treatment. There are some benefits to using intermediaries. They are: (1) direct marketing to consumers of care requires great financial resources, (2) using existing channels is often the cheapest way to get service and consumer together, and (3) funds can often be used more effectively than in developing a new distribution system.

PROMOTION

Promotion is the marketing function many people confuse with marketing. This may be because promotion is the most visible marketing activity. Often the term *marketing* is used instead of *promotion*, but the two words are not interchangeable. *Promotion* includes the marketing mix strategies that communicate aspects of the product and persuade people to buy it (Kotler & Armstrong, 1987). More than just advertising, promotional strategies are necessary for an organization to keep in touch with its customers and publics.

Promotional strategies are not new; they are not phenomena of the 20th century. People have used promotion for thousands of years. Archaeologists have found signs in the Mediterranean region promoting events and offers. Both the ancient Greeks and the Romans used written promotional messages. The Greeks also used town criers and singing commercials for sales promotion. Marks that craftspeople made on their products were also a form of promotion; these marks assured buyers of a certain quality and served the same function as our trademarks and brands. As transportation improved and goods were sold further and further away from where they were made, the mark became more important. In 1450, Gutenberg invented the printing press, which obviously had a major impact on promotion, as materials no longer had to be copied by hand. English-language promotions were first produced in 1478.

To communicate effectively, there are four major tools: advertising, sales promotion, publicity, and personal selling. The specific combination of tools used is called the *communication* or *promotion mix*. It is a subset of an organization's marketing mix. These communication mix tools are traditionally defined by the American Marketing Association as follows (Kotler, 1988):

> **Advertising:** any paid form of non-personal presentation and promotion of ideas, goods, or services by an identified sponsor.
> **Sales promotion:** short-term incentives to encourage purchase sale of a product or service.
> **Personal selling:** oral presentation in a conversation with one or more prospective purchasers for the purpose of making sales.
> **Publicity:** non-personal stimulation of demand for a product, service, or business unit by planting commercially significant news about it in a published medium or by obtaining favorable presentation of it on radio, television, or stage that is not paid for by the sponsor. (pp. 587–588)

Yet, communication goes beyond these tools. The whole marketing mix must be considered and coordinated. For example, all aspects of the product communicate something to customers. Product design, price, and packaging, as well as the attitude and other personal characteristics of the salesperson, convey a message. To have the greatest positive effect, these aspects of a product must communicate a consistent message.

The first step in promotion development is to identify the target audience. Everything else in the promotional mix depends on this decision. For example, what message, as well as where, when, and how the message will be conveyed, depends on the target audience. Even who will send it is determined by this decision. After the target audience has been defined, the desired response must be described as precisely as possible. Because buying is the result of a long process of consumer decision-making, it is necessary to know where the target audience is in relation to buyer readiness.

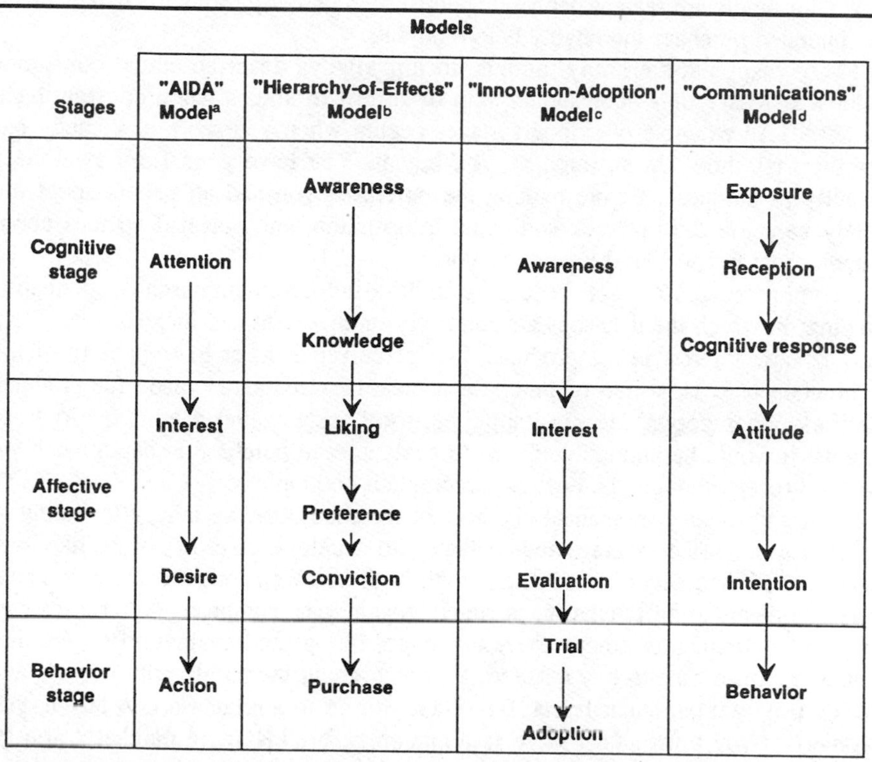
Models
Stages
"AIDA" Model[a]
"Hierarchy-of-Effects" Model[b]
"Innovation-Adoption" Model[c]
"Communications" Model[d]
Cognitive stage
Affective stage
Behavior stage
Attention
Interest
Desire
Action
Awareness
Knowledge
Liking
Preference
Conviction
Purchase
Awareness
Interest
Evaluation
Trial
Adoption
Exposure
Reception
Cognitive response
Attitude
Intention
Behavior

[a] E.K. Strong, *The Psychology of Selling* (New York: McGraw-Hill, 1925), p. 9.
[b] Robert J. Lavidge and Gary A. Steiner, "A Model for Predictive Measurements of Advertising Effectiveness," *Journal of Marketing*, October 1961, p. 61., published by the American Marketing Association.
[c] Everett M. Rogers, *Diffusion of Innovations* (New York: Free Press, 1962), pp. 79-86.
[d] Various sources.

Figure 5-4. Response hierarchy models.

Reprinted with permission from P. Kotler, *Marketing Management: Analysis. Planning, Implementation, and Control*, 6th Edition (Englewood Cliffs, NJ: Prentice-Hall), p. 595.

Buyer Readiness States

There are six buyer readiness states. In the hierarchy-of-effects model, they are awareness, knowledge, liking, preference, conviction, and purchase. Potential customers must be moved through these states, generally in order. This and several similar models describing buyer readiness are found in Figure 5-4. These *response hierarchy models* assume a high level of involvement on the part of consumers. It is assumed that consumers are very concerned about the goods and services they buy. Consumers are seen as deliberate people who gather information and evaluate the intended purchase thoroughly before buying.

These response hierarchy models do not always describe actual consumer behavior. Many times consumers skip or return to stages when considering a purchase. An example of skipping stages occurs when you see a new candy bar for the first time. On an impulse, you buy it. You have gone from awareness directly to purchase. Before making the purchase, you had no beliefs about the candy bar, you did not seek additional information, and you had no idea about whether you would like the candy or not.

Skipping stages occurs frequently in low-involvement purchase decision-making, in which the decisions are relatively unimportant and inexpensive. There may be low interest in the products, low perceived risk, or low visibility of the product in use. This kind of purchase decision is frequently made for products such as paper goods, cleaning supplies, toothpaste, generic goods, and store brands. It would be impossible for us to analyze each purchase in depth when we do our grocery shopping; we would accomplish nothing else.

Returning to our hypothetical purchase of the candy bar, we may, after eating it, go back to the affective stage and evaluate and decide whether or not we like it. A similar disrupted sequence of stages with high-involvement products can occur. When contemplating purchasing a stereo system, car, computer, or furniture, we may move frequently among the knowledge, liking, and evaluation stages. For example, you decide to buy a stereo. You read about them, talk with friends, and decide to buy a particular brand. But when you go to a retail store to buy it, you decide that you must gather more information before making a purchase; you go back to the knowledge stage from the conviction stage.

While these response models do not describe consumer behavior in all situations, the frameworks are useful for organizing promotional efforts. A single message rarely moves a target audience through all stages from awareness to purchase. Most communication managers try to move the target audience one stage at a time. The critical things to know are where the audience is and where it should go next.

Decisions about health care are often high-involvement. People may try to get as much information as possible about physicians and hospitals. They call hospitals, medical societies, and their friends for recommendations. Visits to nursing homes are made. Interviews with staff may be conducted. However, many times the consumer does not have the time or the resources to gather much information. As stated in Chapter 1, lack of information is a problem, and acts against the full working of the marketplace in health care.

Awareness

It is essential to know how aware the target audience is of the product. The audience may be unaware, know only the name, or have limited information. In Case Study 1, 82% of the nurses surveyed had never heard of the district association. Research into awareness of a baccalaureate program described in Case Study 15 also had surprising results. It seems incredible that nurses do not know about a district association or that they are unaware of the value of a BSN. When developing a promotional program, nurses should be wary of assuming that the targeted segment is aware of their product.

The promotional task in both case studies cited above was to build awareness. In some instances, the goal may be to move a target audience from unawareness to name recognition. This may be done with name repetition. Patience is needed for results; building awareness takes time.

Knowledge

While the target audience may be aware of the product, service, or organization, it may not know much more. Objectives in the case studies cited above were to reach people in the targeted markets and increase their knowledge of the program benefits. As its first communication objective, the college decided to achieve product knowledge. It was successful. In contrast, the district association did little to communicate information to nonmembers. Therefore, they were unsuccessful in increasing knowledge and ultimately in adding members.

Liking

Liking is the buyer state that has to do with how the target audience feels about the product. If the audience does not like the product, the reason for an unfavorable opinion must be discovered. If the reason is not known, direct remedies cannot be taken and promotional efforts will be ineffective. For example, if the dislike is due to real problems, those problems must first be corrected. If it is due to perceived but unreal problems, the perceptions must be changed. Then promotional efforts can proceed. When a clinic has long waiting times, rude and inefficient staff, and an unpleasant waiting area, efforts of a "we care" campaign will not be effective. Once the problems or perceptions are corrected, the promotion can proceed.

Preference

If the target audience likes a product, but still does not prefer it to others, the promotional goal becomes building consumer preference. In this case, the product's quality, value, and features are promoted. The success of the campaign should be evaluated by measuring the target audience's preference after the campaign's end.

Conviction

The target audience may prefer the product but still not have the conviction to buy it. Referring to Case Study 15 again, some nurses came to prefer this particular baccalaureate program, but still did not have the conviction to enroll. To reach these nurses, specific strategies and tactics were developed. The promotional goal was to build the conviction that earning a BSN is a good thing to do.

Purchase

Some of the target audience may have the conviction but still not get around to making the purchase. In Case Study 15, *purchase* was defined as enrolling in the program. Enrollment was encouraged and achieved by supporting and reinforcing that the decision to enroll was a sound one. Purchase incentives for other products might include setting a sale price, offering a premium, giving samples, and the like. A discount was offered to employers when they contracted for the smoking cessation program in Case Study 2.

Advertising

The greatest growth of advertising has been in the United States. Several factors contributed to this country's becoming the world leader in advertising. These factors were the development and use of mass production, a system of transportation, and compulsory public education leading to growth of newspapers and magazines. Subsequent development of radio and television further increased and encouraged advertising. United States hospitals now spend about $500 million of their marketing budgets on advertising ("Ailing hospital ads," 1989).

There are five major decisions to be made in developing your advertising strategies. These decisions are setting objectives, allocating budget, developing the message, selecting the media, and setting evaluation criteria.

Setting Objectives

The first step, setting objectives, is based on decisions already made about the target market, positioning, and marketing mix. These past decisions define what advertising must achieve for the overall marketing program. Ads are classified according to whether their aim is to inform, persuade, compare, or remind.

Information advertising is used extensively when a new product category is introduced and primary demand must be built. Thus, when dual-chambered pacemakers were developed, the industry had to inform cardiologists of the benefits. When closed-system intravenous setups were developed, manufacturers had to convince hospital purchasing departments, pharmacies, and nurses of their benefits. An ad featuring a new nursing retention program or a nursing education curriculum must contain information on its unique features.

Persuasive advertising is important when competition increases and when a goal is to build selective demand. This is seen in recruitment advertisements for nurses. Every hospital says it is the very best place to work. Hospitals also try to achieve this favored position in the minds of physicians and patients by using convincing and credible ads.

Comparison advertising has become a form of persuasive advertising. It compares one brand directly or indirectly to one or more competitors. Pharmaceutical companies often use this approach in their ads for over-the-counter drugs. For example, Tylenol may be compared to Bayer aspirin and Advil.

Reminder advertising is important for mature products. It keeps the product or service in the publics' mind. For many years The Presbyterian Hospital in the City of New York had a full page-ad on the inside back cover of the *AJN*. During times of low vacancy, the purpose of the ad was not so much to inform or persuade as it was to remind nurses of Presbyterian.

There are three important objectives to consider in developing the advertising message. These objectives help to focus and direct message development. They are to fit the message to the intended segment, to ensure that the product does what the message promises (truth in advertising), and to match the reasons to buy with the needs and wants of the target market.

Developing the Message

After you identify your target audience and define the desired response, you are ready to develop the message. Advertising professionals go through three steps in ad development. These steps are message generation, message evaluation, and message selection. Message generation is a creative process. People working in this area have different approaches to developing message ideas. Talking with consumers, dealers, experts, and competitors is one way. Another is to imagine both the consumers using the product and what benefits they seek. In developing a member recruitment brochure for a district nurses association, four committee members brainstormed with the consultants. Ultimately they chose, "Your strength is our strength. Our strength is your strength." A good example of the process of message generation is described in Case Study 15. Often many possible messages are suggested; only a few are ever used.

All the generated messages should be evaluated. Twedt (1969) believes that messages should have three characteristics. The message must make the product more desirable or interesting to consumers; it must tell how the product is better than other brands; and it must be believable. Believability is the most difficult characteristic to achieve. Consumers tend to doubt the truth of advertising in general. Studies have repeatedly documented this. You should evaluate your advertising based on these factors. Whenever feasible, studies should be conducted to ascertain if the message achieves your objectives.

Message selection should be done with great care. An effective message can help achieve an increased market share that will substantially improve return on advertising investment. The value of an effective message may be at least 10 times greater than an ordinary, mediocre message (Wright & Bostic, 1983). This is true for customer attitudes, preference for the product, or sales results. Since every advertiser pays the same for time and space in media, the message itself can be competitive, or it can be an expensive disadvantage.

Communications Consultants

Selecting a communications consultant is time-consuming. At best, it is a risky endeavor. Choosing an advertising agency or consultant is something like choosing a physician: It is almost impossible to gather all the information you need. This is because ad agencies are personal service businesses and their most important product is their creative product (Hizar, 1985). It is very difficult to predict accurately how working with the agency will be until you have done it.

Questions to Ask

Hizar (1985) suggests two very important questions to ask when hiring an advertising consultant or agency. Ask them what they think effective advertising is, and what they do to produce it. The answer to the first question is that effective advertising sells. To answer the second question, Hizar gives the following four principles.

Benefit.   Include an explanation of what's in the product or service for the consumer. The ad should tell the consumer about the benefits received. This may sound obvious, but it is missing in many advertisements. Benefits can be rational, tangible, physical, or affective (emotional). Customers tend to believe that they should make rational decisions. However, emotional benefits influence our purchases much more frequently than we think, and should be given more attention.

Demonstration.   After you have selected the benefit to emphasize, you must communicate it effectively. Hizar suggests that the best way to do this is by demonstration of the specific dimension of the product that makes it different from your competitors' products. In demonstrating the benefit, you emphasize what is important to the consumer, and involve the consumer in the communication.

Integration of brand-name benefit.   Create a link between the brand name and the benefit. Brand name and benefit reinforce one another. This gives the consumer a reason to remember the name. The brand name communicates the message. Linkage of name and message is faster when it is done visually as well as aurally. Visual integration is also more effective than just audio integration.

Simplicity.   Make your ad as simple as possible. In order to get your message across, the consumer must pay attention. If the message is too long, and demands time and effort, the consumer will ignore it. You have to make it easy for the consumer to understand your message.

There are other important questions. When hiring an agency, you should find out who owns it. While many large agencies are owned by large, international corporations, be wary of agencies that are owned by advertisers, media, or suppliers, because they are less likely to provide independent consultation.

Membership in the American Association of Advertising Agencies is an important criterion; an agency must be independent to qualify for membership.

Ascertain who is on the management team and how long they have been working for the agency. The answers can tell you something about the agency's stability. If the managers are new, find out why. The background of the managers will give you some indications of the organization's philosophy. For example, if the team includes creative people, an innovative product will probably be more important than it is to a team composed of all marketers.

Ask about the size of the agency in terms of income. Find out what the size has been over the last two years. Size in terms of billings has little relevance to strength or capacity; gross income is the important number. Some agencies describe themselves only in terms of income. Check if there is a steady growth of income. A small but consistent growth each year is a reasonable indication of an agency that is functioning well.

Find out how many full-time employees the agency has and the type of work each does. This information will verify the answers they gave you about income. It takes at least four people to handle a million dollars in billings. A million dollars in media billings with the standard 15% commission produces $150,000 for the agency, but income is higher because of creative and art charges and production mark-ups. Out of this, the agency must pay staff, materials, taxes, and other expenses. Overstaffed agencies do not make a profit, and you should not hire them. Understaffed agencies will not be able to provide the service you need when you need it. Look for an efficient agency.

Find out the names of the companies for whom the agency works and the product lines with which they work. Try to assess how well the agency, based on its experience, will be able to understand your needs. Ask to see several successful campaigns developed by the agency. This will help you ascertain whether the agency's style suits your goals. If you like a particular example, find out who did it. You may be able to arrange to work with that person or team. Who will be responsible for management of your account is also an important question. You need to know with whom you will be working on the business, as well as the creative, aspects of the development of your promotional pieces.

Sales Promotion

Although there are many definitions of *sales promotion,* it is generally accepted to include the use of short-term incentives to stimulate market response. An *incentive* is something of value added to an offer to encourage purchase. Sales promotion generally excludes most forms of radio, television, newspaper, magazine, and outdoor advertising. Direct mail is often used in sales promotion. Sales promotion tools are quite diverse. They range from coupons, contests, deals, premiums, business gifts, trading stamps, samples, and point-of-purchase promotions, to trade shows, catalogs, technical publications, and specialty advertising (giveaway items). However, these tools have three important characteristics: they communicate, invite, and provide incentives for immediate purchase. Sales promotion tools get attention. By providing information, they may interest the potential consumer in the product. And, they include something—a concession, contribution, or an inducement—that gives something of value to the consumer.

Sales promotion activities should be managed with care. It is important to set up a system to identify how money is spent. All expenses, such as special packaging, incentives, and loss of revenue through price reduction, must be included. This kind of information helps make planning and control efficient.

The first step in an efficient sales promotion program is to identify the role of promotion in achieving market objectives. For example, is the sales promotion for market expansion, or is it to defend market share? It is important to look at sales promotion in relation to other elements of the marketing mix, especially advertising. Advertising is often the primary strategy used to attract new customers, but it may be supplemented by sales promotion techniques. Some use advertising to attract new customers and sales promotion as a defensive tactic. Sales promotion is especially effective when used with advertising in introducing new or substantially modified products. These tools boost sales of products that are already increasing. Sales promotion is usually a short-term campaign to increase sales, while advertising is used for long-term retention. Sales promotion tools are not effective for building long-term brand preference. They are used to dramatize product offers and to increase sales quickly.

Sales promotion tools are used by most organizations to supplement advertising and personal selling. They are directed to one or more of three target markets: sales representatives, middlemen, and consumers. In developing the sales promotion program, the target audience should be specified and the desired response quantified. This will facilitate evaluation of the promotion program. An example of a sales promotion targeted to middlemen is seen in Case Study 11, as part of the development of the VIP program for physicians by the Visiting Nurse Service (VNS). In that instance, the physicians were middlemen and the home care consultants were sales representatives. VNS could also develop a sales promotion program for its representatives. For example, they could give a prize for recruiting the largest number of physicians to the VIP program.

A sales promotion program has seven steps. They are setting objectives, selecting tools, developing the program, pretesting, implementing, controlling, and evaluating results.

Setting Objectives

Objectives for a sales promotion program are based on marketing objectives for the product. They are also based on the target market. For example, objectives for consumers include getting users to buy more, getting nonusers to try the product, and converting users of competing brands. The objectives for trade promotion of goods to middlemen include getting retailers to carry new items, advertise the product, increase shelf space, give the product more prominent shelf space, and increase stock. Sales force objectives include achieving more support for products and increasing new accounts through sales representatives.

Drug companies use all these tools for promoting sales of their products. In their ads on television, they encourage patients to ask their doctors about new anti-histamines, estrogen replacements, and ulcer medications. Their salespeople encourage physicians to prescribe the medication by giving them free samples, which are then given to patients. Salespeople also persuade pharmacists to stock the product. To increase salesperson productivity, a drug company may give bonuses.

Service organizations also have sales promotion objectives. Nurses associations use sales promotion to increase membership. They may invite nonmembers to attend meetings, give issues of their newsletters to students and other nonmembers, and reduce conference fees for members. Membership contests are frequently used, with prizes given to members who recruit the most new members. Joint advertising may be done by the association and a hospital or other health care agency. A sales promotion technique used by hospitals is giving new parents a candlelight, gourmet dinner the night before discharge.

The decision to use a sales promotion must have a sound rationale. It should be part of a long-range plan and be based on research whenever possible. Turning to the candlelight dinner again, the objective is to increase use of the obstetrical service. However, if market research shows that there is a large decline in the population of childbearing age, the dinner is not effective marketing; it is a gimmick. A more reasonable approach would be to reduce the maternity service and reallocate the funds to a more profitable and needed service. Conversely, if market research shows that there is a need for the obstetric service, the dinner could be an important part of the marketing mix.

Selecting Tools

Many tools can be used to achieve sales promotion objectives. These tools are used to stimulate early purchase of the product and to gain customer goodwill. To choose among them, consider the target market, objectives, competition, costs, and effectiveness of each tool.

Samples, coupons, price packs, and premiums. These represent the major tools of consumer promotion. Samples are small amounts of a product given to a consumer, generally free. Occasionally, a nominal fee is charged to help offset the costs. Samples can be distributed by direct mail, given out in stores or physicians' offices, offered in ads, distributed at seminars, conventions, and sporting and community events, disseminated through civic and social groups, attached to another product, or delivered door-to-door. Samples are the most effective and most expensive way to introduce a new product. Cosmetic and pharmaceutical companies use this tool extensively. Nurses receive many samples at conventions. Erdman (1985) maintains that if the concept has a failing, it is that not enough companies consider it in their promotional program. Remember that you can also offer a sample of some services to a target market.

Coupons and certificates give consumers a reduced price when the product is bought. They are effective for stimulating sales of a mature product and for encouraging early purchase of a new product. Coupons can be a valuable part of your promotion program. Coupons appeal to people who need to watch their budgets and to those who have a sense of thrift. People tend to accept and handle a coupon as something of value. They are especially useful in getting people to purchase the product the first time. Almost 200 billion cents-off coupons are offered to consumers each year. Major consumer product manufacturers are the most frequent users of coupons, but smaller manufacturers, wholesalers, retailers, and service organizations can use coupons profitably. Publishers of nursing drug handbooks use them for their mail orders. In Case Studies 2 and 10, Corbett and Kelly used coupons effectively for sales promotion of a smoking cessation program and continuing education offerings.

Coupons can be distributed in many ways. Print ads and direct mail are the most common means of distribution. Other ways include putting them on or in a product (sometimes in cooperation with other businesses), putting them in coupon books used by fund raisers, and handing them out at trade shows, special events, or on the street.

Another form of coupon, the rebate, has become especially popular among car and appliance manufacturers. Rebates are usually used for larger amounts of money than are coupons. The average face value for coupons is about 25 cents; rebates can exceed $100. In health care, rebates have been used effectively. A hospital offered a smoking cessation program for a fee to its employees, but if they successfully completed the program and did not smoke for one year, the hospital gave a full rebate of the fee charged.

Price packs give savings off the regular price of a product. They are very effective for stimulating short-term sales. The manufacturer puts the reduced prices directly on the label or the package. A price pack can be single package sold at a reduced price. Johnson & Johnson, while making a comeback after the Tylenol tampering incidents, did an extensive promotion offering two for the price of one. In a variation, price packs may be made up of two related products banded together. Packaging a toothbrush and toothpaste or an antiseptic with bandages are two examples.

Premiums are goods given free or at nominal cost as an incentive to purchase the product. The premium may be the package itself, such as a canister for coffee or flour. In the nursing field, *JONA*'s *Nursing Scan in Administration* offered a binder with a subscription. Offers received after sending proofs of purchase to a company are another form of premium. Household products use this form of sales promotion extensively; you can get all kinds of premiums, from t-shirts and toys to dishes, pots, and pans.

Manufacturers may provide free specialty advertising items bearing the company's name as a means of trade promotion. The specialty advertising industry has flourished for more than 100 years. It sells more than 83 billion dollars worth of imprinted promotions products a year (Ebel, Madden, & Caballero, 1987). Specialty items are used by a plethora of organizations as a token of gratitude or as a means to keep their organization in the minds of the target markets. College alumni and museum donors receive mugs or pens with name and logo; board members and bank customers receive calendars; applicants to nursing education programs receive pens, pencils, tote bags, and key rings.

Conventions and trade shows.   Annual conventions of associations often sponsor a trade show concurrent with their event. Companies that sell their products to the sponsoring industry show their products. At nursing conventions, these often include publishers and pharmaceutical firms as well as medical equipment and supply companies. Conventions are effective for obtaining new sales leads, contacting old and meeting new customers, introducing new products, and increasing sales to current customers (Kotler & Armstrong, 1987). Case Study 3 describes an effective use of this tool.

The booth, graphic presentation, sales personnel, and support materials all communicate important messages about your product. They must be well executed to achieve your goals and objectives. A thorough analysis of the objectives must be undertaken in order to ensure a good return on your investment. Costs of exhibiting at conventions and trade shows can be exorbitant.

To set and evaluate objectives, you need to identify the following: (1) the purpose in exhibiting, (2) the target market, (3) the advantages of local, regional, or national exhibiting, (4) the cost-benefit analysis, (5) the approach your competition uses, and (6) the cost ratio per sale or sales lead (Cavanaugh, 1976). Exhibiting is often presumed to be for the purpose of increasing sales. In some cases, it is not cost-effective to exhibit for this purpose, but exhibiting can do more than promote short-term sales. The purposes for exhibiting can include introducing new products, training sales personnel, promoting corporate identity, securing orders, and conducting market research.

Contests, sweepstakes, and games.   There are many forms of contests. They range from jelly-bean guessing to puzzles, and are used to stimulate salespeople, middlemen, and consumers. The commonality is that someone wins a prize through effort or by luck. Although it may be minimal, contests require some skill. Contestants submit some kind of entry such as a jingle, a guess, or the number of sales they made. The entry that is evaluated as the best wins the prize. Another form of contest is the incentive campaign, in which one competes against personal past performance. Often nurses associations use members as the sales force and hold contests to see who can recruit the most members. Prizes have ranged from tote bags and restaurant meals to trips for two to Scandinavia. Various types of contests are used by vendors of health care supplies and equipment, particularly at convention exhibits.

Sweepstakes are based purely on chance; they do not require skill from the entrant. Sweepstakes call for consumers to submit their names for a drawing. In contrast to a lottery, a sweepstakes does not require money or purchase of a product to enter. Games give consumers something, such as letters or numbers, every time they make a purchase; these help to win a prize. Soft-drink and fast-food businesses often use games for sales promotion.

To develop a successful program, some important decisions need to be made. Timing and duration are primary decisions. It is possible to hold more than one event a year, but it is probably not feasible to do so during traditionally slack periods of the year. Generally, a campaign or contest of less than a month is too short; more than three months is usually too long, because interest wanes. In planning a promotion campaign, a theme should be selected, forms and records developed, and a promotion campaign developed, prizes announced, and rules for participating published.

Important advantages of all forms of contests are the interest and excitement they generate. Contests increase sales and an interest in the product. Disadvantages include the costs of administering and promoting the contest, the taxable status of the prizes, and the possibility that sales stimulation may be short-term. In addition, consumers may become tired or bored with contests because of the large numbers that are held.

There are problems in running an effective contest. Its success depends on the attractiveness of the contest theme, prizes, and rules. If you do hold a lottery or raffle, you should be aware that Federal Trade Commission regulations may apply.

Point-of-purchase promotion.   Point-of-purchase promotions (P-O-P) can be almost anything that is designed to attract a potential customer's attention where and when a buying decision is made. Cosmetic companies use P-O-Ps effectively with their gifts of umbrellas, satchels, glassware, and other premiums, as well as their purchase-with-a-purchase promotions. Slide show and video P-O-Ps are used to great advantage by health care suppliers, publishers, and pharmaceutical companies at nursing conventions.

Direct mail.   A distinct advantage of direct mail is that it can be used in many situations. The Direct Marketing Association compiled a list of 49 reasons and ways to use direct mail. Uses range from building employee morale, creating a need or demand for a product, and announcing a new service, to correcting mailing lists and raising funds. It is a versatile, highly personal, and direct promotional method. Some hospitals recently used direct mail to recruit nurses. Nursing schools also use direct mail promotions.

One advantage of direct mail is that it can be less expensive than other forms of sales promotion. It also affords audience selectivity, is flexible, allows for personalization, and can be time-sensitive. Disadvantages include the image of junk mail and, frequently, a relatively low return on investment.

Developing the Program

After you select the promotional tools, you must develop the rest of the promotion program. Decisions concerning this step are how much of an incentive to offer, to whom to make the offer, how to advertise the promotion, length of the promotion, when to start, and how much money to allocate. The size of the incentive is important. An incentive that is too small will not succeed. A large incentive will produce more sales, but only to a certain point. It is important to find a balance so that the incentive will be sufficient to increase sales, but not so large as to hurt profits. Whenever possible, sales promotion tools should be pretested on a portion of the target market. Pretesting with various incentives will identify the most effective size of incentive. Decisions on how to promote and distribute the promotion must be made. In Case Studies 2, 3, and 10, Corbett, Crawford and Fisher, and Kelly did direct mailings.

As with the size of incentive, the length of the promotion is important. A time that is too short will miss many potential customers; one that is too long will lose its immediacy. Implementation plans should be made for each promotion, beginning with lead time (the time necessary to prepare the program) and ending with sell-off time (the time from launch to end of promotion). The dates are important to all concerned with the product. An anticipated increase in sales or use has important implications for production, sales, and distribution. In order to be effective, you must have sufficient goods or services available, price them correctly, and have a means to distribute the product as needed. If any of the Ps of the marketing mix are lacking, the program will fail.

Budget Allocation

Two methods are used to develop a sales promotion budget. They are choosing the promotions and estimating the cost, or allocating a percentage of the total budget. The latter is the most common way (Kotler & Armstrong, 1987). To develop the budget, consider the cost-effectiveness of the promotion strategy. Spend to achieve objectives; do not just expand last year's budget. Take a percentage of expected sales, or choose the amount you can afford. Strang (1976) recommends that you prepare your advertising and sales promotion budgets together.

Personal Selling

Sales personnel are those employed to sell something to others. Until recently, rarely was the term "sell" used in relation to health care. It was strongly felt that health care services were not "sold"; they were "offered." This is purely a semantic difference. For many years, hospitals have used personal selling to raise money, recruit nurses, and implement community outreach programs. Personal selling at conventions was one of the promotion strategies used by Crawford and Fisher to sell nursing manuals (Case Study 3).

Sales personnel are distinct from intermediaries in a health care organization; the former are employed to sell. In hospitals, they include recruiters, fund raisers, and the sales force in the marketing department. Intermediaries are not employed to sell; their job is to provide a professional, clinical service such as nursing. It is fallacious to say that all nurses are selling the organization. They are not; they are providing nursing care and serving as public relations agents for themselves, the nursing profession, and the employing organization.

Although personal selling is the most costly way to promote products, it is also the most effective method for building preference and conviction leading to purchase, because personal selling has several important characteristics. These characteristics are personal interaction, relationship development, and response. Personal selling involves interactions between buyers and sellers. They observe the other's responses and are able to modify their own behavior to make the most of the situation. Uncertainties and ambiguities can be clarified and questions can be answered.

Many kinds of relationships can develop in personal selling. They may range from short-term sales relationships to life-long, personal friendships. Salespeople use approaches that range from a soft to hard sell. In order to keep a good selling relationship, it is vital to keep the customer's long-term interests in mind. Since personal selling involves interaction, the potential buyer needs to listen and respond. Responses can range from a mere thank-you to purchase.

In addition to selling goods, services, ideas, or the organization, sales personnel can perform five other functions for an organization. These are:

1. Finding and cultivating new customers.

2. Communicating useful information about the organization.

3. Providing services such as consulting on problems and giving technical assistance.

4. Gathering market research and other useful information.

5. Advising on allocation of scarce resources.

Each organization has different needs, and will necessarily place emphasis on different activities. In Case Study 11, the Visiting Nurse Service of New York needed the nurses doing personal selling to spend most of their time finding physician customers, communicating, and selling. They also consulted on problems and gathered information.

The sales force is important to a company's effectiveness. It is therefore essential that the organization design and develop its sales force carefully and thoughtfully. Important issues are sales force objectives, strategy, structure, size, and compensation. The sales force must also be managed. Management includes recruiting, selecting, training, directing, motivating, and evaluating sales personnel. It is beyond the scope of this book to discuss these aspects of personal selling, but interested readers can find a vast literature in both the business and the lay press.

Publicity

Publicity is a major promotion tool. It is part of public relations. For an in-depth discussion of publicity, see Chapter 6.

CONCLUSION

Nurses and their leaders, managers, and executives must have skill in using the processes of marketing and strategic market planning. These processes have become important because of changes in the environment that have brought about increased competition for scarce resources. In order to meet patient wants and needs, nurses must be able to obtain and use marketing information to develop and implement cost-effective strategies. Additionally, nurses must be involved with marketing health care institutions as well as the nursing profession and its services.

REFERENCES

Ailing hospital ads need intensive care. (1989, July 31). *The Wall Street Journal,* p. B1.

Alward, R.R. (1988). Prospective payment systems and implications for the management of nursing resources. In J. Kirsch, *The middle manager & the nursing organization* (pp. 185-203). Norwalk, CT: Appleton & Lange.

Bloom, P.N. (1984). Effective marketing for professional services. *Harvard Business Review, 62*(5), 102–110.

Breindel, C.L. (1988). Nongrowth strategies and options in health care. *Hospital & Health Services Administration, 33*(1), 37–45.

Carmel, S. (1985). Satisfaction with hospitalization: A comparative analysis of three types of services. *Social Science Medicine, 21,* 1243–1249.

Cavanaugh, S. (1976). Setting objectives and evaluating the effectiveness of trade show exhibits. *Journal of Marketing, 40*(4), 100–103.

Cooper, P.D., Maxwell, R., & Kehoe, W. (1985). Entry strategies for marketing in ambulatory and other health delivery systems. In P.D. Cooper (Ed.), *Health care marketing* (2nd ed.) (pp. 30–36). Rockville, MD: Aspen.

Davis, L.J. (1989, April 9). Phillip Morris's big bite. *The New York Times Magazine,* pp. 30–33, 40, 84–85.

Droste, T. (1989). Research and customer satisfaction top agenda. *Hospitals, 63*(1), 38.

Ebel, R.G., Madden, C.S., & Caballero, M. (1987). Proactive image management. *Association Management, 39*(7), 47–49.

Erdman, K.B. (1985). Sales promotion requirements. In E.E. Bobrow & M.D. Bobrow (Eds.). *Marketing handbook: Volume I: Marketing practices* (pp. 377–397). Homewood, IL: Dow Jones–Irwin.

Gibson, K.R., & Pulliam, C.B. (1987). Cooperative care: The time has come. *Journal of Nursing Administration, 17*(3), 19–21.

Heskett, J.L. (1987). Lessons in the service sector. *Harvard Business Review, 87*(2), 118–126.

Hill, C.J., & Neeley, S.E. (1988). Differences in the consumer decision process for professional vs. generic services. *Journal of Services Marketing, 2*(1), 17–23.

Hizar, T.W. (1985). Two questions almost everyone forgets to ask their advertising agency. *Journal of Consumer Marketing, 2*(3), 45–53.

Holbrook, F.K. (1972). Charging by level of nursing care. *Hospitals, 46*(16), 80–88.

Ireland, R.C. (1985). Marketing: A new opportunity for hospital management. In P.D. Cooper (Ed.), *Health care marketing* (2nd ed.) (pp. 38–46). Rockville, MD: Aspen.

Johnson, J.E. (1988). Writing a winning business plan. *Journal of Nursing Administration, 18*(10), 15–19.

Keith, J.G. (1985). Marketing health care: What the recent literature is telling us. In P.D. Cooper (Ed.), *Health care marketing* (2nd ed.) (pp. 13–25). Rockville, MD: Aspen.

Kotler, P. (1986). Megamarketing. *Harvard Business Review, 64*(2), 117–124.

Kotler, P. (1988). *Marketing management: Analysis, planning, implementation, and control.* Englewood Cliffs, NJ: Prentice-Hall.

Kotler, P., & Andreasen, A.R. (1987). *Strategic marketing for nonprofit organizations* (3rd ed.). Englewood Cliffs, NJ: Prentice-Hall.

Kotler, P., & Armstrong, G. (1987). *Marketing: An introduction.* Englewood Cliffs, NJ: Prentice-Hall.

Kotler, P., & Clarke, R.N. (1987). *Marketing for health care organizations.* Englewood Cliffs, NJ: Prentice-Hall.

MacStravic, R.E. (1985). Price of services. In P.D. Cooper (Ed.), *Health care marketing: Issues and trends* (2nd ed.) (pp. 230–235). Rockville, MD: Aspen.

MacStravic, R.S. (1986). Product-line administration in hospitals. *Health Care Management Review, 11*(2), 35–43.

MacStravic, S. (1988). The patient as partner: A competitive strategy in health care marketing. *Hospital & Health Services Administration, 33*(1), 15–29.

McCarthy, E.J. (1981). *Basic marketing: A managerial approach* (7th ed.). Homewood, IL: Richard D. Irwin.

Pope, J.L. (1986). Marketing research for service industries. In V.P. Buell (Ed.), *Handbook of modern marketing* (pp. 36-1 to 36-10). New York: McGraw-Hill.

Schmenner, R.W. (1986). How can service businesses survive and prosper? *Sloan Management Review, 27*(3), 21–32.

Shaffer, F.A. (1984). Nursing power in the DRG world. *Nursing Management, 15*(6), 28–30.

Shapiro, B.P. (1968).The psychology of pricing. *Harvard Business Review, 46*(4), 14–16, 18, 20, 22, 24–25, 160.

Solovy, A. (1989). Limited use for product management in hospitals. *Hospitals, 63*(2), 72.

Strang, R.A. (1976). Sales promotion—fast growth, faulty management. *Harvard Business Review, 54*(4), 115–124.

Surprenant, C.F., & Solomon, M.R. (1987). Predictability and personalization in the service encounter. *Journal of Marketing, 51*(2), 86–96.

Twedt, D.W. (1969). How to plan new products, improve old ones, and create better advertising. *Journal of Marketing, 33*(1), 53–57.

Tyson, P.R. (1977). Modify your services and marketing to recover investment. *Modern Healthcare, 7*(2), 49–50.

Vestal, K.W. (1988). Writing a business plan. *Nursing Economics, 6*(3), 121–124.

Wood, C.T. (1982). Relate hospital charges to use of services. *Harvard Business Review, 60*(2), 123–130.

Wright, J.S., & Bostic, J.R. (1983). The advertising message. In S.H. Brett & N.F. Guess (Eds.), *The Dartnell Marketing Manager's Handbook* (pp. 1039–1050). Boston: Dartnell.

Zeithaml, V.A., Parasuraman, A., & Berry, L.L. (1985). Problems and strategies in services marketing. *Journal of Marketing, 49*(2), 33–46.

CHAPTER 6

Public Relations

Public relations can provide an effective approach for achieving optimal results within the political and economic constraints of the current marketplace by stimulating interest in the nursing profession. The local community, news media, businesses, local politicians, government officials, and social action groups all can take an active or reactive interest in nursing's activities. Planned, skillful use of public relations in marketing nursing services can facilitate achievement of goals and objectives. More specifically, public relations is a marketing function that can assist the nurse manager and nursing staff to achieve unit and divisional goals and objectives. The process and tools of public relations can help make the most of what you have; this is essential in today's changing marketplace. *Public relations* is concerned with the activities that earn and maintain favorable publicity for a company, agency, or individual. The management function includes evaluation of the public's attitudes, identification of an individual or organization with the public interest, and planning and implementing programs to gain public understanding and acceptance of an individual, organization, product, service, or idea. Public relations practitioners are the caretakers and enhancers of an organization's and profession's image. They are charged with the job of forming, maintaining, or changing public attitudes. All nurses are potential public relations practitioners. This chapter will help you develop your public relations skills and assist you in working with an agency's public relations department.

HISTORY OF PUBLIC RELATIONS

Public relations has its origins in ancient history. Its three main elements—informing people, persuading people, and integrating people with people—are as old as society (Bernays, 1952). Bernays gives a history of the development of public relations from prerecorded time through ancient history, the Dark Ages, the Renaissance and the Reformation, the Enlightenment, the French Revolution, and into modern times.

154

In the New World, public relations was used from the beginning. While many colonists came seeking religious freedom, some sought adventure and economic opportunities. They were often persuaded to emigrate through public relations activities used by land companies. The colonists brought with them a belief in a free press. Freedom of opinion was an important issue; it became the issue that united colonists against King George III. Samuel Adams of Boston used the press skillfully against the British. In doing so, he became a master political strategist (Bernays, 1952). The colonists were not the only ones at the time to use public relations. Louis XVI's ambassador to Philadelphia planted stories supporting French policy (McCarry, 1989).

Public relations was used so successfully by the abolitionists that many politicians were forced to change their positions on slavery. At the beginning of the Civil War, Abraham Lincoln stated, "In this and like communities, public sentiment is everything. With public sentiment nothing can fail; without it, nothing can succeed. Consequently, he who molds public sentiment goes deeper than he who accepts or makes decisions" (Bernays, 1952, p. 44).

P.T. Barnum, who said, "There's a sucker born every minute," used the press to gain a great deal of publicity for his circus. He made his circus, and its arrival in town, a newsworthy event. Barnum kept the story in the press by writing to newspapers and signing fictitious names. In 1871, he launched the slogan "Greatest Show on Earth"; the slogan is still used by the circus. The use of advance men or press agents to publicize the circus helped it develop a nationwide reputation.

The period between 1865 and 1900 was a time of rapid industrial growth and great social change. Small businesses grew into huge corporations. During this time, public relations served a contact function (Kotler & Andreasen, 1987). The corporate goal was to influence favorably the press and legislators. Next in the evolution of public relations came increased realization that planned publicity could be invaluable. In the time between 1919 and 1929, companies added publicists to their staffs. H.L. Mencken stated in 1925 (p. 309) that "every politician, movie actress, and prize fighter in America has a publicist." Indeed, even the Boy Scouts in Toledo, Ohio had a publicist (Mencken, 1926).

The Depression and World War II brought profound changes in the way businesses operated. They had to sell themselves to the public, and needed to modify their attitudes and actions to conform to public demands. Business realized that it had to do the following:

1. Adhere to the principle that private business must always be in the public interest if it is going to survive.

2. Recognize that the public interest changes and the business must change with it.

3. Understand that the place of business in the American system must be sold to the public.

4. Use public relations to help achieve the above. (Bernays, 1952, p. 103)
A very broad, diverse group of businesses sought professional public relations guidance. Jewelers such as Cartier, broadcasters such as NBC and CBS, chain stores, and many others hired public relations consultants. Because public opinion was identified as important, public relations companies and consultants had to be able to conduct the necessary research.

In 1937, Bernays surveyed institutions of higher learning and found them offering a wide range of courses on public relations. Public relations grew and matured during the period from 1929 to 1941. The need to develop and integrate theory and praxis grew from the political and socioeconomic events of the time. Public relations consultants were hired to (1) analyze the client and the publics on which the client was dependent, (2) identify causes of problems between the client and its publics, and (3) identify actions to be taken to improve the relationship. The public relations consultant was often hired on a long-term basis, as well as for short terms to handle specific problems or crises.

In fact, the American Nurses Association (ANA) hired Bernays' firm on a long-term basis during this time (Bernays, 1947). Bernays' report to the ANA, which was based on survey research, counseled that change was slow and that public relations was not a panacea. Bernays' recommendations to the ANA had to do with public relations and image; they are still pertinent. However, this was and still is only part of nursing's problem. Public relations and image management cannot be expected to make fundamental changes in society. It has taken decades for the social changes that have brought about civil rights and women's rights. Women still do not have equal status with men in the workplace, and nursing continues to be a woman's profession.

As measurement of public opinion and theory of mass communication developed, public relations became more sophisticated. Progressive companies hired lobbyists, publicists, and researchers. Soon, public relations departments were established within companies in order to coordinate and integrate these functions. Social consciousness was a hallmark of the 1960s and 1970s. Organizations now had to heed society's demands regarding civil rights, human rights, women's rights, ecology, conservation, consumerism, and safety. As an outcome of the Vietnam War and Watergate, ethics also became an issue in the late 1970s and the 1980s. Many public relations practitioners now see their role as assisting the organization to be socially responsible.

PUBLIC RELATIONS IN THE MARKETING MIX

More than simply a communications function, public relations strategies are most effective when viewed and conducted as part of the marketing mix used by the organization. Marketing mix is one of the basic concepts in marketing theory (see Chapter 5). It is the mixture of controllable marketing elements—product, promotion, place, and price—that is used to achieve organizational goals. A successful marketing mix is "having the right product in the right place at the right time with the right promotion at the right price" (Kotler, 1980, p. 17). Public relations is one of the aspects of promotion, but it deals with promotion of the organization or practitioners rather than a specific product or service. Public relations can be seen primarily as a communication tool to advance the objectives of the organization or professional; nevertheless, it is more than simply a communications function. Public relations reinforces an institution's mandate and credibility with the public, thereby assisting in the achievement of goals and objectives, and it provides ways and means of connecting an organization and its publics, facilitating two-way communication. It is most effective when viewed, planned, and implemented as part of the marketing mix.

The influence the public relations function has in an organization depends on the view the board of directors and the chief officers have of the function, and where it is placed in the table of organization. Some public relations departments are managed by vice presidents who are involved with policy and strategy formation. The advantages of this are: (1) better anticipation of potential problems, (2) better handling of these problems, (3) consistent public-oriented policies and strategies, (4) greater number of and more professional communications (Kotler & Andreasen, 1987). Other public relations departments are headed by managers who produce publications (e.g., the annual report), and handle news and special events. These managers often have little influence on corporate policy.

THE NURSING ORGANIZATION'S PUBLICS

Regardless of where the public relations function is positioned within the health care organization, the nursing division can and should use the department and the process of public relations to its advantage. This necessitates first identifying the publics with whom the nursing division should interact. Patients, employees, physicians, directors and trustees, management, and various community groups are *primary publics* who are especially important. *Secondary publics* include vendors, government regulatory groups, and competitors. *Tertiary publics* are general-purpose groups that seek to advance the interests of their members; examples are labor unions, churches, clubs, associations, media, and social action groups (Kotler, 1980). You will notice that, in public relations, the term *public* is used more broadly than in Chapter 2.

All the mentioned publics have an impact on achievement of the goals of the nursing division. They have relationships with one another as well as with the nursing division. Any particular public may have a great influence on the attitudes and behavior of other publics toward the division or organization. For example, a nurse who has a high degree of satisfaction will be enthusiastic about her job and the institution. She may recruit her friends, which will reinforce the staff's self-esteem based on a positive image. This in turn will affect nursing performance and influence the attitudes and behaviors of other hospital publics.

On the other hand, dissatisfied nurses are likely to have attitudes and behaviors that have a negative impact on the care they give and on the overall function of their units. They may complain to family and friends. The patients, recipients of less than optimal care, may complain to the physician and will certainly complain to family and friends. Unfortunately, many patients do not use formal channels for complaints. Soon the nursing division and the hospital may have a community-wide reputation for uncaring service, and patients and nurses will choose competing hospitals the next time nursing care is required or a position is sought. Revenue is lost, recruitment costs and difficulty increase, and the image of the organization is tarnished.

PUBLIC RELATIONS PROCESS

The rest of this chapter describes the steps of the public relations process. These steps are similar to any other problem-solving process, and include identifying publics, doing research, establishing goals, developing strategies, implementing strategies, and evaluating outcome. The first step in the public relations process is to identify the public that you want to reach. Consider all your publics. Careful assessment of goals and objectives must be made. A first-line manager in a hospital may decide to develop public relations strategies focusing on patients' families or physicians. Indeed, in Case Study 12, both families and physicians were targeted. In Case Studies 4 and 6, Davis and Frost describe how they targeted the Boy Scouts and Girl Scouts in their social marketing.

The second step is to measure the image and attitudes of the target or relevant public. This is often a difficult task, but one that must be done. Frequently our assumptions are not supported by research studies. In our marketing research for Case Study 1, we found that the local nurses' association did not have an image problem as much as an awareness problem. Contrary to popular belief, nurses did not join specialty organizations instead of the state nurses association (SNA). Those who belonged to specialty organizations tended to belong to the SNA, but those who did not belong to the SNA did not belong to specialty organizations either. Competition for nonmembers came from leisure and family activities.

To assess the image of an organization or the attitudes of a public, some market research must be done. Marketing research is the design, collection, analysis, and reporting of data and findings pertaining to a specific marketing situation (see Chapter 4). For the hospital nursing division, competing forces can be outside nursing, but within the hospital, or they can be outside the institution.

A literature search is a good place to begin investigating image and attitude. The search may alert you to problems and pitfalls. You may find little or a gold mine of information relating to your particular problem. From there, you can go on to develop qualitative and quantitative studies. These can be simple or sophisticated, as is appropriate to the question, time, expertise, and funds that are available. Qualitative methods range from the solicitation of feedback from various publics, to focus groups, in-depth interviews, nominal groups, and Delphi techniques. Quantitative studies are valuable tools for assessing image and attitudes in relation to both internal and external markets. They can be done using management information gathered by the division or organization, such as patient questionnaires, exit interviews with staff nurses, and physician or patient complaint reports. Consider the goals and objectives of the study and the resources available. In light of the difficulties of doing market research studies, employment of market research consultants may be desirable (see Chapter 4).

Through periodic researching of primary publics, the nurse manager will acquire some hard data on how these publics view the organization. The data will be the basis for a public relations plan, which will be used to establish image and attitude goals for key publics.

Establishment of image, knowledge, and attitude goals for key publics is the third step of the public relations process. These goals are specific to public relations and are distinct from marketing goals. For instance, a public relations goal might be to promote a positive image of a new well-baby clinic staffed by nurse practitioners. It is important that the goals be measurable. Establish criteria for the systematic assessment of results. An example of a measurable goal would be that 25% of patients know before their first appointment that the clinic is staffed by nurse practitioners. Use the goals throughout the campaign. The publicity campaign should usually be completed before other promotional activities, such as paid advertising, are begun. Simultaneous use complicates the task of evaluation.

Development of cost-effective public relations strategies is the fourth step. Many options are available for you to improve, change, or maintain the attitudes of a particular public. Work to increase your options before you select the one you will use. Your first task here is to understand why the attitudes have come about. You can then develop an appropriate strategy geared to the specific causal factor. After you know what audience you want to reach and the response you want, you *then* decide upon the message. The media, or tools, are chosen last.

Tools for Implementation

The fifth step in the process is the implementation of actions. There are at least eight public relations tools to use in implementing your public relations plan (Kotler, 1988). They may be categorized as: (1) written material, (2) audiovisual material, (3) corporate identity media, (4) news, (5) public service activities, (6) events, (7) speeches, and (8) telephone information services.

Written Material

The function of written material is to provide information for the ultimate purpose of building confidence in the organization and its leaders. The material must be readable, interesting, professional, and have aesthetic appeal. This applies to all written material, from memoranda and letters to articles for publication. How written material is presented makes a statement about you and the group to which you belong, be it nurse administrators, practitioners, or entrepreneurs.

Publication in both the professional and lay presses increases the visibility of the nurse and the employing health care agency. All levels of nurses should be encouraged to write for publication (see Case Study 5 for one example). Writing courses and workshops are widely available if help is needed to develop writing skills. Effective publications give an institution a dynamic, creative, innovative, and progressive image. This positive image can assist in the recruitment of staff and patients.

Brochures. Brochures, also called pamphlets, flyers, or folders, are an effective way to provide important information to a targeted public. They can provide information about an organization, product, health problem, conference or seminar, and professional practice. Brochures are useful for selling as well as for public relations. Nurses frequently use them for recruitment and patient education. The brochure must be appropriate to, and consistent with, your goals and objectives. To what use are you putting the brochure, and to whom is it directed? Is it to be used to increase membership, promote a conference, sell a service? Is it a public service? These are important decisions upon which all the other decisions are based.

Brochures must be well-designed to be effective. A poorly produced brochure can do more harm than good. It is important that it be attractive. If it does not look good, people will not read it. Take great care in preparing brochures (see Exhibit 6-1). Hiring a graphic artist and a printer is often a cost-effective measure.

How the brochure will be distributed must also be decided early in development. If it is to be mailed, an important decision is whether to use a self-mailer or an envelope. This decision must be based on your target audience and the purpose of the brochure as well as on direct costs. Self-mailers—brochures with one outer panel to be used for return address, postage, and recipient's name and address—are cheaper and easier to mail. They are cheaper because envelopes do not have to be purchased, stuffed, and sealed, nor do self-mailers have to be stapled, taped, or glued. The use of envelopes looks, and is, more expensive. Upscale market segments are more effectively reached with the use of envelopes.

The cost of production must be appropriate to the target public. A poor-quality mimeographed or xeroxed product will usually not help achieve your goals. Overspending on glossy pictures, fancy graphics, and a four-color printing process may also have a negative impact if it causes the target public to be concerned about the goals and fiscal management of the organization or professional.

EXHIBIT 6-1   Brochure Checklist

1. Front cover
   a. Is it clear, clean, and concise?
   b. Is it attractive and eye-catching?
2. Typeface
   a. Is the typeface consistent (limited number of styles used)?
   b. Is it consistent with the message and image you want to convey?
3. Layout
   a. Is it consistent in style (margins, paragraphs, etc.)?
   b. Is the art good?
   c. Are photographs labeled?
   d. Is white space used to best advantage?
   e. Is color used appropriately?
   f. Is the amount of text appropriate?
4. Paper
   a. Is the weight appropriate?
   b. Is the color and texture appropriate?

In writing the content for the brochure, remember that less is more. The content must be presented in a clear, concise way. Be wary of too much text. On the other hand, too little text may look skimpy and may also project a poor impression. Blank space is important. It is a design element and provides relief to the eye. Adjusting the type size can help control blank space.

Edit the text to eliminate technical jargon and unnecessary or negative words. Keep the style and point of view consistent. *Always* avoid sarcasm. Humor should be used with great care and forethought. Headings should be easily understood and succinct, not clever or cute. The title must be strong and demand attention.

The size and format of the brochure depend on the length of the text and how the brochure is to be distributed. A wide variety of sizes and formats can be used. If the brochure is to be mailed in envelopes, a format that fits a standard envelope is the most cost-effective; having envelopes made to order adds to the cost. Standard envelopes come in several sizes, so you are not limited to a #10 business envelope. Also, consider postage costs when making decisions about size.

Choosing the paper is an important decision. Use 70- to 80-pound paper. Lighter weight papers may show print from one side to the other, and often have a cheap, slippery feel. Paper that is heavier than 80-pound is difficult to fold and adds significantly to the costs. The texture of the paper is also a factor to consider. The use of photographs limits your choice of paper somewhat, as photographs do not reproduce well on heavily textured paper. It may be appropriate to use the same color paper as that of your stationery.

Color should be used judiciously. Use it only on the most important parts, such as the logo, artwork, headings, and subheadings. Large areas of text printed in a strong color are harder to read than those printed in black. Reproducing photographs of people in the cool colors of blue, green, and purple make the people look sick and unattractive. Four-color brochures are very expensive.

If brochures are for a long-term project, the number to order should be based on the estimated use for six months. Adding a few hundred, or even a few thousand, does not add significantly to the cost. It is much cheaper than doing a second printing because you ran out. Many brochures are revised after the first printing because of errors, changes, or dissatisfaction. When you revise the brochure for a second printing, order enough to last one or two years.

Newsletters. Publication of a newsletter is a popular way to reach your public. A variety of professional practices, businesses, and associations, such as health care, construction, landscaping, financial/investment, medicine, law, and nursing, use newsletters. Hospitals have published internal newsletters for years. Many nursing divisions and associations publish newsletters. A newsletter allows communication with publics on a regular basis. It demonstrates that you care about constituents all the time and not just sporadically. In Case Studies 1, 5, 9, 15, and 18, the authors used newsletters in their marketing plans.

Before beginning a newsletter, carefully assess the costs and benefits. While it has much to offer in the way of publicity and other public relations benefits, a newsletter requires substantial, *regular* investment of time, money, and effort. Therefore, it should not be among the first public relations projects implemented. Only after a smoothly running organization is established, with staff, policies, and procedures in place, and brochures, logo, and stationery available for image support, consider a newsletter. Be certain that a newsletter is the best public relations tool to choose. Decide what is to be accomplished with the newsletter, that is, what you wish to communicate. Define the newsletter's purpose, goals, and objectives; put them in writing. It may be a good idea to publish the purpose in the newsletter.

The next step is to decide on the target audience to be reached by the newsletter. This is important so that the newsletter can be designed and developed appropriately for it. If the newsletter is for a private practice, the patients will be a primary target audience. Patient feedback, patient records, and your personal experience can help identify the needs and wants of the average patient. A survey would also provide pertinent information. Segments of patients, such as adolescents, women, parents, athletes, or senior citizens, could be targeted. Another public to consider is potential patients. These people may be found in community groups, among new arrivals in town, or in other locations identified through market research or through networking. Referring professionals may also be a primary target market. Secondary and tertiary publics might be appropriate recipients of the newsletter. For instance, consider local business people and suppliers.

Make a realistic assessment of resources before committing them to a newsletter. Enough material for at least three issues, plus the finances to support one to two years of publication, should be available. This is a long-term endeavor; positive results may not be seen for two years. It is best to plan conservatively. Start with an annual, biannual, or quarterly publication. When things are going well, the publication can be expanded. Upgrading and expansion are always better than cutting back, running late, or downsizing (see section on demarketing in Chapter 5). These maneuvers can have an adverse effect on image.

Audiovisual Material

Audiovisual material can be an effective public relations tool. The same considerations should be given to audiovisual as to written material. It must be put together with great care in order to achieve objectives.

Slides. With the advent of videocassette recorders (VCRs) and other sophisticated audiovisual equipment, slides have become undervalued. However, slides can contribute enormously to a presentation. They are the best way to show diagrams, graphs, and illustrations. In order to be effective, they must be well designed, easy to read, of good optical quality, and have limited amounts of data. Too often slides do not meet these criteria; the speaker then loses the audience to boredom or confusion.

If funds are available, hire a graphic artist and a photographer who specialize in projection media. Ask to see slides they have produced. Very few commercial photographers know the specifications and limitations for effective lecture slides. Use 35mm film and a 2 × 2 horizontal slide format. Slides made from other film may be difficult to use because they are not a standard format. With Polaroid technology, it is easier to prepare your own slides.

Keep the content of the slide simple and to a minimum. Only enough information to illustrate one major idea should be on a single slide. Use key words instead of sentences. If a large amount of information is necessary, break it down for two or three slides. A slide is most useful if it shows something that cannot be explained as well without the slide.

For clear tables, do not crowd the slide. Again, two or more slides are better than one complicated slide. Use graphs rather than tables whenever possible; information presented in graphic form is more quickly understood. Keep graphs simple and use captions sparingly. Simplify illustrations. Omit unnecessary detail; use bold lines and round numbers.

Slides are often prepared from a template measuring 3 × 41½ inches. Type must be large enough to be seen. The Orator and Gothic typing elements on IBM typewriters or primary typeface works well when used with single spaces between letters in a word, and triple spaces between words. Keep the layout simple, with a lot of open space. The space between the lines should be at least the height of a capital letter. Avoid using more than seven double-spaced lines per slide. Some experts limit slide text to no more than six lines (Bauer, 1976). The number of words in a line must also be limited. Bauer recommends no more than 45 characters, including spaces; Meyer-Hartwig, Bleifeld, and Hegewald (1977) limit each line to seven words.

Use color for emphasis. Black print on a clear or pastel background works best. Colored letters on dark backgrounds do not provide the necessary contrast. White letters on black backgrounds are difficult to read and should be avoided. Be sure type is clean. A black carbon ribbon should be used; a fabric ribbon causes a slide to look fuzzy and out of focus when it is projected. Rub-on letters may be the best solution and are available from office suppliers. Companies that make transparency blanks also make letters for this purpose in various styles and colors. Handwritten visuals are not appropriate at a professional meeting.

Many graphics programs can be used to make slides on a computer. Hewlett-Packard Graphics Gallery, Harvard Graphics, Lotus Freelance, and Microsoft Chart are some of the most popular programs for IBM computers. Apple computers also have excellent graphics capabilities. Using these programs, you can compose simple text slides of typeset quality as well as graphs. The material can be printed on paper and then photographed. For more complex slides or special color formats, there are expensive devices that will compose the slide directly from a special high-resolution monitor. For occasional use, some mail-order services will take your diskettes with the slide data and return high-quality slides by next-day mail. These services are expensive and charge about $12 per slide.

Organize and code the slides for presentation. This is usually done by putting a dot in the lower left-hand corner of the slide as it faces you. The dot will then be in the upper right-hand corner when inserted into the projector tray. Using pencil, number slides in consecutive order. Put your name on each slide. This helps to eliminate projectionist's errors in loading the projector.

Plan the appropriate number of slides for the needs of the presentation and for the allotted time. Do not use more than one slide per minute. Note on the written speech where slides are shown. Rehearse the whole presentation, timing your delivery.

When the slides are ready, evaluate them for effectiveness. Enlist a friend to help. Project the slides in a large auditorium. Seat your friend in the back to assess the slides for legibility and clarity. Evaluate the slides; check that the labeling is adequate and that there are no excessive details. This will also help accustom you to the appearance of the giant enlargement a few feet from you.

Videotapes.   Videotapes are effective in reaching many audiences. They are a colorful, exciting way to get your message across. The brilliant image on the screen grabs the viewer's attention. There is an aura of magic. Videos are used for promotional activities and instructional or training programs. In Case Study 6, Frost effectively used video.

There are many advantages to video. Video commands attention. It presents processes more effectively than any other medium. Thus, it is useful for teaching skills, dealing with the affective domain, problem-solving instructional situations, instructing in the social sciences and humanities, discussing subtleties of unfamiliar cultures, and safely observing phenomena that may be hazardous to view directly (Simonson & Volker, 1984).

Major disadvantages of video are the cost, the difficulty of production, and the length of time required for production. Other limitations include the fact that small monitor screens limit audience size unless multiple monitors or projection systems are used. The amount of lettering or graphics for video is limited to about one-half that of film or slides. Also, rapid changes in technology make obsolescence of video systems a continuing problem.

Production involves three phases: planning, production, and editing. Of these phases, planning is the most important. Critical decisions made during the planning period will affect the whole project and its outcome. The first critical decision is whether a video is the most effective medium to use. To make this decision, consider your goals and objectives. Video may not be appropriate to achieve your goals; for instance, slides may be a more effective and less expensive way to enhance a live presentation. Printed materials may be the appropriate way to present large amount of statistical data. A typed, traditional news release may be the most cost-effective way to get your message to the media.

Production of video is expensive. While there is a tremendous range of fees for camera crews, editing facilities, and producers, Stecki and Corrado (1988a) cite prices for a video news release ranging from $3,650 to $50,000 for production and distribution; the average cost is between $15,000 and $20,000. Average cost for producing a television commercial is $200,000 (Kanner, 1988). The costs of videos depend on the quality of the final product. Plan on at least $1,000 per minute for a basic training tape, and up to $3,000 per minute for a polished marketing tape with professional talent and original music. Developing a budget includes planning the costs of the script, director, camera crew, professional actors, editing, and other costs.

A script is difficult and time-consuming to write. Scriptwriters often spend years in college and in apprenticeships. Although the cost of a scriptwriter is $500 to $1,000 a day, this may be a worthwhile investment. Specific shooting and editing directions in a well-written script can save money later on. Alternately, you can write the script yourself, but it is wise to have it reviewed by a professional scriptwriter.

The director is key to keeping the production on time and within budget. A director supervises the shooting (photographing) and editing of the video, and costs $500 to $1,000 for each day of work.

The number of camera crew members required, the format of the tape, and the necessary light and sound equipment influence the cost of the crew. A two-person crew with one camera and minimal lighting equipment costs $900 to $1,250 for a 10-hour day (Stecki & Corrado, 1988a). For each four to five minutes of finished tape, plan on one day of shooting. In addition, if the tape is shot in a studio, add studio rental costs of $350 to $500 a day.

Although adding to costs, professional actors and narrators can often be more effective than in-house spokespeople. Narrators can cost from $350 for a short, off-camera role to $750 for on-camera work. Costs of celebrities can be much higher. In a video for association recruitment that we reviewed, student members were used as actors. The students did not look like they were having a good time—in fact, not one smiled. Another pitfall of this video was the use of a male narrator. As an association for nurses, with an overwhelming majority of women members, a female voice would have been more effective. While this video cost $20,000 to produce, association leaders state that it failed to achieve its goals.

Editing costs depend on tape format and on the special effects desired. Simple editing costs about $200 to $275 per hour. Each minute of finished tape requires about one hour of editing. Special effects can cost an additional $200 to $400 an hour. A flashy opening logo can add $5,000 to $10,000 to the cost (Stecki & Corrado, 1988a).

Many incidentals can increase the final cost. Music can add $50 to $1,000. Duplicate videotapes can cost from $10 to $30 each, depending on the format, length, and number ordered (Stecki & Corrado, 1988a).

Deciding who you are going to hire to produce a videotape is critical. You can hire a company to do the whole job—scripting, shooting, and postproduction—or you can use different firms for each phase. It is best to hire a consultant or experienced producer to help conceptualize your program and help you find the right crew for the work. The information you get from the consultant can mean significant savings during production.

Alternatively, you can put the crew together yourself. Published sources such as video directories and video journals are good places to start. Talk with people in your organization, or other organizations, who have produced videos. They may be able to make suitable recommendations. You are looking for a team that can make your video as effective as possible at reasonable cost. Therefore, look for people who have experience producing the kind of video you are making. An inexpensive firm specializing in low-budget training tapes is not the place to go for a slick television commercial; likewise, a high-powered, upscale communications company is not necessarily the best or most appropriate choice for the production of a modest training video. Stecki and Corrado (1988a) advise that using location crews with experience in television news is cost-effective because these crews work faster than those who produce commercials. Stecki and Corrado also advise that you hire a video photographer rather than just a camera person. A photographer knows about camera positioning, lighting, and other aspects of aesthetics; the camera person works with the technical part of producing images. When hiring for scripting and/or directing, look for someone who understands your goals. Remember that a simple, clear, and direct message can have enormous power. Overdone videos are rarely successful.

One-inch video equipment is most commonly used for both shooting and editing. The high-quality picture, due to the larger surface area, has made this equipment the state of the art. It is standard for television. Disadvantages are that the equipment is expensive and not easily portable, making it difficult to use on location. Sony's three-quarter-inch U-matic format has been the standard for field production (Stecki & Corrado, 1988b). As you know, rapid technological advances are being made. These advances have made possible half-inch systems whose quality approaches that of the one-inch systems. Sony's Betacam is currently the most popular camera in the half-inch format. To make a master tape that is of higher quality, the material is later transferred to a one-inch format.

VHS, VHS-C, and Beta cameras are used to make home video tapes. These machines are not appropriate for high-quality, sophisticated productions. However, their relatively low cost—$1,300 to $2,000 list price with selling prices of about $1,000 ("VCRs," 1987)—and their high portability, along with a picture of sufficient quality, make them an alternative for in-house training programs. All cameras do not produce the same quality videotape. Before buying one, be sure to do your homework on them.

Shooting a video is time-consuming. For taping on location, a one-camera crew must unpack and set up a minimum of a camera, tripod, tape deck, monitor, and three or four lights. Each time the location changes, all of the equipment must be disassembled, packed, transported, unpacked, and set up again. The number of locations that can be used in a day is therefore limited. As the number of locations increases, so does the cost.

A production assistant is very useful for the small, but important, chores such as keeping track of shots, arranging props, obtaining releases, and getting coffee and lunch for the crew. While it is possible to use someone on your staff for this job, it is more effective and efficient to hire an experienced production assistant who can help with other jobs and also knows how to stay out of the crew's way (Stecki & Corrado, 1988b).

Choose participants carefully. Always get releases from individuals who have speaking parts or whose faces are seen. It is a good idea to get releases from all participants. What the participants wear is important. Generally, conservative color and style in clothes work best. Red should be avoided because it becomes fuzzy on duplicates. See the section on television for other suggestions.

Video is interesting and exciting because of the rapidly changing images. When images do not change, video becomes boring (for example, the proverbial talking heads). Frequently changing images means a new image approximately every six seconds. This means that you need 10 images per minute, or 100 for a 10-minute tape. In order to have enough tape for the final product, you must shoot a great deal more than you will ultimately use. Shoot every scene from a variety of perspectives. Use wide shots and close-ups, zoom in and out, change focus, take fade-outs, and so on. Having enough tape makes editing easier.

Taking still pictures at the shoot is a good idea. You may need photographs for publicity, advertising, or a newsletter. Stills taken from video are usually not satisfactory, because they are grainy and do not reproduce well.

Every frame must be time-coded. This is a system of identification for each frame of video. Time-coding makes editing easier because it enables you to find each frame you want. It saves time and money in the editing process.

Editing, or postproduction, should take place in stages. This is where your hard work in the planning stage pays off. The final piece takes shape and your creativity is seen in this phase.

Stecki and Corrado (1988b) suggest that in order to save editing time and money, a step called pre-editing be done first. A pre-edit is done by using your script, time-coded video, video player, and paper and pencil. With your director, go through the whole video and select the segments you want to include. Then write the codes on the script where you want them to appear. Doing this can save valuable editing time.

The same authors also suggest doing an off-line edit. Off-line editing is done with an editor on less sophisticated equipment than is needed for on-line editing, although both processes are electronic editing. For off-line editing, the program is put together from abrupt cuts identified by exact time codes. These are later fed into the on-line equipment. On-line editing costs $200 to $500 an hour, while off-line editing costs only $50 to $100 an hour.

During the final editing, you will be working with both audio and video. How you approach this task will depend on the nature of your program. For example, if you are using an off-camera narrator throughout the entire piece, it may be easiest to first lay down the entire sound track and then edit the pictures to the sound. The sound track will establish the length. Listening to the narrator will give you good indicators as to when you should change the picture. This probably will not work if the participants in the video are doing the talking; in that case, both audio and video have to be edited simultaneously in some spots and individually in others.

There are many special effects you can use. However, they add significantly to the cost. Many producers use special effects only on the program opening and logo. The logo is often used on all subsequent tapes produced by that organization. Consider carefully if flashy effects are appropriate to your goal; how is the tape to be used and what is the subject? Glitz is probably not consistent with a life-and-death topic. Special effects are also not recommended for video news releases, because most news programs do not use them. Work with the editor. Seek out creative advice. Together you can make the video an exiting, effective, public relations piece.

Corporate Identity Media

Corporate identity refers to the way an organization chooses to present itself to all its publics. Management of corporate identity influences the organization's *image,* the public's perception of the organization (Margulies, 1977). Mismanagement of corporate identity can have disastrous consequences, whereas its skilled, thoughtful management can have many positive effects. Whether corporate identity is an asset or a liability, it is part of the organizational fabric. It is not a discrete program, standing on its own.

Corporate identity media become valuable public relations tools when they are attractive, memorable, and distinctive. Logos, stationery, brochures, signs, business forms and cards, buildings, and uniforms visually identify the organization. Ambiance is also an identifying characteristic of an organization. It is determined by lighting, temperature, noise level, smell, activity level, comfort, accessibility of services, and personnel appearance and attitude. In a hospital, the quality of the services, such as nursing, dietary, housekeeping, and security, communicate important messages to the publics.

The most common reason for undertaking a corporate identity program is to increase important publics' familiarity with the organization. By increasing familiarity, the organization's reputation is enhanced. Less effort is required to evaluate a familiar product; it is perceived by consumers as less risky. Humana put its corporate name into each hospital's name to achieve this goal. See Case Study 13 for a discussion of this example.

Factors related to the intangibility of health care may make corporate identity a crucial difference in decisions having to do with choice. Often patients do not have the ability or time to evaluate attributes of services and care providers, or to compare providers with one another. There usually are no other cues available, such as price or care features; the patient must make a decision based on little experience or knowledge. There is often some risk associated with health care, which is frightening. Finally, health care is a rapidly changing service. Coupled with constantly evolving technology is the fact of individual provider differences in the quality of service.

All these aspects of health care make a strong corporate identity an important way to maintain loyalty. By conducting a survey, The Mount Sinai Hospital in New York City found that individuals who had contact with the institution thought highly of it; those who had no contact with Mount Sinai did not think of it at all, or gave it incorrect or weaker ratings. Mount Sinai undertook a major campaign in 1986 in response to this situation (Mount Sinai, 1987). The campaign that was implemented produced changes in awareness, attitudes, and behavior. The next year, a second study using a similar sample showed that Mount Sinai had moved from seventh place to first place in terms of public awareness. As the hospital of choice, Mount Sinai moved from fifth place to first place. Use of the doctor referral service quadrupled and has remained high.

Change in the corporate identity must be managed carefully, and must be based on research and in-depth analysis of the organization and how the organization is perceived by its various publics. Inauguration of a new corporate identity must be planned in great detail, and the plan executed in a coherent manner (Ackerman, 1987; Margulies, 1977; Selame, 1985). A corporate identity program requires expertise for maximum effectiveness. See Chapter 5 for discussion of use of communications consultants.

People are consciously aware of many corporate identities. The logos of Mercedes-Benz, BMW, and IBM represent more than a product. Perhaps Ralph Lauren is at the apex in selling a lifestyle or culture rather than just a product. Likewise, the robin's-egg blue of Tiffany's box is a coveted symbol of treasures. Generally, people use conscious assessment as a way to evaluate professionalism, style, and quality. Five factors may influence consumer evaluation of a product: exposure effects, unconscious associations, aesthetics, familiarity, and conscious associations (Hutton, 1987). These characteristics are discussed in relationship to logos.

Logos. The term *logo* (a short form of *logotype*, which has a Greek origin) is the commonly used word for an arbitrary letter, symbol, or sign used to represent an entire word. In business, and in common usage, a logo represents an organization or profession. It has long been known that simple, repeated exposure to a stimulus can cause people to show a preference for that stimulus. Examples of this can be seen in the changes in fashion over the years. When first introduced in the 1970s, long skirts were rejected as frumpy by many women, but they soon became the fashion norm. During the 1960s and 1970s, pearls were not fashionable. Recently fashion leaders wore pearls and, all of a sudden, they looked right once again. People in photographs taken 25 years ago look odd in their bubble hairstyles and 1960s clothes. The eye has gotten used to different proportions, colors, and structures. This is a problem for nurses' uniforms, the styles of which generally seem to be five years behind the times. The exposure effects of fashions and logos are the same. Repeated exposure to a logo may cause a preference for it without conscious effort or awareness.

The form of the logo is critical. People make unconscious associations with logos. A mutually reinforcing name and symbol encourage associations and increase recognition. Examples are the use of the rock by Prudential Insurance Company, and Apple Computer's rainbow-colored apple. Another example is the name problem of the Harlem Savings Bank of New York City (Selame, 1985). The name gave the bank an image of a small, local, old-fashioned institution. As part of the marketing plan, a corporate identity program was instituted, and the name was changed to Apple Bank in honor of the Big Apple (New York City). An apple logo was adopted. The logos of International Paper, Woolmark, and United Fund are very well known in this country and are recognized by many. Good examples of logos that have world-wide recognition are those of IBM, Coca-Cola, and Kodak.

There are two important considerations that have an impact on aesthetics. The first is that the design should be consistent with the product, service, or organization. A modern, pacesetting image requires a modern logo. If the desired image is traditional, a modern, flashy logo would lack credibility and would not be

---

EXHIBIT 6-2   Characteristics of an Effective Logo

1. Is it consistent with the image of the organization?
2. Is it consistent within itself?
3. Is it crisp, clear, and clean?
   a. Does it reproduce well?
   b. Does it work well in a range of sizes?
   c. Is it easy to read and identify?

---

consistent; a traditional logo is required. See Exhibit 6-2 for a checklist for effective logo development.

News

For most people *publicity* is synonymous with *public relations*. It is the securing of editorial space, as opposed to paid space, in media that are read, viewed, or heard by an organization's publics, for the specific purpose of achieving public relations goals. Publicity can be used to advantage to increase visibility, help change a poor public image to one that is positive, and generally promote marketing goals. It is often thought of as advertising that is free, and it has three distinct advantages over ads. First, it has a high level of credibility, because it appears as news and not as sponsored information. Second, it catches people off guard. Because it is presented as news, it reaches people who avoid advertising. Third, it has a high potential for dramatization, similar to advertising, but in the guise of a newsworthy event.

Nurse administrators may have to promote nursing to the public relations department. They should develop an ongoing working relationship in order to have some control over how nursing is presented to the public. Give your public relations department stories that present nursing in a professional light and that symbolize the division the way you want it represented. Ask for editorial control, or at least review all articles about nursing.

News releases.   The *news* (or *press*) *release* is the single most important way to reach the public. It is the cornerstone of many public relations program. News releases are fast, effective, efficient, and the least expensive method to get your story directly to the press, although they should not be used to the exclusion of other public relations tools.

Getting releases used in the print or electronic media is a very difficult task. This is especially true on the national level. The sheer volume of news releases that editors receive contributes to the difficulty. For instance, *Business Week* receives 10,000 news releases a week in its New York editorial offices. The editor of the magazine's industrial edition receives 400 releases a week (Lovell, 1982). *The New York Times, The Wall Street Journal*, the *Los Angeles Times*, and the *Chicago Tribune* receive equally high numbers of news releases. For small- and medium-size publications, the scale is similar. A local television news program in New York City receives 200 releases a day. An editor spends less than half a second determining if a release is worth more time. Most are not. Eighty percent of news releases are perceived by editors as having marginal value at best; they estimate that 90% are discarded (Graves, 1988).

As you write news releases, keep in mind the editors and reporters who will read them. Your objective is to write the news in a way that will appeal to the editor. The challenge is to make your point clearly and concisely without being overbearing. The best markets for press releases commonly have their editors rewrite any they use.

Because of the number of releases received by media, you should always have a good reason to write one. Major management, financial, research, or product developments are appropriate for organizations to write about. Writing about major grants and research results is appropriate for nonprofit organizations such as hospitals and schools of nursing. Releases on minor personnel changes, departmental reorganization, unveiling of plaques, esoteric or insignificant research results, and small awards are not news, and will ensure that all releases from that source will be discarded. Before writing a release, make sure that the topic is of interest to the general public. Consider what the information means to the reader, how the reader is affected by the information, how the reader can apply the information, and what action the reader should take after reading the news.

To find news, consider the nursing staff. Is there a nurse with an unusual background or anyone doing something exceptional? Has a staff member developed an innovative solution or approach to a problem? Consider events, activities, history, standards, and goals related to the nursing division that might interest the public.

After deciding that you have an appropriate topic for a release, gather factual information about the subject. This is important in order to avoid major errors. Interview personnel if you need additional information. Remember that in this case, the interviewer and the interviewee work for the same organization and want to present it in the best light possible. It is a good idea to give personnel interviewed the opportunity to read the release for technical accuracy.

Target your press releases. Know the kinds of stories a publication prints and who reads the publication. Do not send releases to every publication on a routine basis, but write as many versions of the release as necessary; this may result in more widespread coverage. A story may have more than one aspect to it. For example, a research study may have financial as well as product aspects. A release discussing the financial impact of DRGs can be written to the financial editor;

another release discussing DRGs' effects on length of stay and patient outcomes can be written for the health care editor.

State your news in the first sentence. The first six or eight words have to interest the editor, or the release will land in the trash. Most editors prefer news releases that are "short and sweet." One hundred words is the best length, 300 is the maximum. If background data are needed, provide a fact sheet. Grammar is important. Refer to Strunk and White (1979) for help. Progression from paragraph to paragraph must be logical and must make sense. Write in a clear, clean, and concise way. Your goal is to get the attention of the editor, not to impress with fancy language. Editors are busy people and they must be able quickly to read and understand what you are saying. Do not write in the passive voice; the active voice is easier and more interesting to read. Avoid the use of qualifiers and superlatives such as *tremendous, first, only, superb, unique, absolutely, definitely, impossible, superior,* and so on. Value judgments have no place in a release. They lead to exaggeration, which discredits the sender. The quality of writing is improved by repeated editing and rewriting.

Type all releases using an easily read typeface. Use 8½-by-11-inch bond paper with your letterhead and 10- or 12-pitch type. Do not use 15-pitch type. If you use a headline, center it and use capital letters; do not underline it. Indent each paragraph. Use 1- to 1½-inch margins. Never send a release without a date. The phone number and contact person should be at the top; the date should be in the lower left corner. To end a release, type, "-30-," "# # #," or "ENDIT," centered below the last paragraph. A dateline is not needed. "For immediate release" can be put at the top, but is not necessary. If a release is mailed, it is obviously ready to appear in print unless an embargo date indicates otherwise.

After your release is published or broadcast, follow up with a letter of appreciation to the editor, or producers and hosts. Pass on the positive comments you have received about the story. If appropriate, make a suggestion for a follow-up story.

If an error is made in the presentation, discuss the problem in a matter-of-fact way with the editor or producer. A solution may be to develop a second story. This may be more to your advantage than a simple retraction. Before pressing for rectification, make a careful assessment of the impact of the error. It may make sense to allow the matter to drop in exchange for the goodwill of the editor and future releases. Pursue the matter with media management only if your reputation has been damaged and you believe that you must clear your name. If you do go to management, it is probable that your contacts with that medium will be severed (Sachs, 1986).

Letters to the editor.   An effective way to get your viewpoint to the public is to respond to news items and articles with letters to the editor (see Exhibit 6-3). You can add to public debate, clarify positions, correct errors, cite historical positions, and so forth. This is an opportunity to give your opinion.

EXHIBIT 6-3   Letter to the Editor

Letter to the Editor, dated July 10, 1988, as printed in *The New York Times,* July 18, 1988.

To the Editor:

The American Medical Association's proposal to create "registered care technologists" to alleviate the current shortage of nurses is unrealistic and dangerous. Hospital patients are sicker than ever before. Increased patient acuity demands increased levels of *skilled* care. Nurses are primarily concerned about the quality of care provided to sick people under this proposal.

Since the early 1980s, nursing has been concerned about the current shortage. Across the country, nurse educators, nurse administrators, and practicing nurses have been working to recruit talented, bright people to nursing. Activities have included meeting with guidance counselors, attending high school career days, giving talks, developing funding sources for scholarships, and devising programs to make the logistics of going to nursing school easier. Nurse administrators work assiduously to retain nurses in the profession with programs such as career ladders, and flex-time. Individual nurses have worked within the professional associations and on their own to recruit and retain nurses.

However, recruitment to nursing is difficult when salaries are low and the work, while very rewarding, is hard. Nursing suffers from an image which severely constricts recruitment possibilities. The quote by the doctor equating nursing with changing sheets and replacing bedpans reflects the image problem. You can be sure that the patient whose bed is made by a nurse is in the bed, and is too sick to get up. Empty beds are made by aides or housekeeping personnel. While making the bed and talking to the patient, the nurse makes an assessment of the patient's physical and mental status. Is the skin intact? How is the circulation, range of motion, respiration, mood? Checks are made on any tubes, drains, and dressings. Emotional support is given, and teaching may be done.

The physicians who put forth this proposal suffer from the misconception that anyone can do nursing, and, if no one can, it will not be missed. A high school graduate with a few months of training cannot replace a nurse. Furthermore, what would make people take a job like this? The pay would be low, and there would be little or no possibility for advancement. This position is a dead-end job.

Since this "registered care technologist" would be certified and registered "under an arm of the state medical boards to assure minimal standards of practice and protect the public good," it could be presumed that physicians will train and supervise these new workers, or are they committing nurses to train them? Educators can attest to the fact that it is not possible to train individuals in such a short time to work at the required level. Institutions employing student nurse interns insist that they have at least two semesters of clinical courses. This is true of Associate degree and Baccalaureate students. Who will supervise these new workers, will the physicians do it, or do they expect nurses to do so? Will they propose also a new "registered care technician supervisor"?

This proposal is a sad commentary on nurse-physician relations. Even though the American Nurses Association has consistently stated that this is not a viable solution to the nursing shortage, the AMA has put forth this ill-conceived, seriously flawed proposal. Because of the added costs with no control of quality, it is not in the best interest of patients, tax payers, and third-party payers.

As with teaching and education, our society has undervalued nursing. The public must demand that nurses be hired in adequate numbers at appropriate salaries. Only in this way will a sufficient supply of nurses be assured. Public support of nursing is necessary for the profession to grow and to do what it does best: *provide nursing care.*

Sincerely,

Caroline Camuñas, EdM, RN
Joan Gittins Johnston, EdD, RN
Catherine Mallard, EdM, RN
Elizabeth Vecchione, EdD, RN

Reprinted with permission.

Write letters to the editor in a clear, succinct style. Do not use jargon or technical language. Remember that you are writing to the general public. Know the kinds of letters the newspaper or magazine prints, and gear your letter to that audience.

Generally, it is a good idea to keep the letter short. Space is at a premium. However, if, in order to make your point, the letter must be longer than the paper usually prints, write it that way. The editor may print all of it, or only a portion. In either case, you will be contacted for permission before the letter is published.

Since this is a letter you are writing, format it as you would a business letter. Type it single-spaced. If appropriate, use your business letterhead. Include your telephone number so you may be contacted. Because of space considerations, limit the number of people signing the letter. One or two signatures are best. Certainly, do not use more than four.

Media interviews.   If you are in a position to deal with reporters, you must be comfortable and skillful in working with them. A common perception is that the media has an anti-business, anti-organization attitude. This perception has come about because the public holds professionals increasingly accountable for performance and outcomes and because the media usually works for the public good rather than for the person being interviewed.

To achieve effective outcomes when dealing with the press, two criteria are essential: have a sound attitude and always be carefully prepared. A sound attitude means to be yourself without arrogance or undue humility. Understand that you are competent in your field and that the reporter is competent at interviewing. The interviewer's goal is to elicit provocative, interesting, and sometimes controversial answers. In order to prepare for an interview, understand who the audience is, anticipate likely questions, research the facts, and structure effective answers. Learn to quote appropriate literature. Avoid interviews when you are unprepared. Rehearse your answers, but do not memorize them or use notes. Provide a press kit with pertinent background information and statistics and the correct spelling of names, titles, and terms. Credit sources of facts and figures you quote. By making yourself a resource to the media, you can potentially influence the attitudes of millions of people.

You must develop your story effectively. A primary goal is to tell the simple truth. You must not lie under any circumstances. The public can be very forgiving, but it will not understand, nor will it tolerate, lying. Remember that you can lose your credibility only once. Do not deny knowledge, and do not exaggerate the facts. On the other hand, you do not have to disclose all the facts. If you do not know the answer to a question, say so. Offer to get the information, and then follow up.

It is important to present what you have to say in a way that is interesting from the public's point of view. Make your most important point first, in order to get attention. The first thing said is usually remembered and is generally not cut if time or space run out. When asked a direct question, you should give an amplified, direct answer using language that the public understands. Technical terms and jargon are not appropriate for effective communication with the general public.

The most personal contact is best remembered, so use personal terms whenever possible. Your individual accountability increases the perceived accessibility and personalness of your organization. By using the pronoun "I" and reflecting pride, you are increasing the humanity of the organization and creating a positive impression. Involving staff, first-line and middle managers, as well as nurse executives, in interviews can be an effective way to enhance the image of the organization. They should be well-prepared to answer and discuss questions. However, nurses must be limited to answers that are appropriate to their level in the organization. If they give information to which realistically they have no access, their credibility will be lost.

There are some major things to avoid in dealing with reporters. Never make off-the-record statements or comments. Doing so can put you and the reporter in an uncomfortable position. If you do not want a statement quoted, do not make it. This includes anything said before or after taping of the interview. Likewise, do not repeat, even to deny, language that may be offensive or words you do not like; you can be quoted out of context as having used them. Finally, do not argue or lose your temper with the reporter. Answer questions to present your story fairly, accurately, and adequately.

Press kits. *Press kits* are usually folders containing background materials reporters need to write a story. Included in the kit are background data, photographs, press releases, and anything else that may be pertinent. Press kits can be developed for new services, issues, opinions, events, and so forth. For a report about a person, the press kit might contain a résumé, photograph, and introductory press release. For general use, press kits may be too expensive and presumptuous (celebrities generally have press kits). However, if, for example, you are a nurse entrepreneur, it may be convenient to have a modified press kit containing a black-and-white glossy portrait and a résumé.

Radio and television talk shows. Locally produced radio and television talk shows are always looking for interesting, informative, and perhaps controversial topics and speakers. Talk shows are different from news interviews. The latter are generally taped ahead of time and edited; only a brief portion is aired. In contrast, talk shows are usually broadcast live and each segment lasts 15 to 30 minutes. You talk directly to the audience.

It is possible to get on a show by invitation because you came to the attention of the producer through press releases and publications. Rees (1980) became a guest because of a press release from the university about her doctoral dissertation. That press release had a snowball effect and ultimately did a lot to improve nursing's image. In 1988, nurses were invited to debate the registered care technician proposal on talk shows. Recently, many nurses have discussed the nursing shortage.

To get on a show, familiarize yourself with that program. Study the style and format. Make sure that it is the appropriate showcase for your presentation. Talk directly to the producer (Rees, 1980; Sachs, 1986). You can make this contact through a sponsor or agent, publisher, or organization. If you personally make the contact, you will have to demonstrate to the producer that you are a legitimate expert with appropriate credentials.

The producer's primary goal is to interest or entertain the audience. Therefore, your topic must be socially relevant. You must be an expert in the subject and make a clear and interesting presentation. Skill and ease in answering questions are necessary. This is especially important because some talk shows take questions from studio and home audiences. In order to determine if you fit the requirements, the producer will interview you.

Thoroughly brief the producer on your topic. A written summary is helpful. Keep in mind that you are not making a presentation to professionals; gear your information to the lay public. This briefing should enable the producer to complete a list of questions for the host and should prevent misconceptions. It should help you get your point across when you are on the air.

Be well prepared. Know who the other participants are, and what their positions are on the topic. Anticipate questions you may be asked and develop answers to them. Do not memorize, and do not rely on written answers, but know important facts. Be spontaneous. If you prepare notes for a radio program, make the notes on sturdy paper that will not rustle when you turn the pages while on the air.

For television interviews, it is important to look your best. Wear glasses if you usually do. More makeup than usual will prevent a washed-out, tired look. Avoid wearing hats, highly polished jewelry, or black or white clothes. Busy patterns, such as plaids and checks, get distorted on camera. Wear clothes in which you are comfortable. Control nervous habits or mannerisms. Avoid hand wringing, playing with jewelry, and touching your face or hair. Keep your hands resting comfortably on your lap or on the chair arms. Do not make full, wide gestures. Crossing legs at the ankles is the most graceful way to sit. Act as if you are on camera all the time, even when you are not speaking.

Keep your voice at the same volume as the host. Focus on and talk to the host, not to the camera. Relate to the host and the studio audience. Do not look at yourself in the studio monitor. Respond to the questions in a relaxed, confident, spontaneous way. Try to give answers in 10- to 30-second intervals. This allows the host to question or make comments. Answer only when you are sure that you understand the question. If you do not understand it, ask for clarification, more information, or paraphrase the question and ask if that was meant. Be polite to any callers, even those who try to provoke you. Being rude to a caller, even one who is obnoxious or asks ridiculous questions, makes you look bad.

Write a thank-you note to the producer and the host. Courtesy makes good public relations. A note helps to build a relationship and may bring about another appearance on the show.

Self-evaluation is the first measure of success. Successful interviews are fine-tuned with experience and time. Reactions of the host, studio audience, and production staff after the show are the second measure of success. The third measure is the at-home audience's response, in the form of letters and telephone calls (Rees, 1980).

Public Service Activities

Public goodwill can be enhanced by giving money and time to good causes. Many large corporations such as Humana, Mobil, Texaco, Johnson & Johnson, and IBM give generously to support programs on public television, and arts programs such as opera, ballet, and concerts. Other companies support the Olympics and the Special Olympics. Since 1987, Proctor & Gamble (P&G) and

Publishers' Clearing House co-sponsor a promotion to aid the Special Olympics. P&G product coupons are included in a Publishers' Clearing House mailing. For every coupon redeemed, P&G donates 10 cents to the Special Olympics program.

Many other companies have given generously to fight illiteracy, substance abuse, homelessness, and child abuse. Employees are often encouraged to participate by donating time or money. These activities are perceived as evidence that the company is part of, and cares about, the community. The company is a good citizen.

Contributions. Many people contribute to health, education, art, athletic, and religious organizations. Sharing with neighbors in time of difficulty has been an American characteristic since early colonial days. Giving may be expected in many communities. In general, not contributing has little effect, but some businesses and professionals have been ostracized by their communities for not supporting a local activity (Smith, 1984).

Assess your situation carefully. Financial support of local organizations may not be an obvious marketing necessity, but it may pay off in public relations as well as in personal satisfaction. In some situations, giving may be a political necessity; for instance, contributing to the nursing scholarship fund or participating in raffles in support of the fund, when you are on staff at the medical center. Consider whether you should give in your name or in the name of your practice or professional affiliation or organization. Religious donations are generally private and made in one's personal name.

Associations, clubs, and organizations. Membership in associations, clubs, and organizations can be invaluable. Support of professional nursing associations at the national, state, and local levels is a professional responsibility and obligation. By giving your support, especially if you attend meetings or become more active, you will become known in the nursing community in your area. Active participation can help you develop leadership skills and provide other valuable experiences. Your personal and professional reputation can be enhanced significantly.

Whether membership in country clubs and other organizations is a good marketing or public relations activity is dependent upon your community and your business. Ask yourself if these activities will put you in contact with your target audience. From a public relations perspective, benefits from membership in these organizations take a long time to develop. Do not expect to see any substantial results or relationships in less than a year.

Events

Events can be created to attract the attention of target publics. They can be for wide external publics or for small publics within the organization. Conventions and conferences can be hosted, and important historical events and anniversaries can be celebrated. Art exhibits, cake sales, book sales, dances, fashion shows, and similar events can increase the newsworthiness of the organization (see Case Study 5). Consider using radio, television, and newspaper public service announcements (PSA). A *PSA* is an announcement made in the media without charge. When preparing a PSA for an event, make it short and simple. Give only the bare facts, because most PSAs are 15 seconds long. The announcement should be typed triple-spaced on your letterhead. This makes it easier for the on-air person to read. On the upper right-hand side, list your name and phone number as the contact person. The media should receive the announcement no less than 10 days before the event. Public service announcements must have wide appeal. If they do not, they will not be used. For the same event, avoid trying to use a PSA in addition to buying paid advertising space. The media will not give you free time if you are willing to pay for it. The Federal Communications Commission recently changed the required amount of time radio and television stations must devote to PSAs, making it more difficult to get PSAs on the air.

Speeches

Skillful public speaking is a useful and effective public relations tool for nurses. It is useful for internal communications and for community talks, conferences, conventions, news conferences, and national and local talk shows. There are, of course, some who seem to have been born with good voices, the capacity to turn an apt phrase, the ability to personally engage listeners, and the skill and judgment to use appropriate humor. The rest of us have to learn to give speeches by practicing, as we once started in nursing by giving saline injections to an orange.

To write an effective speech, it is essential to know the audience. Learn everything you can about its members—their education, professions, positions, interests, and commonalities—to assist you in tailoring the speech to meet their needs. Consider what they already know about the subject and what they expect to learn. Is the purpose of the speech to inform, persuade, solve problems, or make decisions? Talk in terms that are relevant to the audience.

Avoid gimmicks when writing a speech. For example, every speech does not have to begin with a joke. Jokes often turn out not to be very funny and detract from the speech. Likewise, quotes from Shakespeare or other historical figures may add little. The speech usually gets twisted around to fit the quote. Borrowing from contemporaries can be just as problematic. Unattributed quotes are unethical. Even when correctly attributed, liberal use of quotes can be settling for second best. Find an original way to say what you want to say.

Keep the message simple. The purpose of a speech is to enlighten, not to confuse. Talk in terms that the audience understands. Review the meeting agenda and who is speaking before and after you. Try to find out what they are going to say and tailor your speech appropriately, particularly for a panel presentation.

When the speech is written, practice giving it. Read the paper aloud to yourself. Awkward phrases and ambiguities will become apparent. Polish the speech until you are satisfied; then begin practicing the whole presentation, using audiovisual materials. With enough practice, the speech will become so familiar that only an occasional glance at the manuscript will be necessary. All speeches are better delivered when they are not read directly. Practice public speaking and get constructive feedback from someone who is not familiar with your topic, as well as from experts in the field. Take courses and hire a speechwriter or a coach for your important speeches. The investment will pay off.

When you agree to deliver a speech about a topic on which you are also submitting a written presentation, you must prepare two different texts. One is the manuscript you are submitting, in a format appropriate to the publication, journal, or proceedings. The other text is the oral presentation, tailored to the audience to whom you will speak. Check for a smooth flow of the text with any audiovisual material. You may have to make different graphs and tables, because those developed for an article are often unsuitable for oral presentations. Visual aids must serve a purpose.

Telephone Information Services

The last public relations tool, the telephone, is not usually thought of, and is used much less frequently than are other tools. Telephone information services frequently enable an organization to provide information and better service to customers and potential customers. General Electric has a hotline for callers having problems with their appliances; at Thanksgiving, they have a number to call with questions about roasting the turkey. Many hospitals provide health messages or counseling of different kinds, such as for rape victims, those contemplating suicide, substance abuse patients, and physician referrals. Providing such services in a courteous manner helps build a positive image. These services suggest to the public that the organization cares about them and is available and ready to serve them. Telephone information services were used to advantage by Davis, Thole, and Ware in Case Studies 4, 15, and 19.

Evaluating Public Relations Results

The final step in the public relations process is evaluation of the results. Although evaluation is often difficult, it is not impossible, especially if criteria were established for the original goals. The major response measures are exposure, awareness, comprehension, attitude changes, and sales or use of services. Exposure, awareness, and comprehension are difficult to evaluate. Publicity fosters more reading and believing than advertisements. You may have a scrapbook full of clippings and articles, but no indication of how many people have been reached. A more accurate measurement requires the use of survey methods before and after the publicity campaign. The best measures of effectiveness are sales and profit impact. For a hospital, this could be related to recruitment of personnel, utilization of services, increase in volunteers and donations, to name a few examples.

Consumer satisfaction and actions after purchase are based on expectations of the product or service and on the perceived performance of the product. This is called expectations-performance theory. Cognitive-dissonance theory can also be applied. The latter theory states that there is likely to be some discomfort associated with every purchase. Of concern to the health care provider are the amount of discomfort and what the consumer will do about it. Consumers can continue to use the organization or health care provider or they can go elsewhere for service. No matter how large or well-known the organization, it is subject to consumer erosion.

Evaluation then brings you back to the first step of the public relations process. It is important to establish an ongoing program using public relations as part of the marketing mix. There are opportunities in any economy as long as there are unsatisfied needs.

Career Development

One application of the public relations process is the enhancement and advancement of your nursing career. Public relations can help you get the position or promotion you want. However, no public relations plan alone can achieve your goals. Appropriate preparation in both education and experience is necessary; you must be able to deliver what you promise. A public makes decisions based on performance and perceived performance. In the end, an image is a combination of performance, the perception of performance, and the packaging. The packaging helps to sell the product, which in this case is you and your performance.

In order to use the public relations process and tools to your advantage, to help advance your career, first identify the publics with whom you interact. In most nursing organizations, your primary publics are your patients, the nursing staff, peers and colleagues, nursing administration, employees of other departments, physicians, family and friends of patients, and volunteers. These are the publics that are most important to you. Many of your publics are related to one another as well as to you. Each may have a great deal of influence on the attitudes and behavior of others. For example, if you are a head nurse and your unit is well-managed, and you are enthusiastic about your work, your supervisors will see you as an effective head nurse and will reinforce you in a positive way. You will subsequently be reinforced by your staff, peers, and by physicians. You will be respected for your contribution to the achievement of organizational goals.

On the other hand, if you are unhappy and you are not taking constructive steps toward positive change, your attitude is likely to have a negative impact on your behavior. This can result in your providing lower quality management and decreasing the effectiveness of the unit. Patients, staff, peers, physicians, and nursing administration will be dissatisfied. Soon, you and your unit will have a reputation for uncaring service. You will have lost a great deal in possible promotions, authority, and image. Remember, if your image is tarnished, it diminishes the image of nursing.

Assessing the image and attitudes of your identified publics is important in achieving your career goals. Be sure to include the macroenvironment in your assessment. Consider it carefully so that you can establish realistic image, attitude, and career goals. Set achievable, measurable criteria for their achievement. Use the goals in your daily life. Understand where you are, where you want to go, and what your publics' attitudes are. You can then develop specific strategies and tactics that will help you improve, change, or maintain the attitudes of a particular public. Some of these tactics are discussed below.

Written Material

You can increase the confidence your superiors have in you by providing well-written information. For the staff nurse, this is writing clear and concise nurses' notes, care plans, discharge summaries, and instructions. All managers and administrators must write succinct, to-the-point, and appropriate memoranda, letters, evaluations, and the like. The importance of quality in middle managers' and nurse executives' written material is evident in proposals and justification of budgets. Pay attention to format. Make the content interesting and professional. Your presentation of written material makes a statement about you, your attitudes, and your abilities. A note written in red ink on scrap paper in a moment of anger may make a superior think twice about how you might function in difficult situations. Do not use affectations. Know the norms of your institution.

Publication increases your visibility and demonstrates your expertise. For guidance, consult with someone experienced in writing for publications. Writing courses and workshops can provide invaluable assistance, as can books on writing. There is much assistance available to help you develop your writing skills. See the end of this chapter for a list of books and articles useful for sharpening your writing skills.

Audiovisual Material

Audiovisual aids should be given the same consideration as written material. Well-prepared diagrams, charts, and graphs can help you get your point across and will enhance your image. However, they must be of high quality. Poorly designed and executed audiovisual materials leave long-lasting negative impressions.

Personal Identity Media

Corporate identity media may seem impossible to apply to an individual, yet some of the media tools are the easiest to use. They are your packaging—that which visually identifies you to your publics. The way you look should inspire confidence; the look should be professional and convey the message that you can do the job. Consider your clothes. Are they neat, clean, and well-fitting? Is the length appropriate? Are the clothes themselves appropriate? Do they convey the message that you are a little girl, a vamp, or a competent professional? How do people dress in the role to which you aspire? Pay attention to the norms of your organization. Assess your grooming and your makeup. Study the popular press. It is replete with information about image and appropriate work clothes and makeup.

Other things can also help you make a favorable impression. Be punctual. No matter how well you do your job, you do not do it when you are not there. It is an irritation to, and shows a lack of concern for, your fellow employees when you are frequently late. Do not conduct your social and personal business while on duty. Complete all aspects of your assignments in a timely fashion; if you cannot, tell the appropriate person and have a good reason for not being able to do it. Carelessness about details is not in the best interest of the organization, and will detract from your performance and your image.

How your attitude comes across gives as important a message as do the objective qualities of your work. Introducing yourself by name and title lets people know who you are, building your image as a credible professional. Also, it is just plain courtesy. Do not be anonymous; value yourself and your publics. Fonteyn considered these questions carefully and used this tool in a careful, considered, and effective way (see Case Study 8).

News

News may be a difficult tool to use for career development, but possibilities do exist. If there is a public interest story in your work area, suggest it to nursing administration. It may be possible to use it in some way, perhaps in an internal newsletter if not in the popular press. Remember, what is good for nursing and the organization is good for you.

Events and Public Service Activities

Your participation in events and public service activities sponsored by your employer or other community organization can enhance your image. Volunteer to serve on committees, boards, and task forces. Be sure to follow through. This makes you visible, known, and respected. It provides opportunities to hone, as well as to demonstrate, your skills and knowledge. New skills can be learned and viewpoints can be broadened. By participating, you establish yourself as a concerned, committed, responsible professional.

Speeches

Speechmaking is a useful and effective tool to have in your repertoire. Credibility can be better established through speechmaking than by any other method. Understand the members of your audience, and plan a speech that is appropriate to them. Talk about subjects that involve them. If necessary, develop skill by taking courses and by practicing speechmaking. Volunteer to present talks at work and in the community. Religious groups, health care agencies, and other civic groups, as well as state and local nursing associations, can provide opportunities to polish your skills while you give a valuable service (see Case Study 5). Seek out constructive criticism after your presentation.

Telephone Services

The telephone is not usually thought of as a personal public relations tool, but answering the telephone by identifying yourself and your position or area paves the way for effective communication. Providing information in a courteous way helps to build a positive image. It will facilitate communication, make the day go smoother, and decrease frustration and stress.

CONCLUSION

The best marketing and public relations programs will ultimately fail if the health care provider or organization does not deliver what it promises and what the public expects. We must constantly earn loyalty. An image is not acquired simply through public relations planning. Image is largely a function of the actual deeds, products, and services of an organization and individuals. Nurses can use public relations to effectively promote their products (image and reality) to any and all of their publics. The marketing of nursing, with all its components, is the responsibility of nurses.

REFERENCES

Ackerman, L.D. (1987). Managing your corporate identity. *Public Relations Journal, 43*(5), 29.

Bauer, E.J. (1976). Pro's guide to A-V. *Successful Meetings, 26*(1), 31, 134.

Bernays, E.L. (1947). A better deal for nurses. *American Journal of Nursing, 47*(11), 721–722.

Bernays, E.L. (1952). *Public relations.* Norman, OK: University of Oklahoma Press.

Graves, F.C. (1988). The news release updated. *Hospital Public Relations Advisor, 1*(11), 1–3.

Hutton, J. (1987). Workshop how to: Think corporate identity. *Public Relations Journal, 43*(5), 25–26, 28–29.

Kanner, B. (1988, June 6). On Madison Avenue: Bells are ringing. *New York,* pp. 20, 22, 23.

Kotler, P. (1980). *Principles of marketing.* Englewood Cliffs, NJ: Prentice-Hall.

Kotler, P. (1982). *Marketing for nonprofit organizations* (2nd ed.). Englewood Cliffs, NJ: Prentice-Hall.

Kotler, P. (1988). *Marketing management* (6th ed.). Englewood Cliffs, NJ: Prentice-Hall.

Kotler, P., & Andreasen, A.R. (1987). *Strategic marketing for nonprofit organizations* (3rd ed.). Englewood Cliffs, NJ: Prentice-Hall.

Lovell, R.P. (1982). *Inside public relations*. Boston, MA: Allyn & Bacon.

Margulies, W.P. (1977). Make the most of your corporate identity. *Harvard Business Review, 55*(4), 66–72.

McCarry, C. (1989). Two revolutions. *National Geographic, 176*(1), pp. 50–55.

Mencken, H.L. (1925). *Americana: 1925*. New York: Knopf.

Mencken, H.L. (1926). *Americana: 1926*. New York: Knopf.

Meyer-Hartwig, K., Bleifield, W., & Hegewald, U. (1977). *How to compose slides for lectures*. New York: Gerhard Witzstrock.

Mount Sinai. (1987). Take good care of yourself. *Mount Sinai People, 6*(3), 1, 4.

Rees, B.L. (1980). Television talk shows: An untapped resource for nursing. *Nursing Outlook, 28,* 562–565.

Sachs, L. (1986). *Do-it-yourself marketing for the professional practice*. Englewood Cliffs, NJ: Prentice-Hall.

Selame, E. (1985). A new corporate identity. In E.E. Bobrow & M.D. Bobrow (Eds.), *Marketing handbook: Volume 1, Marketing practices* (pp. 398–415). Homewood, IL: Dow Jones-Irwin.

Simonson, M.R., & Volker, R.P. (1984). *Media planning and production*. Columbus, OH: C.E. Merrill.

Smith, R.F. (1984). *Entrepreneur's marketing guide*. Reston, VA: Reston.

Stecki, E., & Corrado, F. (1988a). How to make a video, Part I. *Public Relations Journal, 44*(2), 33–34.

Stecki, E., & Corrado, F. (1988b). How to make a video, Part II. *Public Relations Journal, 44*(3), 35–36.

Strunk, W., & White, E.B. (1979). *The elements of style* (3rd ed.). New York: Macmillan.

VCRs. (1987, January). *Consumer Reports, 52* 17–26.

SELECTED READINGS FOR SHARPENING WRITING SKILLS

Bates, J.D. (1985). *Writing with precision*. Washington, DC: Acropolis.

Brosnan, J., Kovalesky, A., & Lewis, E.P. (1980). Perishing while publishing. *Nursing Outlook, 28,* 688–690.

Hanson, S.M. (1988). Write on. *American Journal of Nursing, 88,* 482–483.

Kolin, P.C., & Kolin, J.L. (1984). *Professional writing for nurses in education, practice, and research*. St Louis, MO: Mosby.

Mirin, S.K. (1981). *The nurse's guide to writing for publication*. Rockville, MD: Aspen.

O'Connor, A.B. (1979). *Writing for nursing publications*. Thorofare, NJ: Slack.

Robinson, A., & Notter, L. (1982). *Clinical writing*. Bowie, MD: Brady.

Stauch, K.P., & Brundage, D.J. (1980). *Guide to library resources for nursing*. New York: Appleton-Century-Crofts.

Strunk, W., Jr., & White, E.B. (1979). *The elements of style* (3rd ed.). New York: Macmillan.

Swanson, E., & McCloskey, J. (1986). Publishing opportunities for nurses. *Nursing Outlook, 34,* 227–235.

Twedt, D.W. (1977). A marketing strategy for marketing knowledge—or how to publish and prosper. *Journal of Marketing, 41*(2), 69–72.

Warner, S., & Schweer, K.D. (1982). *Author's guide to journals in nursing and health related fields.* New York: Haworth Press.

CHAPTER 7

Product Line Management

Product line management (PLM) is one of the business terms that crept into the nursing world and its literature in the 1980s. Although the term *service line management* is also found in the health care literature, we refer to the concept as *PLM*. This marketing management system began in the manufacturing industry when managers were assigned to coordinate development and promotional activities for related groups of products. In the early 1970s, hospitals began to investigate the usefulness of this type of management for their services. Now nurses manage product lines in and out of hospitals.

After diagnostic related groups (DRGs) were adopted as the basis for a hospital prospective reimbursement system, hospital output was increasingly described as DRG products, defined in terms of diagnoses and resource consumption. Although it was not practical from a management or a marketing perspective for hospitals to have hundreds of products, DRGs could be clustered to form 20 or 30 product lines. However, not everyone agrees that a DRG is a product, and other criteria have also been developed for hospital product lines. In this chapter we focus on how product lines and their management have developed in the health care field. The evolving role of nurse managers in PLM is also discussed.

PRODUCT LINE AND PRODUCT MIX

We have already defined a *product* as anything that is produced to fulfill a specific need or want. Goods, services, and ideas are products if they are produced to be offered in an exchange. Note that when we use the word *product* in this book, we are usually referring to services, because nursing is a service profession. On occasion, nurses produce goods as well, for example, nursing manuals and books that are sold (for an example, see Case Study 3).

Product lines are groups of products that are closely related by function, by customer usage, by distribution channels, or by price (Kotler, 1988). The key words in the definition are *closely related*. This close relationship of the products in the line can be based on a wide range of variables. Thus, in the health care field, as in the manufacturing industry, the similarities can be in the needs of consumers, in the use of the product, in how and where the products are exchanged, and even in price range. Each product line should be a separate profit center for accounting purposes, so that revenues and expenses can be monitored and analyzed.

Product line management has been used longer and more extensively by some for-profit companies than in the nonprofit arena. Its greatest use is in the manufacturing industry. The product lines of a for-profit company such as General Motors are well-known, and include the Buick, Cadillac, Chevrolet, Oldsmobile, and Pontiac lines of automobiles. Each product line is related primarily by distribution, and secondarily by customer loyalty and price. Function and appearance now play less important roles in differentiating these product lines. Universities are examples of nonprofit organizations that can be organized by product lines, with deans serving as administrators of each line or college. Place and subject matter (function) differentiate the business lines within the university. Price may also vary by school if, for example, a university's medical school tuition is more expensive than its law school's tuition.

Although lines of hospital business were not always identified by this terminology, groups of related products were traditionally offered to health care customers. A review of the current hospital literature shows that hospital product lines are usually related by clinical service; for example, ophthalmology, orthopedics, and cardiology. Specific medical diagnoses, clustered DRGs, demographic characteristics, and place where service is provided are other ways of forming product lines in the health care industry. Thus, there might be a diabetes, pediatrics, or outpatient product line. Hospital and nursing product lines are discussed in greater detail later in the chapter.

Product mix is the set of all products that an organization or individual offers to consumers. Product mix is defined by its length, width, and depth. *Length* describes the number of products or product lines made available. *Width* describes the products offered in each product line. *Depth* describes each product item or distinct unit that can be differentiated from other products in the line, by purpose, price, target market, or other variables (Kotler & Clarke, 1987).

To illustrate these terms, think of a small hospital that has four product lines based on the organizational structure. The four product lines are inpatient services, outpatient services, staff development, and patient education. The width of the outpatient line is comprised of outpatient clinics, the emergency service, and ambulatory surgery. The depth of the ambulatory surgery product item is four operating rooms. Products are also classified as *core* or *ancillary products* depending on their contribution to the organization's mission and its financial base.

PRODUCT LINE MANAGEMENT (PLM)

From a marketing perspective, the interest in product lines lies in the way they are managed. In this section, we present the meaning of product line management, the reason it was developed, how it has evolved, the responsibilities of the product manager, and some general advantages and disadvantages of this management system for organizations.

Product line management is a system of planning, organizing, directing, and controlling a group of related products from development through delivery to consumers. Although this sounds relatively straightforward, there is some confusion in the marketing arena and its literature about what PLM really means.

Product or *brand management,* as it is also called, began in 1927 when the Proctor & Gamble Company (P&G) assigned a manager to coordinate the development and promotion of a single product called Camay soap (Kotler, 1988). The product manager competed as fiercely with Ivory soap, another P&G product, as he did with other manufacturers' products. Not until 1987 did P&G reorganize to manage by its 39 product categories, such as laundry detergents, cake mixes, and diapers, rather than by individual brands such as Camay soap. The P&G brand management system was widely copied in the consumer products manufacturing industry, although with some variations. It was called *product management, brand management, and product line management.* Many product managers had more than eight products to coordinate, although they were not always called product *line* managers (McDaniel & Gray, 1980). Regardless of the number of products they managed, many reported to product group managers, who in turn reported to marketing managers or marketing vice presidents rather than to operational vice presidents. To understand product management and PLM, it is important to remember that both of these terms refer to systems developed to address marketing problems, and are really marketing management systems.

Product planning decisions require input from many functional areas of the organization. Without a product manager, however, there was no single manager responsible for integrating the decisions as the product moved through development stages to the consumer. The product manager evolved in the manufacturing industry to coordinate the management of functional departments such as product development, engineering, manufacturing, marketing, and sales. Although the functional managers continued to make product decisions, the decisions were better, as well as more timely, if they were coordinated by a product manager. Ultimately, higher quality products arrived in the marketplace in a more cost-effective manner.

Dominguez (1970) best describes the complex role of the product manager:

> The product manager is the central focus for all information relative to his product or product line. He is the repository of all such data, the source of information about his product, the planner, the profit controller

and motivator, and the center of a large sphere of product influence that permeates every aspect of the business operation necessary for the accomplishment of his primary duty—the successful introduction, marketing and sale of profitable products and the continuous review and analysis of his product or product lines to assure continued overall profitable growth and marketing position. (pp. 4, 5)

The product manager is clearly responsible for coordinating the product, from market analysis, planning, and development (implementation) to evaluation and corrective action. Kotler (1988) specifies six tasks in this management cycle:

1. Developing long-range, competitive product strategy.
2. Preparing the annual marketing plan and forecasting sales.
3. Working with advertisers and promotion agencies to develop ads, sales programs, and campaigns.
4. Stimulating interest in the product among the sales force.
5. Continuously gathering and analyzing data on the product's performance, consumer attitudes, problems, and new opportunities.
6. Improving the product to meet consumer needs and wants.

Advantages and Disadvantages of PLM

Product line management has several advantages over other administrative systems. One of the greatest advantages is that all aspects of a product line are coordinated by one manager. A product manager can be more sensitive to the consumer market, and can react more quickly to suggestions, criticisms, and environmental changes than can a group of individual functional department managers. The communications and coordination of functional specialists are simplified. Marketing mix decisions can be balanced and customized to make them more cost-effective. One final advantage is that PLM improves customer relations. In general, fewer promises are made but not kept when the product line manager controls all communication with customers.

There are also disadvantages to adopting PLM. According to McDaniel and Gray (1980), the greatest of these is the imbalance that frequently exists between the product manager's authority and responsibility level. Too often, the authority is insufficient for the responsibilities. As mentioned in Chapter 2, a matrix organizational structure results when PLM is imposed on a functional structure. Having more than one boss may lead to conflicts in authority and responsibility between product line managers and the functional managers, when the latter perceive a loss of their control to product line managers. Communications are more complex and require more of the managers' time. Finding product line managers with a broad range of skills may be difficult. With PLM comes an assumption that there will be winning and losing product lines, and this leads to another disadvantage: internal competition for resources and recognition among product line managers (Wodinsky, Egan, & Markel, 1988). Finally, Tucker and Burr (1988) point out that the increased administrative costs of adding product line managers to the functional structure must be balanced against the benefits of flexibility, individualization, and faster decisions.

HOSPITAL PRODUCT LINES

Hospitals and medical centers have traditionally offered a variety of product lines to their consumers. However, product lines were not specifically identified by this terminology, and were usually managed in functional organizational structures. Inpatient and outpatient services, education, training, and research can be thought of as products exchanged with patients, families, communities, medical staff, and employees, as well as with the academic and professional communities in the case of education and research products. Place of distribution, price, and patient characteristics differentiate inpatient and outpatient services, while function and category of consumers are pertinent variables in education and research product lines. An example of four basic hospital product lines, published by Kotler in 1982, included: (1) diagnosis and cure products—inpatient care, emergency care, outpatient clinics, laboratories; (2) illness prevention products—cholesterol counseling and screening; (3) health education products—smoking cessation programs; and (4) restorative products—psychiatric and rehabilitation centers.

Current health care literature describes a great variety of product lines offered to consumers at the end of the 1980s, and recounts many attempts to use PLM as well, although in forms quite different from those used in manufacturing. Health care services most often managed as product lines include women's health, emergency, cardiology, maternity, chemical dependency, geriatric care, laboratory, radiology, oncology, wellness, and outpatient surgery (Steiber, 1987). The four product lines described by Steiber as the most successful are outpatient services and surgery, emergency, maternity, and cardiology. Other product lines referred to in health care literature are pediatrics, rehabilitation, diabetes center, diagnostic center, sports medicine, physical medicine, fitness, digestive disorders, and health promotion centers. This long list illustrates some of the variables used to differentiate product lines: sex, age, place of service, medical diagnosis, type of patient, type of procedure, severity of illness, and the consumer's place on the continuum from wellness to illness.

To be managed as a separate product line, Tucker and Burr (1988) caution that a health care service should have the following characteristics:

1. An identifiable external market interested in an exchange for the service.
2. Competitors that can be identified.
3. Control of price, location, quality, and other marketing mix factors.
4. Measurable financial returns from the exchange.

The first two criteria are not as difficult to satisfy as the last two. Frequently, product line managers do not have as much control over revenue and expenses as they need, due to internal and external factors, such as conflicts with functional managers, autocratic superiors, vendor contractors, and third-party regulators. In addition, the health care management information system may not provide the financial and operating data the product line manager needs to monitor results. In health care, all product lines cannot be expected to be profitable, as they are in the manufacturing industry. Nor can they be automatically discontinued if they lose money. The mission of the organization or health care provider and its political and regulatory climate are more important than profit in developing and eliminating product lines (Solovy, 1989).

HOSPITAL PRODUCT LINE MANAGEMENT

Product line management began to receive much more attention and use after DRG prospective reimbursement was introduced in New Jersey in 1980 and nationwide beginning in 1983. This system forced hospitals to think of health care products rather than functions, because payment was based on the discharged patient (product) rather than on elements of care (functions). The competition engendered by declining length of stay and decreasing occupancy rates in hospitals fostered a marketing perspective not present in the earlier sellers' market that hospitals with high occupancy rates had enjoyed. As hospitals hired marketing professionals and developed marketing departments, the management systems used in other industries were adapted for use in the health care industry.

Hospital PLM does not have a consistent meaning. MacStravic's (1986) definition of *product-line administration* helps to illustrate this. He states that product-line administration in hospitals has three basic elements that can be used alone or together: planning, management, and marketing. Product line planning involves using product lines as the basis for analysis and forecasting when making hospital product decisions. Why MacStravic separated the planning function from management is not clear, but he defines PLM as organizing, directing, and controlling the hospitals' operations through product line categories. He emphasizes the importance of cost control, implemented primarily through monitoring physicians' costs in managing patients. The focus of product line marketing is on meeting goals set for each product line. The marketing process includes product line planning, and is enhanced by PLM, as it identifies, attains, and maintains a specific market position. This differentiation between PLM and product line marketing illustrates the confusion in terminology and concepts related to PLM in the hospital industry.

At least four PLM models and a variety of hybrids have emerged in the health care field, and are described by Cole and Brown (1988). In the *strategic business unit (SBU) model,* there is a product and market orientation. Management structure is decentralized and shifts product packaging, along with profit and loss responsibility, to the SBU manager. Each SBU has a distinct mission and its own competitors. In this model, clinical services are usually SBUs, and major diagnostic categories are product lines. *Strategic product family model* is another name for the SBU model. The *distribution model* has a physician and market orientation that focuses on developing distribution channels for its products. Existing functional line managers take on additional responsibility to increase utilization as product line managers. The *market management model* is market oriented, seeking to find opportunities to meet consumers' needs. Because success is measured by attainment of revenue goals and the development of new services, a sophisticated sales force is created. The *coordinated care model* has a consumer orientation that focuses on case management and integrates the hospital's diverse programs into a cohesive theme. Success is measured by volume.

From the variety of PLM models operating in hospitals in the United States and Canada, we see that the concept has been put into operation in a variety of ways. Answers to the following questions will help you to understand a specific PLM system you may encounter in the health care industry.

1. What is the purpose for using PLM in this organization?
2. What is the prevailing marketing philosophy or orientation in the organization?
3. Does the product line manager have operational control or coordinating responsibility for the product line?
4. To whom do product line managers report?
5. Who reports to the product line manager?
6. Is each product line a separate profit center? (These are also called responsibility, revenue, or cost centers.)
7. Who is held accountable for revenues and expenses for the product line?
8. What qualifications are required for the product line manager's position?
9. Are physicians product line managers?
10. Are nurses product line managers?
11. Are business administrators product line managers?

Because of the various interpretations of PLM, it is difficult to assess how widespread its use actually is in the health care field. In 1987, Steiber reported that 16% of 251 hospitals responding to a SRI Gallup survey had separate departments for product management, although 43% of the hospital marketers worked closely with the PLM function. In a 1988 survey of hospital executives (Traska), only 19% of the respondents had attempted to use PLM; although when this group was surveyed in 1986, 49% had expected to try PLM in attempting to reduce the risk of hospital closure. The implementation of PLM increased with the size of the hospital. Between 30% and 40% of hospitals with more than 300 beds used product management, although the study does not report in what variety of forms.

Droste (1988) analyzed why some hospitals have been reluctant to try PLM (for this study, defined as management of clinical services as separate profit centers). She found that establishing these separate profit centers required major structural and corporate culture changes, as personnel, budgets, and other responsibilities shifted from functional department heads to product line managers. Rather than risking intrahospital turf battles, many hospitals were targeting specific market segments without restructuring the organization. These targeted services were called product lines, centers, centers of excellence, and other names. The product managers had marketing responsibility for, but not budgetary control over, the service. Another finding of this analysis was that hospitals had difficulty finding qualified product managers. Hospital personnel lacked specific PLM and marketing knowledge and skills, while the outsider with an MBA was perceived as a threat to the hospital executive who knew less than the MBA about product management. A third problem revealed in Droste's analysis was the confusion in interpreting the meaning of PLM for health care.

As we pointed out earlier, PLM was developed in the consumer products manufacturing industry. The emphasis there is on developing multiple lines of products to force out competitors by filling the shelves of retail stores (Plantenberg, 1988). It was not designed for complex high-touch/high-tech service organizations, such as the health care facilities of the 1990s. According to Plantenberg, hospital PLM outcomes are affected by four key groups who are often in conflict over goals and operations:

1. Attending and staff physicians control admissions, length of stay, and use of most diagnostic and therapeutic services.

2. Hospital administrators determine the strategic plan and oversee organizational goal attainment.

3. Staff managers are responsible for product line planning, finance, and marketing.

4. Directors of operating units, such as nursing units, laboratory, and radiology departments, manage the human, capital, and material resources essential for service delivery.

Plantenberg singles out the nursing division as the source of many of the problems with PLM, because of the large number of personnel over whom the nurse executive has line authority. This influences decisions when there is a conflict between nursing personnel and the product line manager over resources, policies, or practices. (We will discuss this later in this chapter.)

To avoid the risks and confusion that accompany reorganizing from a traditional functional structure to PLM, Plantenberg recommends that PLM be introduced with one product line that is targeted at a clearly defined group of consumers, following market research that supports this approach. Brand names to identify the products and the product line should be developed and tested on the potential market. All employees with consumer contact must be carefully oriented to the product line and be able to discuss it knowledgeably before it is promoted to external markets. Other product lines can be developed after the first is successful. Plantenberg warns that PLM should not be applied to all hospital products. Even when DRGs are bundled into product groups, the potential is for more than 50 product lines, an unmanageable number.

HOSPITAL PRODUCT LINE MANAGERS

The product line manager is the coordinator of key elements of the hospital organization: operating units, physicians, functional department heads, and executives (Reynolds, 1984). Operating units manage resources and costs, and include the nursing units, laboratory, radiology, and the like. The workload of the units is largely determined by the admitting and clinical practice patterns of another key element, the attending physicians. Physicians not only control most admissions but also influence length of stay. In addition to units and physicians, product managers coordinate marketing and budgeting activities for functional department heads and help hospital executives attain strategic goals.

It is apparent from the hospital literature that, just as there is no universal meaning for PLM, likewise there is none for product line manager. Responsibilities and reporting relationships are not consistent because these managers are meeting objectives specific to the employing organization. In general, health care product line managers are responsible for product development and marketing, meet financial goals for the product line, manage physician relations, and coordinate the functional areas that deliver service to patients. Reynolds (1984) points out that though product line managers may have little line authority, they usually have major responsibilities, and require great interpersonal skills to be effective in the position.

To resolve the conflicts that may arise among the product line managers, PLM staff, and other key groups, Plantenberg (1988) suggests that the assistant administrator who has the greatest motivation, knowledge of, and affinity for that product line has the greatest probability of success as its manager. He argues that the dysfunction of a matrix structure can be avoided by maintaining established lines of authority. We fail to see how this resolves the conflict for the professional nurse, working in the product line, who is torn between reporting relationships to the nurse executive and to the assistant administrator, now a product line manager. Plantenberg argues against registered nurse product line managers, because of their potential conflict in reporting to both the vice president of nursing and the hospital administrator with ultimate responsibility for the product line. A lack of management training motivation, and lack of aptitude for management are cited by Plantenberg in arguing against the physician as product line manager.

No statistics are available that describe the background of product line managers in United States and Canadian hospitals. We do know that physicians, hospital administrators, and nurses are filling these positions, as are individuals with masters degrees in either business or public administration.

Johns Hopkins Hospital provides an example of using physicians as product line managers (Nackel & Kues, 1986). Eight product centers, also called business units, are organized around major clinical services. The management team for each product center includes a unit director and a nursing director who report directly to the physician manager. This team of three is accountable for revenues and expenses of the business unit. The chief nurse executive has a staff position, related on a dotted line basis to the eight business units. (Functions of this nurse executive were not described.)

Since the mid-1980s, nursing publications have been reporting on nurses in product line manager positions for a wide range of programs, including outpatient, ambulatory surgery, same-day surgery, telemetry, cardiac rehabilitation, diabetes, patient education, home health, perinatal, primary care, and wellness centers. Nurse managers also report to product line managers who are hospital administrators and physicians.

NURSING PRODUCT LINES

In the last half of the 1980s, nurses began to identify product lines they could manage for employers or for themselves, in the case of nurse entrepreneurs. One product line consisting of several nursing manuals, and how it was marketed, is described in Case Study 3. Johnson et al. (1987) organize the inventory of nursing products offered by Washington Hospital Center into four product lines: (1) operations management, (2) consultation services, (3) publications, and (4) education. See Exhibit 7-1 for their list of products. Notice that nursing care is not included there as a product or product line.

As discussed earlier, nursing care delivered by employees of a hospital or other health care organizations should be described as a production function (Anderson, 1985) or an intermediate product (Piper, 1985) rather than as a hospital product or a nursing product. Hospital or nursing products are more accurately defined in terms of patients' needs, such as improvement in state of health, prevention of health risks, or a better quality of life (Stanton, 1986). Thus, all hospital employees and physicians, as well as patients and their significant others, contribute to production of the hospital product lines. However, nursing care can be called the product of a professional nursing corporation, a nursing supplemental agency, or nurse entrepreneurs who directly sell their services to individuals, hospitals, HMOs, or other agencies. Types of nursing services provided through nursing corporations and independent practice are programs for wellness promotion, stress management, weight loss, smoking cessation, childbirth education, and many more. Nurses manage, and sometimes own, corporations for geriatric,

EXHIBIT 7-1   Inventory of Nursing Products:
Washington Hospital Center

Operations Management
Quality Assurance Plan for Nursing
Absenteeism Reporting System (Lotus)
Budget Variance Reporting System (Lotus)
Human Resource Use Reports
Nursing Research Proposal Critique Tool
Guidelines for Revenue Producing Activities
Patient Classification and Charging System
Guidelines for University Collaboration and Student Placement
Policy, Procedure, and Protocol Format

Consultation Services
Hemodialysis Skills—Staff Education and Training
How to Open an Oncology Unit
Preoperative Teaching Program for Open Heart Patients,
    Continuing Education, and Patient Education Services
Primary Nursing in the Surgical Intensive Care Setting
Nursing Administration and Management

Publications
Discharge Teaching for Transplant Patients
Infant Stimulation—Baby Play (Videotape)
Leading a Balanced Life: Handbook for Diabetics
CenterNurse—A Nursing Newsletter

Education

Community Education
    Food—Facts and Fallacies
    Focus on Poison Prevention
    Early Cancer Detection and Preventing Risks
    Drugs—Not a Dead Issue
    Blood Pressure Screening

Patient Education
    Medication Care Teaching Tools
    Printed Pamphlet Series
        Colonscopy
        Endoscopic Retrograde Choledocho Pancreatogram
        Barium Enema

　　　Upper Endoscopy
　　　Upper GI

Staff Education
　　　Physical Assessment
　　　Leadership
　　　Preceptorship
　　　IV Therapy Certification Program
　　　Chemotherapy Administration for RNs
　　　Self-Learning Modules
　　　　　Infection Control
　　　　　Operating Room Paperwork
　　　　　Kardexing
　　　A Practical Approach to 12 Lead EKG Interpretation
　　　Medical ICU Course (University Credit Granted)
　　　Surgical ICU Course (University Credit Granted)
　　　Neonatal ICU Course (University Credit Granted)
　　　Perioperative Course: Basic Operating Room Techniques (University
　　　　　Credit Granted)

Graduate Nursing Education
　　　Nursing Administration Course

Source: Johnson, J.E., Arvidson, A.C., Costa, L.L., Hekhuis, F.M., Lennox, L.A., Marshall, S.B., & Moran, M.J. (1987). Marketing your nursing product line: Reaping the benefits. *Journal of Nursing Administration, 17*(11), 29–33. Reprinted with permission.

hospice, and childbirth care, as well as a host of other services that can be managed as product lines:

Strasen (1987) offers these suggestions to nurses and other health care professionals making decisions to reorganize patient care services by product lines:

1. Define product lines as broadly as possible so that the number of lines is manageable.

2. Define product lines so that they are meaningful to the health care professionals providing the services.

3. Define a product line so that resources used for each case are relatively homogeneous.

4. Define each product line using statistically valid data.

Using these criteria, we see that much analysis needs to be done before adopting a product line management approach to health and nursing care. If you are going to benefit from PLM, managing products as a group should yield measurable advantages over single-product management.

OPPORTUNITIES FOR NURSES

Product line management has been described as a growth opportunity for nurse managers. Certainly the coordination of operational units and physicians' services is a familiar role. Many nurses are experienced expense managers; fewer have had responsibility for the revenue side of the budget. Nurses are educated to understand the physiological and psychosocial needs of patients and could readily develop a marketing perspective, particularly in regard to patient services. The patient advocate role is familiar, but more emphasis is needed on patient satisfaction. In addition, perceiving physicians, other nurses, and the community as our markets needs more development.

On the negative side of the ledger, hospital administrators who hire MBA-prepared product line managers, in lieu of either nurses or physicians, may rationalize their decisions based on two areas of deficiency in health care professionals' education: finance and marketing. Neither of these fields are part of the average clinician's educational background. Recent graduates of nursing administration masters programs should have studied financial management, and have at least been exposed to marketing principles, but expertise in these areas is most often acquired from management experience. The nurse manager with a combined nursing administration graduate degree and a masters in business administration may be in the strongest position to compete for a product line manager assignment in health care.

CONCLUSION

Although product line management has been adopted by a number of health care organizations, it has not proven to be a marketing management panacea for the industry. Moreover, there are many forms of this management system, and its associated terms have no universal meaning. Nevertheless, nurses are now working as product line managers, and we see this field as an opportunity for more nurses in the future.

REFERENCES

Anderson, R.A. (1985). Products and product-line management in nursing. *Nursing Administration Quarterly, 10*(1), 65–72.

Cole, G., & Brown, C. (1988). Product-line management: Concept to reality. *Topics in Health Care Financing, 14*(3), 62–75.

Dominguez, G. (1970). *Product management.* New York: American Management Association.

Droste, T. (1988). Product-line management: Misunderstood, feared. *Hospitals, 62*(13), 30, 32.

Johnson, J.E., Arvidson, A.C., Costa, L.L., Hekhuis, F.M., Lennox, L.A., Marshall, S.B., & Moran, M.J. (1987). Marketing your nursing product line: Reaping the benefits. *Journal of Nursing Administration, 17*(11), 29–33.

Kotler, P. (1982). *Marketing for nonprofit organizations* (2nd ed.). Englewood Cliffs, NJ: Prentice-Hall.

Kotler, P. (1988). *Marketing management: Analysis, planning, and control* (6th ed.). Englewood Cliffs, NJ: Prentice-Hall.

Kotler, P., & Clarke, R.N. (1987). *Marketing for health care organizations.* Englewood Cliffs, NJ: Prentice-Hall.

MacStravic, R.S. (1986). Product-line administration in hospitals. *Health Care Management Review, 11*(2), 35–43.

McDaniel, C., & Gray, D.A. (1980). The product manager. *California Management Review, 23*(1), 87–94.

Nackel, J.G., & Kues, I.W. (1986). Product-line management: Systems and strategies. *Hospital & Health Services Administration, 31*(2), 109–123.

Piper, L.R. (1985). Managing the intermediate product. *Nursing Management, 16*(3), 18, 20.

Plantenberg, T.M. (1988). The problem with product line marketing. *Journal of Health Care Marketing, 8*(3), 30–32.

Reynolds, J. (1984). Product managers must decide what products to market and how. *Modern Healthcare, 14*(9), 176, 178, 180.

Solovy, A. (1989). Limited use for product management in hospitals. *Hospitals, 63*(2), 72.

Stanton, L.J. (1986). Nursing care and nursing products: Revenue or expenses? *Journal of Nursing Administration, 16*(9), 29–32.

Steiber, S. (1987). Marketing budgets increase a modest 4%. *Hospitals, 61*(22), 52–53.

Strasen, L. (1987). *Key business skills for nurse managers.* Philadelphia, PA: Lippincott.

Traska, M.R. (1988). Fear of failure and what hospitals did about it. *Hospitals, 62*(13), 20, 22.

Tucker, S.L., & Burr, R.M. (1988). Strategic marketing planning. *Topics in Health Care Financing, 14*(3), 44–55.

Wodinsky, H.G., Egan, D., & Markel, F. (1988). Product line management in oncology: A Canadian experience. *Hospital & Health Services Administration, 23*, 231–236.

CHAPTER 8

Ethics in Marketing

It may seem unusual that a book with a pragmatic approach to marketing includes a chapter on ethics. Ethics is a theoretical subject. It is the branch of philosophy that deals with values relating to human conduct, the rightness and wrongness of certain actions, and with the goodness and badness of the motives and ends or outcomes of such actions. Ethics is concerned with doing good and avoiding harm. The need for ethical conduct is so important that most, if not all, professions have developed ethical codes or standards of conduct. Professional nurses have the *Code for Nurses*. The American Marketing Association has a code of ethics; there is a *Code of Advertising Ethics* and a *Marketing Research Code of Ethics*. These codes are supposed to guide the individual in choosing right behavior, thereby avoiding causing harm. The good or the ethical is not always apparent or an easy choice; gray areas are increasing in industry and professional services. This is so important that the area warrants critical examination in a marketing book for nurses.

Since the early 1970s—the era of the Vietnam War and Watergate—the public has been very concerned with the moral behavior of all professionals. Every professional, whether lawyer, nurse, physician, educator, legislator, or business executive, must behave in an ethically responsible manner. This concern is so prevalent because of the all-too-frequent unethical behavior of people in responsible positions.

For decades, executives at the Manville Corporation suppressed evidence proving that asbestos inhalation was killing their employees (Gellerman, 1986). Recent examples of unethical behavior are the Ivan Boesky and Dennis Levine episodes of insider trading, the selling by Chrysler of used cars as new, the Iran-Contra scandal, and the Pentagon purchasing system. The list goes on and on, with scandals of bribes and kickbacks in government, the marketing of unsafe birth control devices, banking and financial rip-offs, and manufacturing behavior that leads to tragedies such as that of the space shuttle Challenger.

Within health care, major ethical problems and controversies are frequently in the news. These situations revolve around care for the dying patient, Baby Doe cases, health care costs, organ procurement, reproductive technology, surrogate parenting, AIDS, human gene therapy, and abortion (see Exhibit 8-1). As technology and knowledge increase, ethical difficulties are bound to become more pronounced. This is because not only can we do more, but the stakes are higher. Increasingly, health care providers are being held accountable for the ethical basis of their actions.

EXHIBIT 8-1   Ethics: Major Health Care Problems and Controversies

1. Caring for the dying patient:
   a. Differences between acts and omissions
   b. Differences between withholding and withdrawing
   c. Differences between intended death and foreseeable death
   d. Differences between ordinary and extraordinary.

2. Baby Doe cases: What kind of life-sustaining treatment, if any, should be used to preserve the lives of severely mentally or physically defective newborns?

3. Health care costs:
   a. Substantive questions involving competition for scarce resources—
      (1) Access to care
      (2) Distribution of resources
      (3) Right to health and health care
   b. Health care may be justifiably limited (rationed) in order to use resources more effectively or to increase equity
   c. Prospective payment questions—
      (1) The direct interest of society at large in how much care each patient uses
      (2) Initial pressure to eliminate useless care
      (3) Possible pressure to eliminate marginally useful care
      (4) On what basis, if any, should care be reduced?
         (a) efficiency?
         (b) equity?
         (c) ability to pay?

4. Procurement of human organs for transplantation:
   a. Welfare and rights of patients
   b. Should life-saving human tissue be distributed on a market basis or equal access?
      (1) Health insurance programs coverage of transplantation surgery

        (2) Cost of post-transplant immunosuppression therapy ($4,000–$10,000 per year for cyclosporin)

        (3) Shortage of organs

        (4) Shortage of transplant centers

        (5) Allocation of organs based on ability to gain the attention of the mass media, public officials, health care professionals

        (6) Logistics of timely retrieval and transportation of organs

    c. Questions regarding multiple transplants—

        (1) Should multiple organs from a single donor be used to save multiple lives or just one?

        (2) When should organs be used at a local center and when should they be available to the network?

        (3) Should physicians consider the issue of equitable distribution of organs and transplantation?

    d. Issues surrounding living donors—

        (1) Acceptable risks to a living donor

        (2) Circumstances under which a donor should give part of an irreplaceable organ such as a liver

    e. Restrictions on donated organs—

        (1) Upper age limit for donors

        (2) Limits on using flawed organs as temporary transplants until healthy organs are found

    f. Use of organs from anencephalic infants

    g. Fetal tissue transplant research.

5. AIDS:

    a. Mandatory screening—

        (1) Cost

        (2) Feasibility

        (3) Loss of confidentiality

        (4) Discrimination in
            (a) work
            (b) housing
            (c) education
            (d) insurance

        (5) Disposition of test results: Who should be informed of positive results? Families? Sexual partners?

    b. Drug research—

        (1) Controlled trials

        (2) Experimentation on fatally ill patients

   (3) Early treatment before appearance of clinical symptoms
  c. Ethics of refusal to care for AIDS patients?
  d. The high cost of drugs such as AZT (zidovudine)
  e. Making drugs available before FDA approval.
6. Human gene therapy.
7. Reproduction technology (ethical problems compounded by combination possibilities):
  a. In-vitro fertilization
  b. Artificial insemination
  c. Embryo transfer
  d. Embryo freezing
  e. Surrogate parenting
  f. Research with early human embryos
  g. Pregnancy reduction
  h. In-utero or postnatal testing for genetic diseases.
8. Role of hospital ethics committees in health care decision-making.
9. Abortion.

ETHICS AND NURSING

Nursing research (Crisham, 1981; Ketefian, 1981a, 1981b; Mayberry, 1986; Murphy 1976, 1978) has consistently suggested that the workplace strongly influences the individual's judgments. Decisions are often made more difficult by administrative policies and organizational structure. Nurses' responses to situations are similar to those seen in business; that is, they generally display obedience to authority and need to maintain harmony within the institution and with those in authority. According to Murphy (1978, p. 102), this need is pursued "even when the rights of patients are being violated."

An expanding body of literature supports an ethical component in nursing management. (Aroskar, 1984; Bowie, 1982; Fry, 1983; Newton, 1982; Silva, 1983). In a survey of ethical issues in administrative decision-making, Sietsema and Spradley (1987) found that nurse executives experience ethical dilemmas in their practices. Issues presenting ethical dilemmas identified by the survey are (1) allocation and rationing of scarce resources, (2) access to care for the indigent, (3) staffing level and mix decisions, (4) employee selection, hiring, demotion, termination, and promotion, (5) treatment versus nontreatment, (6) downsizing, (7) diversification of services, (8) marketing/advertising services, (9) developing/maintaining standards of care, (10) incompetent nurses and physicians, (11) employee relations, and (12) labor negotiations with professional nurses. Each of these ethical issues is concerned with marketing (defined broadly as the exchange of values).

Sietsema and Spradley's (1987) respondents based dilemma resolution on their own and others' personal values and beliefs. They consulted frequently with colleagues in hospital administration. The only ethical code the group used as a resource was the *Patient's Bill of Rights*. However, this approach does not acknowledge the nurse manager's responsibilities beyond the patient to the health care staff, the organization, and the community.

Nurse managers must establish a work environment that supports ethical decision-making. Socialization for awareness of moral conflicts is necessary, as are the organizational influences supportive of rational, ethical decision-making. These two factors must be present if nurses are to assess and respond rationally to moral problems in a manner that is in the best interest of all nursing markets.

Whether it is nursing theory and practice or marketing theory and practice, there is a dialectical relationship between theory and practice. That is, each defines itself and its nature in relation to the other. There is an ongoing interaction, enabling each to contribute to the growth and development of the other. We are using *theory* in the broadest, least exact definition possible. Theory here is a way of looking at the world and making sense of it. Therefore, the more one understands of theory, the more highly developed is practice. This holds true when applying marketing theory to nursing. It is also true when dealing with ethics. Some of the discussion included in this chapter may seem remote to nursing, but we have included it to enhance knowledge. The future may find that it is not really so far removed from nursing.

Dilemmas occur whatever the nurse's position may be. For the nurse manager, these issues are becoming more complex. As complexity grows, answers are more difficult to find. Opportunities to think through and discuss the consequences of courses of action are essential. When we avoid discussions of ethics in relation to nursing and management decisions, we evade very complex issues, and also develop particularly limited viewpoints, or what Hedin (1989) calls a "sterile ethical field." This may seem to help us find answers and make decisions; it may also result in behavior that contradicts our values and principles. What we consider ethical may change considerably when we look at the entire, broad context rather than limiting our view to the immediate environment. Nurses must ask those difficult questions that take into account wider contextual reality. Discussion of ethical dilemmas with colleagues is necessary. Other ways to assist in building ethical problem-solving skills are ethics rounds (Davis, 1982), formal courses, and reading.

In this chapter, we discuss ethical problems encountered in marketing and how to incorporate a consciousness of ethics into an organization or practice. Nurses can use this information as food for thought, as a basis from which to make managerial and marketing decisions, and as a means to form opinions as citizens. As nurses use marketing strategies, their need for assessing the ethical implications of their decisions will increase.

LESSONS FROM BUSINESS

Ethical considerations often make decision-making difficult. Eliminating them from the process would simplify the task of management. In his classic book, *Capitalism and Freedom*, Milton Friedman (1962) suggested doing just that. He argued that the interaction between business and society should be left to the political process. Friedman (p. 133) stated, "Few trends could so thoroughly undermine the very foundation of our free society as the acceptance by corporate officials of a social responsibility other than to make as much money for their shareholders as possible." This is a deceptively simple, naive approach. Business is part of the social system, and must be held responsible and accountable for its actions in the same way as other segments of society. It is also impossible to separate the economic aspects of major decisions from the social consequences. Business people have to evaluate the economic and social consequences of decisions as best they can in a limited time and with limited information (Cadbury, 1987; McCoy, 1983).

In fact, research has shown little support for Friedman's stance. Baumhart (1961) reported that 73% of his respondents agreed that corporate executives must act in the interest of employees and consumers as well as in the interest of shareholders. The group to whom executives felt the greatest responsibility in Brenner and Molander's study (1977) was the customers; stockholders were second and employees were third. Society at large and elected government ranked fifth and seventh.

Baumhart (1961), in a classic study of business ethics, identified the major ethical problems faced by business people: (1) gifts, gratuities, bribes, and call girls, (2) price discrimination and unfair pricing, (3) dishonest advertising, (4) miscellaneous unfair competitive practices, (5) cheating customers, unfair credit practices, and overselling, (6) price collusion by competitors, (7) dishonesty in making or keeping a contract, and (8) unfairness to employees and prejudice in hiring. Five of the eight problems have to do with marketing activities.

Brenner and Molander (1977) found the same undesirable practices, but the order of importance had changed for several items. Laczniak and Murphy (1985) concluded that marketing is the functional area of business most closely related to ethical abuse. Ethical maxims used by business (see Exhibit 8-2) are not sufficient to handle the ethical judgments required.

EXHIBIT 8-2   Ethical Maxims Used by Business

The golden rule:

Act in the way you would expect others to act toward you.

The utilitarian principle:

Act in a way that results in the greatest good for the greatest number.

Kant's Categorical Imperative:

Act in such a way that the action taken under circumstances could be a universal law or rule of behavior.

The professional ethic:

Take only action which would be viewed as proper by a disinterested panel of professional colleagues.

The TV test:

A manager should always ask "Would I feel comfortable explaining to a national TV audience why I took this action?"

Reprinted with permission. Laczniak, G.R. (1983). Framework for analyzing marketing ethics. *Journal of Macromarketing, 3*(1), 7.

Because marketing is charged with communicating and with satisfying customers, it is the management function most open to public scrutiny. When marketing is used in health care, the ethical implications become enormous. In fact, some health care professionals believe that health care is a basic right and that marketing has no place in health care (or nursing).

These questions of health care as a right or as a private service that can be marketed will have to be resolved in the near future. The necessity of controlling costs will probably force resolution. In 1989, we spent $600 billion, or over 11.5% of the United States gross national product (GNP), on health care. It is estimated that at current rates this figure will double by the year 2000. Distribution of these monies in an ethical way is a point of contention between proponents of private enterprise and those who see health care as public responsibility. Among the arguments put forth by proponents of private enterprise are that: the United States Constitution does not make provision for health care; health care is a private consumption product; our current system has brought great strides in health care; we have the finest system in the world.

Opposing this stance is the view that health care is a social good. Health care as we know it today was not, and could not have been, even imagined when our

Constitution was written in 1789. In this argument, universal health care is implied by the Fourteenth Amendment. We currently have a system of diverse quality of care, highly dependent on public funding. While we have some of the world's most sophisticated treatments, we also have a multitier system that limits access to care for those on the bottom tier. For the poor and medically indigent, access to care is difficult at best, impossible at worst. For example, the United States ranks 20th in the world in infant mortality. The poor suffer most from this; the middle class has an infant mortality rate comparable to the rest of the developed world.

While the United States spent 11.1% of its GNP for health care in 1986, Sweden spent 9%, and Britain spent 6.2% (Lohr, 1988). It is ironic that the United States, the richest country, spends more on health care than any other nation, and yet has segments of population whose health care is typical of the Third World. How can we resolve these problems and make the system equitable and just for all? Can marketing, with its emphasis on meeting consumer wants and needs, help to solve them? Britain is turning to marketing to change the National Health Service to meet patient needs. Marketing in and of itself is neither ethical nor unethical: people make marketing decisions, and some of these choices may be unethical.

ETHICAL ISSUES IN MARKETING RESEARCH

All researchers must consider ethics in the design of studies when human beings are used as subjects. Great care must be taken in order to assure that rights are protected. Conflicts often arise during the development of rigorous scientific investigations. The marketing researcher must be alert to potential conflicts among parties involved in a study.

Four groups are affected by the research process: the general public, the respondents in a specific study, the client (the company ordering the study), and the researcher (Tull & Hawkins, 1985). Hunt, Chonko, and Wilcox (1984) found that marketing researchers identified the following ethical problems as the most difficult, in order of difficulty: research integrity; treating clients fairly; research confidentiality; social issues; personnel issues; treating respondents fairly; treating others in the company fairly; interviewer dishonesty; gifts, bribes, and entertainment; treating suppliers fairly; legal issues; and misuse of funds.

The category of research integrity accounted for 33% of all responses, and included deliberately withholding information, falsifying numbers, altering results, misusing statistics, ignoring pertinent data, compromising research design, and misinterpreting results in order to support a personal or corporate point of view. Although these practices are all dishonest, they are not universally viewed as such; this leads to ethical dilemmas.

Protection of the Public

Needs of all of nursing's publics must be considered when collecting and using marketing research data. Some areas of concern have to do with incomplete reporting, misleading reporting, and nonobjective research (Tull & Hawkins, 1985). The effects of these activities are often interrelated, and each can also affect the client-researcher relationship.

Incomplete Reporting

Although there are safeguards that regulate clinical research and advertising for drugs and medical devices, there are no legal requirements to disclose negative marketing information on most other products to publics and markets. However, there are ethical pressures and necessities to do so in all cases. Withholding damaging information about a product, procedure, or service is misleading to potential consumers, as it denies them the information needed to make an informed decision. A reputable research report should always include such information, and it should be shared with potential consumers.

Misleading Reporting

Misleading reporting is closely related to incomplete reporting, in that it involves obfuscating potential consumers. Data are presented in such a way that potential consumers will reach conclusions that are not supported by the results of the study. Advertising campaigns are sometimes guilty of this.

Nonobjective Research

It is easy to see that making up data or deliberately misrepresenting research methods and results is unethical, but there are also less obvious means that can be used to arrive at a desired finding. This generally means using standard research techniques in a nonobjective way. Tull and Hawkins (1985) give the example of a researcher using the average income, rather than the median, in order to inflate a community's income. This is an example of utilitarianism; the end was thought to justify the means, because the community was a poor one and wanted to attract some businesses.

Protection of Respondents

Two ethical issues affect the relationship between marketing researchers and respondents. These issues are using research as a sales ploy, and the invasion of privacy. These problems are so prevalent that legislation has been passed to cope with the problems.

Marketing Research as a Sales Ploy

Asking people to participate in marketing research as a guise to sell a product is illegal as well as unethical. The Federal Trade Commission (FTC) established that it is illegal to use "any plan, scheme or ruse as a door-opener to gain admission into a prospect's home, office, or other establishment, which misrepresents the true status and mission of the person making the call" (Frey & Kinnear, 1979, p. 296). This practice, sometimes called *sugging*, is a continuing problem that plagues legitimate researchers world-wide.

In sugging, people are called on the telephone and asked to participate in a marketing survey or a brand identification program. The so-called researchers say they are independent and have no sales motive. Typically, the questionnaire is very brief, consisting of three to four questions. High-pressure sales pitches follow (Frey & Kinnear, 1979). Personal interviews and some mail surveys have been surreptitiously used for sales or for development of mailing lists.

Privacy and Informed Consent

The general public demands control of the amount of personal data that are made available. Important elements in this concept are: (1) informed consent, by which an individual can waive the right to privacy, (2) maintenance of anonymity and confidentiality, and (3) privacy.

Every individual has the right to decide how much personal information to share with others. The Constitution grants all the right to live life as they see fit, to have beliefs, and to speak freely without fear of observation or publicity beyond that which is sought or submitted to. What an individual chooses to divulge is a matter of personal choice, and may vary among individuals and even by the same individual at different times or places. Many people are becoming very wary of sharing their thoughts, feelings, and personal facts because of the potential for invasion of privacy with the increasing use and capacity of computers. This wariness also reflects a lack of trust of business and government.

Care must be taken by marketing researchers to ensure that potential respondents are able to choose freely, and that they do not feel real or imagined pressure to participate in marketing research. Marketing researchers must not abrogate the individual's ability to decide whether to participate and what to divulge. Informed consent must be obtained. *Informed consent* means that, from the individual's point of view, he or she has sufficient information to make a decision about participating. In general, respondents in marketing research studies need to know the types of questions or the tasks required, the areas covered, the time and physical effort demanded, and the ultimate use of the data obtained.

Important concepts are anonymity and confidentiality. *Anonymity* means that the respondent's identity is known to only a limited number of people, and will be protected from dissemination. Confidentiality requires the same attention in marketing research as it does in patient care.

Right to Seek Knowledge

On the other side of the coin are the rights of the market researcher to learn and to gain new information. The researcher should feel free to conduct any study that does not physically or psychologically harm respondents. Competently done research results in more effective marketing; that is, better products, improved advertising, better distribution, and fair pricing.

An alternate view, that the researcher commonly has a right to seek knowledge, is called the *no-harm, no-foul approach*. This position maintains that "one's privacy cannot be invaded if one is unaware of the invasion and the invasion causes no harm" (Tull & Hawkins, 1985, p. 63). Strict attention must be paid to anonymity and confidentiality. In this view, informed consent is not required. However, no physical or psychological harm should come to respondents.

Protection of the Client

In this usage, the term *client* refers to the organization that hires a marketing research firm or consultant. The client must be protected from: (1) abuse coming from specialized knowledge, (2) unnecessary research, (3) unqualified researchers, (4) disclosure of identity, (5) treating data as nonconfidential and nonproprietary, and (6) misleading presentation of data (Tull & Hawkins, 1985).

Abuse in position.   Most managers hiring a research firm or consultants are at a distinct disadvantage. They do not have the specialized knowledge and experience of the market researcher. Therefore, the manager may have difficulty making good marketing decisions. Opportunities exist for the researcher to take advantage of the client.

It is the responsibility of the market researcher to guard against using faulty designs and methods to meet time and cost demands of the client. Pressuring respondents and failure to verify that interviews were actually conducted are examples of unethical conduct. Failure to pilot a new questionnaire and to ensure the validity and reliability of research instruments are other examples.

Unnecessary research.   Managers frequently ask researchers to conduct a study that is unrelated to the problem, has already been done and has known results, or is economically unjustifiable. Often it is in the researcher's interests to conduct the study again. Although the American Marketing Association's *Code of Ethics* does not speak to this issue, Tull and Hawkins (1985) maintain that the researcher has a professional obligation to tell the client that the proposed research is unwarranted. After this is clearly stated, if the client still wants the study done, the researcher can do the study with a clear conscience. Unnecessary marketing research should also be avoided by in-house nurse researchers.

Unqualified researchers.   This problem involves the request for research that is beyond the capabilities or expertise of the marketing firm or consultant. The researcher should inform the client that the proposed study requires use of skills the researcher does not have. In order for the client to avoid delays, increased expenses, and decreased accuracy, the research should refer the client to another firm or consultant. Likewise, nurse researchers should not use methods in which they are not skilled.

Anonymity of client.   Research is carried out to assist in identifying and solving marketing problems. Competitors of the client may stand to gain if they know about the study. The researcher has an obligation to preserve the anonymity of the client. Unless the client agrees, no one, including respondents, should know who is sponsoring the study. Anonymity must also extend to other clients of the research firm.

Confidential and proprietary information.   Data, analysis, conclusions, and interpretations gained from a particular marketing study are the exclusive property of the client who ordered and paid for the research. While it is obvious that a research firm should not give the study to a client's competitor, it is less obvious what should be done when basic demographic data gathered for one client is needed in a study for another client who does not compete with the first client. Tull and Hawkins (1985) suggest that the data cannot be used without the explicit consent of the client who ordered and paid for it. If permission is given, the clients should share the cost. The research organization should not have competitors as clients if there is any chance that the confidential relationships with clients will be jeopardized.

Misleading presentation of data.   There are a number of ways in which a research agency can mislead the client, by the way research reports are written and delivered. The client needs to understand the outcomes so that rational business decisions can be made. Obfuscation by using overly technical jargon, failing to round numbers properly, using overly complex analytic procedures, and reporting incompletely can mislead by creating an illusion of precision that is beyond the capabilities of the study.

Protection of the Market Researcher

There are several behaviors on the part of clients that are unethical and from which the market researcher needs protection. These include improper solicitation of research proposals, disclosure of proprietary information on research techniques, and the misrepresentation of findings.

Improper solicitation of proposals.   Research proposals or bids are requested for two purposes: to assist in deciding whether to conduct the research, and to assist in deciding which research agency to use. The proposals should be evaluated on their own merit. Only if other criteria (often related to size and capabilities of the firm) are made known to the researcher in advance should they be used. A proposal received from one agency should not be given to another firm or an in-house department for implementation.

Disclosure of proprietary information or techniques.   Research firms often develop unique techniques to deal with special problems. Examples of these techniques are models for predicting success of new products and simulation techniques for predicting effects of changes in marketing mix variables. These techniques are proprietary; they belong to the developer. It is unethical for the client to make them known to other research firms or to use them without the explicit consent of the developer.

Misrepresentation of findings.   It is unethical for the client to misrepresent the findings of a study. Such conduct is not only misleading to the public, but is also potentially damaging to the research agency. The researcher could be accused of careless research or dishonesty in reporting results.

ETHICAL ISSUES IN PRICING

Price and Profit

Price is the amount of money (or its equivalent) for which something is bought, sold, or offered for sale. As discussed in Chapter 5, price is theoretically determined to maximize profit. In the everyday work world, pricing decisions are made in four ways: (1) a cost-plus basis, (2) a target rate of return, (3) a competition-oriented basis, and (4) analysis of demand for the product or service.

In order for price to be ethical, it should be either equal or proportional to the benefit received. The benefits are difficult to ascertain for many products. Important questions are: what are the benefits and how are the benefits perceived by the consumer? For example, if you spend $150 on designer eyeglass frames, as opposed to $50 for unbranded ones, what additional benefit are you getting? The wearer of the designer glasses gains status that justifies the added cost. While this example is rather prosaic, an appropriate question follows: Are there aspects of charging a higher price, given some perceived benefit such as status, that justify this price as moral, even when there may also be some form of wrong? In other words, is it wrong to charge a price that gives a very large profit even when customers are willing to pay that price? This last question figures prominently in the news reports and debates over the extremely high price of AZT (zidovudine), the drug used to treat AIDS.

In economics, *profit* is defined as pecuniary gain resulting from the employment of capital in a transaction. It is often described as the excess of total revenue over total expenses. It may also be defined as the return received by the organization as the result of participating in a successful exchange relationship.

Profit from health care has been an unacceptable concept to some professionals as well as to a segment of the public. These individuals believe that nonprofit hospitals provide the best services. An often unspoken assumption has been that the purpose of for-profit health organizations is not for the public good. Some feel that it is wrong to make a profit on someone's misfortune—one's illness—although this perception is slowly changing.

It is difficult to determine reasonable profit; judging if a profit is ethical is even more complex. A reasonable profit is one that rewards a company for its contribution, allows it to accumulate a surplus or to pay competitive dividends, enables it to compete in financial markets with other financial instruments such as stocks, bonds, and certificates, allows reinvestment for growth of the organization, and considers the degree of risk taken (Kehoe, 1985). From a utilitarian point of view, a reasonable profit serves the greater good of society, but other factors must also be considered. Some questions should be asked. In making the profit, was society injured in any way? Were employees adequately and fairly paid for their contributions? Could anyone purchase the product, or were the poor, minorities, women, or the elderly excluded from purchasing the offering? Did the organization participate in price fixing or deceptive advertising? Is the agency socially responsible or does it pollute the environment? Does it offer unsafe services? These and other questions must be considered when judging whether or not a profit is ethical.

Kehoe (1985) states that, of the marketing mix variables, price is the most difficult to investigate from an ethical perspective. Profit goals of the organization, federal and state laws, and the many factors within the system that are susceptible to abuse all contribute to the price of a product. The structure and values of health care make pricing it more difficult than pricing consumer goods, or even than pricing hotel, restaurant, and travel services. One has only to look at the efforts of costing out nursing care to see how difficult this is. How much should we charge for teaching the diabetic patient self-care? What is it worth to avoid serious postoperative complications?

Because health care deals with life, death, and quality-of-life issues, its pricing is fraught with ethical dilemmas as well as accounting difficulties. The list of unethical pricing practices is very long. Some ethically questionable activities include pricing branded products higher than generics (a practice prevalent in pharmacies), and the practice of psychological pricing (intending that the consumer perceive $295 as closer to $250 than $300, for example). Some practices, such as price fixing, are illegal. Consumers expect pricing to be done on an ethical basis.

Organizational Influences on Unethical Pricing Behavior

Organizational influences on unethical pricing behavior are manifested in at least five ways. The first is an overemphasis on profit, or *surplus* as it is called in nonprofit organizations. In health care, this has the potential to become a very sore point. Because of DRGs, the hospital has a profit motive for discharging patients early. If physicians, utilization coordinators, and nursing line managers decide that profit is to be considered ahead of ethical considerations, an 80-year-old patient may be sent home before self-care is possible. Nurse managers in hospitals must be wary of this.

Second is the existence of ethical standards without an effective quality assurance program. Management must monitor quality. The health care industry saw the need for control of quality years ago when it first began to develop audits. Quality assurance programs and other control mechanisms are especially important if line management is profit-oriented.

Third is permitting the law to be a surrogate for corporate ethics. Minimum standards are established by law, but these are *minimums;* it must be remembered that just because something is legal, it is not necessarily ethical. Slavery was at one time legal; it was never ethical. Apartheid is legal in South Africa; it is not an ethical way of living. The highest ethical behavior should be expected in all situations, even when the law is vague or permissive, because of the vulnerabilities of patients.

The fourth influence on ethical behavior and pricing behavior is ambiguous corporate policies. Policies must clearly define ethical behavior in pricing decisions. All employees should know for certain that policies are to be followed. Specific behavior on the part of employees must be spelled out, as must the consequences if the policies are not upheld.

Fifth is amoral decision-making. This entails ignoring the ethical implications of the decision and its impact on people. Again, this is prevalent when profit is the pervasive criterion in decision-making. An example is setting artificially inflated prices for medications or health care services in a captive market, such as a community in which the majority is retirees on fixed incomes. Another example is the extremely high price one drug company charged AIDS patients for AZT. Public response was so negative that the company lowered the price.

Situational Influences on Unethical Pricing Behavior

Situational influences on unethical pricing practices are also found in the health care industry. These practices tend to occur when a market is at overcapacity or is characterized as an oligopoly. For example, the fact that hospitals are generally the only employers of large numbers of nurses works against the nursing profession to keep salaries depressed. Where there is a choice of employing health care institutions, collusion in setting wage scales is common. Nurses' salaries in an area's hospitals tend to be similar. Patients face the same situation when there is only one source of health care, or when providers collude in setting charges.

In situations where the quality of services is hard for the consumer to evaluate, unethical pricing practices occur frequently. Because of the nature of health care, providers must be aware of the potential for abuse when developing and controlling price structures. For example, in community health nursing, charges should be based on the nursing time, expertise, and overhead involved rather than on what the market will bear.

ETHICAL ISSUES IN ADVERTISING

Because advertising is the most visible element of the marketing mix, the ethics of advertising have been criticized frequently since the late 1950s, when Packard (1957) and Galbraith (1958) wrote their popular books, *The Hidden Persuaders* and *The Affluent Society*. Advertising is not, in itself, by nature and scope, unethical (Arrington, 1982). Ethical problems arise from the relationship of the advertising agency and its client and between the advertiser and the consumer (Ferrell, 1985).

Major Criticisms of Advertising

There are several major ethical criticisms of advertising. Advertising can: (1) violate a person's inherent right of autonomy; (2) lead to addictions, such as cigarettes, alcohol, and gambling; (3) be dishonest, because the goal is to make money, not spread truth; (4) degenerate into vulgarity; (5) stereotype women and minorities; (6) make extensive and inappropriate use of sex appeal, especially in advertising items such as clothing and perfume; and (7) be an "ethical morass" when directed to children (Turk, 1979).

Opportunity and peer interaction often work together to produce unethical behavior in advertising (Ferrell, 1985). As with other areas of business management, peers and top management have significant influence on most of the ethical decisions regarding advertising. It is therefore imperative that the organization have in place policies regarding ethics.

ETHICAL ISSUES IN INTERNATIONAL MARKETING

International marketing may seem to be far removed from the day-to-day world of nurses, but, with instant communication and a global marketplace, nurses must be aware of the ethical implications of decisions and actions in international marketing. Unethical marketing activities take place in the international arena all the time. As nurses and as citizens, we must be able to evaluate these activities. For direct application, this knowledge may not be necessary today, but it may be essential with tomorrow's technology. Also, many health care organizations, such as Humana, are international (see Case Study 13). The number will no doubt increase.

Developed nations are frequently criticized for marketing harmful products to the Third World. Harmful products are of two types: those that are banned in the United States or other developed countries, and those that are unsuitable to developing countries. An example of a product banned in the United States, but sold abroad, is the insecticide DDT. Infant formula is an unsuitable product to sell in developing countries, because often mothers cannot read and therefore cannot make the formula correctly; also, because there is a widespread lack of potable water, making prepared formula is unsafe.

The Marketing Mix

Ethical problems affect all aspects of the marketing mix in the multinational marketplace. Examples of these problems are discussed according to elements of the marketing mix. Ethical questions are raised for your deliberation as you consider a marketing approach to your nursing practice.

Product

Drugs.   Pharmaceutical manufacturers have been accused of unethical practice in the development and sale of contraceptives in Third World countries. In developing oral contraceptives, clinical trials were done in Puerto Rico and some developing nations rather than in the United States. Is it ethical to risk the lives and health of poor women? The benefit to the countries involved was the control of the growth in population. However, an important question was whether the women had been given sufficient information for them to give *informed* consent to participate in the research.

While the FDA has refused approval of the drug Depo-Provera for sale in the United States, Upjohn continues to sell the drug to the Third World. If we believe the drug is unsafe for personal use, how can we continue selling it to others? Other reliable, safe means of birth control are available.

Cigarettes.   While former Surgeon General C. Everett Koop worked toward a smoke-free society, and as each year fewer Americans smoke, tobacco companies are actively working to increase market share and market size abroad. Is it ethical to increase exports of a product that causes disease, disability, and death? In many of the countries where trade officials are working very hard to break down barriers, resources are too scarce to cope with the health problems (morbidity, mortality, and lost productivity) that tobacco addiction brings. Since we do not look kindly upon the importation of addicting substances, how can we justify exporting this one? In fighting for relaxation of trade barriers for cigarettes, the United States government is wasting bargaining leverage for other products such as textiles and semiconductors. It is also exchanging its image of world leader for that of "Ugly American" because of the aggressive marketing of cigarettes (Schmeisser, 1988).

Price

Dumping. American firms have accused Japan of dumping microchips and other products in the United States. *Dumping* is selling a product at less than cost to increase market share. This action could be seen as beneficial because it lowers the cost to consumers, but it can also be seen as injurious to the American microchip industry. Most, if not all, countries (including the United States) have been accused of dumping at some time. Dumping is considered unethical, because it violates rights and justice principles and may violate the utilitarian standard (Fritzche, 1985).

Recruitment. Recruitment of nurses from some foreign countries is relatively easy, based on price. Salaries in the United States are high in relation to those in most countries. However, we must ask if recruiters disclose the cost of living and disposable income factors in the United States. On the other side of the exchange are questions about the recruits' understanding of American culture and their ability to speak English, both of which have an impact on the quality of care given. What support is given to these nurses to help them adjust? Does reliance on recruitment of foreign nurses foster a failure to develop nursing as an attractive career for Americans, and compromise the quality of care for future patients in this country? In view of the world-wide nursing shortage, is foreign recruitment a fair practice? How would we look upon the British or Canadians recruiting American nurses for work in England or Canada?

Promotion

Bribes. Payoffs and bribes are illegal to facilitate trade within the United States and within some foreign countries. Their use is also illegal for international commerce under the Foreign Corrupt Practices Act of 1977. The problem with bribes is that a few benefit at the expense of society in general. Companies with adequate resources flourish; less capitalized companies are shut out of the competition for business. Bribes carry with them no redeeming social value.

When health care providers deal with companies such as pharmaceutical and medical suppliers, they should avoid even the semblance of taking a payoff. Be wary of accepting financial support for programs. You may find that doing so unduly influences your policies, and is not in the best interest of patients in the long run. Additionally, salespeople may expect more, in terms of your using their product, than was stated when you accepted the token gift or negotiated a contract (MacPherson, 1987).

Advertising.   As American tobacco companies lost customers in the United States and Canada, they became very aggressive in Asia. Their activities have been equated with the Opium Wars of the 1840s (Schmeisser, 1988). With the help of the federal government, these companies are demanding and winning the right to advertise cigarettes in countries where such advertisements have previously been prohibited. These advertisements do not include health warnings. Long-term threats to public health are being created.

It is the federal government that negotiates trade policy, and thereby promotes smoking in other countries. A serious ethical question here is whether the United States government should promote the sale of a hazardous product abroad. Can we condone this behavior when we recognize the societal costs and are decreasing the use of cigarettes in our own country? The American Public Health Association, the American Heart Association, the American Lung Association, and the American Cancer Society have joined forces to limit the exportation of tobacco products.

ETHICAL ISSUES IN MARKETING DECISIONS

Research has consistently demonstrated that several factors shape the ethical behavior of persons in organizations (Baumhart, 1961; Bartels, 1967; Brenner & Molander, 1977; Hunt, Chonko, & Wilcox, 1984). These factors are: the individual's personal code, the attitudes and actions of superiors, the behavior of peers, the organization's policies, the ethical practices of the industry, and financial circumstances. Because of the many factors contributing to unethical conduct, policies must be developed to ensure ethical decision-making. Unethical marketing decisions often have significant personal, organizational, and societal costs.

Personal costs incurred from unethical marketing decisions are high. A manager who makes an unethical decision can be held liable if the action is illegal as well as unethical. Decisions in product liability cases indicate that managers who knowingly decide to market unsafe products are subject to the same criminal charges and liability as are the organizations for which they work. For example, in international commerce, the Foreign Corrupt Practices Act of 1977 prohibits the bribery of foreign officials to obtain contracts for overseas business. For each payment of a bribe, the organization is subject to a $1 million fine. The manager who makes the decision to pay the bribe is subject to a $10,000 fine for each bribe paid and a maximum of five years in prison.

Organizational costs are also substantial. Society extracts severe economic penalties from an organization that engages in unethical practices. A prime example is the experience of the Swiss-owned Nestlé Company in selling infant formula to Third World countries. In this situation, Nestlé marketed infant formula aggressively, apparently ignoring the fact that the product would most likely be used unsafely, because of unsanitary environmental conditions (especially lack of potable water) and the fairly high illiteracy rate of the mothers. These conditions did in fact lead to improper use of the product and high rates of infant malnutrition and mortality. A large amount of international media coverage was given to this problem. The Nestlé Company incurred significant financial losses, negative publicity was a public relations nightmare, and worldwide boycotts of other Nestlé products led to further significant losses of sales.

This episode had an impact on the industry as well. Shareholder protests were filed in 1975 at the annual meetings of American infant formula companies. Universities and the Rockefeller and Ford Foundations took positions sharply criticizing the lack of response of the companies. Religious organizations coordinated shareholder's campaigns. Governments of Third World countries passed legislation severely restricting the sale of baby bottles, nipples, and pacifiers, as well as formula, because of the health hazard they present (Sethi & Post, 1985).

Many societal costs from unethical marketing practices are incurred. Most, if not all, unethical practices have victims. In the Nestlé case, considerable harm was inflicted upon the infants and their families. When people buy unsafe products, when they buy products because of misleading advertising, or when they buy fixed-price products, they are victims of unethical marketing practices. Groups that are especially vulnerable are the young, elderly, poor, illiterate, mentally or physically handicapped, and recent immigrants. These groups cannot afford the costs, cannot cope with the problems, and must either bear the costs under hardship or gain assistance from society.

Another cost to society is the disadvantage unethical firms cause ethical companies. Eventually, as in the Nestlé case, the industry suffers. Society may be unable to purchase wanted products at fair cost. All this leads to a significantly tarnished image of business, and especially of marketers. Respondents to a 1983 Gallup Poll ranked salespeople and advertising practitioners at the bottom of the ethics scale. Twenty-three professions were ranked higher (Laczniak & Murphy, 1985).

Improving Marketing Ethics in Organizations

Baumhart (1961) found that the single most important factor in the ethical climate of an organization is the attitude and behavior of top management.

Subsequent research supports this finding. In fact, it is one of the few undisputed findings of business ethics research (Laczniak & Murphy, 1985). Top nursing management must be ever-mindful of their influence on other managers and staff. All nurses must tend to ethics in the everyday life of the organization.

Policies of the organization must reflect an ethical position. For instance, profit cannot be the primary criterion for evaluation of performance. Profit and efficiency are important to any business, but they must be balanced by other values. These other values assist in the definition of boundaries for activities to achieve profit and efficiency objectives. Policies can be used to spell out other important ethical and socially responsible behaviors.

An example of the well-being of the customer taking precedence over short-term profit is the action of Johnson & Johnson (J&J) several years ago, when faced with contaminated Tylenol capsules. Seven people died after taking capsules containing cyanide, after an individual, who was in no way connected with the company, poisoned the capsules in retail stores. Within the week, J&J began a total product recall, which cost the company an estimated $50 million after taxes (Gardner, 1982). When further tampering occurred, J&J stopped making capsules. It also spearheaded an industry movement to develop more effective, tamper-proof packaging.

In sharp contrast is Ford Motor Company's behavior when confronted with the Ford Pinto's dismal safety record. The Pinto had a fuel system problem that produced fires when the car was involved in a collision. More than 500 deaths were linked to this problem, leading some to describe the Pinto as a fire trap on wheels. Ford was aware of the problem before the statistics revealed it (Dowie, 1977), but Ford had conducted a cost-benefit analysis and had decided that the more cost-effective way to handle the problem was to deal with the accidents rather than recall and repair the cars. This decision showed a flagrant disregard for customer welfare and the domination of the profit motive.

There is an interdependency between organizations and their employees. Organizations that fail to develop mutually accepted and shared ethical values tend to be unable to withstand stress. The sharing of these values is a positive force, not a constraint (McCoy, 1983).

Robin and Reidenbach (1987) advocate an approach that introduces and maintains ethical and socially responsible values in the organization. Values are consistently applied in the development of marketing strategies and throughout the marketing process. This approach begins with a mission statement to guide the work of the organization and development of the organization's ethical profile. The primary purpose for the organization's existence is expressed in its mission statement. The ethical profile provides broad, general guidelines for identifying ethical stances and for developing more specific objectives. It is a statement concerning how the organization chooses to interact with its publics. Similar in importance and function to the mission statement, the ethical profile projects an image to all the publics of the organization, whether internal or external. The ethical profile and the mission statement must be consistent. A lack of consistency will lead to confusion on the part of the general public, stockholders, managers, and employees, while consistency will make for easy, clear communication.

The profile is based on the strategic planning that underlies development of the mission statement. Consider ideas coming from opportunities, threats, organizational history and mission, current corporate image, personal preferences of owners and management, and any other resource that seems appropriate. Ethical profiles can be developed from any or all of these sources or situations.

An example of corporate behavior springing from an ethical profile is McDonald's concern for chronically or terminally ill children and their families that led to the establishment of Ronald McDonald's Houses. These houses were established near major medical centers to enable families to stay with sick children during treatment. McDonald's saw a need and responded to that need as an opportunity to help a segment of its market. Likewise, the Nurses Network of Pelham (Case Study 6) saw a need for respite care, and responded to that need with a program that satisfied the needs and wants of handicapped children and the community, as well as the nurses' needs. Proctor & Gamble (P&G) also used its special resources in an ethical and socially responsible way several years ago during the investigation of toxic shock syndrome linked to the P&G Rely tampon. P&G assisted the Centers for Disease Control by loaning them personnel with needed expertise. In looking for market opportunities that are consistent with your mission and ethical profile, assess the problems surrounding you as well as those of consumers, suppliers, and competition.

Threats to an organization can come from any situation or group that affects the marketing exchange. Anything that may discredit the organization is a threat. Proactive behavior to prevent a potential threat from becoming an actual threat can serve the company well. Many companies use environmental threats as a springboard to action. These efforts work to their advantage as well as to the advantage of the general public.

An organization's history, mission, and current image can also provide material for an ethical profile. While it has generally been the financial industry that has most depended on tradition to develop an image and ethical position, tradition can also be a rich source for health care organizations. Some institutions have been pioneers while providing high-quality services to patients. An example is the Visiting Nurse Service of New York. This kind of history can clearly help structure an ethical profile.

In order for the ethical profile to be useful in the day-to-day life of an organization, it must be easily translated into actions by the employees. Robin and Reidenbach (1987) give the following examples as appropriate statements to support customer orientation, product and service quality, and environmental concern:

> Treat customers with respect, concern, and honesty, the way you yourself would want to be treated or the way you would want your family treated. Make and market products you would feel comfortable and safe having your own family use. Treat the environment as though it were your own property. (p. 55)

Exhibit 8-3 shows one company's (Medtronic) working profile, that they have called corporate objectives. Medtronic publicizes its corporate objectives well, in part by publishing them on internal media and by giving them to the general public on business cards. Their approach has been successful in sales, image, and productivity.

EXHIBIT 8-3   One Company's Corporate Objectives (Working Profile)

To contribute to human welfare by application of biomedical engineering in the research, design, manufacture and sale of instruments or appliances that alleviate pain, restore health, and extend life.

To direct our growth in the areas of biomedical engineering where we display maximum strength and ability; to gather people and facilities that tend to augment these areas; to continuously build on these areas through education and knowledge assimilation; to avoid participation in areas where we cannot make unique and worthy contributions.

To strive without reserve for the greatest possible reliability and quality in our products; to be the unsurpassed standard of comparison and to be recognized as a company of dedication, honesty, integrity and service.

To make a fair profit on current operations to meet our obligations, sustain our growth and reach our goals.

To recognize the personal worth of employees by providing an employment framework that allows personal satisfaction in work accomplished, security, advancement opportunity and means to share in the company's success.

To maintain good citizenship as a company.

MEDTRONIC

Reprinted with permission.

CONCLUSION

Nurses are familiar with dealing with the ethical problems of patient care. However, not all problems of ethics confronting nurses are clinical. As health care becomes more competitive because of scarce resources, and as nurses participate in business and marketing decisions, nurses must examine related moral issues. Health care institutions cannot make decisions based solely on economic criteria. The public is holding everyone, individuals and organizations alike, accountable for the ethical implications and outcomes of decisions. That health care facilities exist to deliver health care cannot be overlooked or forgotten in the quest for market share or profitability. Institutions need to be able to identify the values that undergird their decisions and policies, and so must the nursing division. Society is holding professionals at all levels accountable for a multifaceted bottom line that includes quality and ethics as well as finances.

REFERENCES

Aroskar, M.A. (1984). Ethics are important in allocating health resources. *The American Nurse, 16*(1), 5, 20.

Arrington, R.L. (1982). Advertising and behavior control. *Journal of Business Ethics, 1*(1), 3–12.

Bartels, R. (1967). A model of ethics in marketing. *Journal of Marketing, 31*(1), 20–26.

Baumhart, R.C. (1961). How ethical are businessmen? *Harvard Business Review, 39*(4), 6–19, 156–176.

Bowie, N. (1982). "Role" as a moral concept in health care. *Journal of Medical Philosophy, 7,* 57–63.

Brenner, S.N., & Molander, E.A. (1977). Is the ethics of business changing? *Harvard Business Review, 55*(1), 57–71.

Cadbury, A. (1987). Ethical managers make their own rules. *Harvard Business Review, 65*(5), 69–73.

Crisham, P. (1981). Measuring moral judgment in nursing dilemmas. *Nursing Research, 30,* 104–110.

Davis, A.J. (1982). Helping your staff address ethical dilemmas. *Journal of Nursing Administration, 12*(2), 9–13.

Dowie, M. (1977). How Ford put two million firetraps on wheels. *Business and Society Review, Fall*(23), 46–55.

Ferrell, O.C. (1985). Implementing and monitoring ethics advertising. In G.R. Laczniak & P.E. Murphy (Eds.), *Marketing ethics* (pp. 27–40). Lexington, MA: Lexington Books.

Frey, C.J., & Kinnear, T.C. (1979). Legal constraints and marketing research: Review and call to action. *Journal of Marketing Research, 16,* 295–302.

Friedman, M. (1962). *Capitalism and freedom.* Chicago, IL: Chicago University Press.

Fritzsche, D.J. (1985). Ethical issues in multinational marketing. In G.R. Laczniak & P.E. Murphy (Eds.), *Marketing ethics* (pp. 85–96). Lexington, MA: Lexington Books.

Fry, S. (1983). The social responsibilities of nursing. *Nursing Economics, 1*(1), 61–64, 72.

Galbraith, J.K. (1958). *The affluent society.* Boston, MA: Houghton Mifflin.

Gardner, J.B. (1982, November 8). When a brand name gets hit by bad news. *US News & World Report,* p. 71.

Gellerman, S.W. (1986). Why "good" managers make bad ethical choices. *Harvard Business Review, 64*(4), 85–90.

Hedin, B.A. (1989). Nursing, education, and sterile ethical fields. *Advances in Nursing Science, 11*(3), 43–52.

Hunt, S.D., Chonko, L.B., & Wilcox, J.B. (1984). Ethical problems of marketing researchers. *Journal of Marketing Research, 21*, 309–324.

Kehoe, W.J. (1985). Ethics, price fixing, and the management of price strategy. In G.R. Laczniak & P.E. Murphy (Eds.), *Marketing ethics* (pp. 71–84). Lexington, MA: Lexington Books.

Ketefian, S. (1981a). Critical thinking, educational preparation and development of moral judgment among selected groups of practicing nurses. *Nursing Research, 30*, 93–103.

Ketefian, S. (1981b). Moral reasoning and moral behavior among selected groups of practicing nurses. *Nursing Research, 30*, 171–176.

Laczniak, G.R., & Murphy, P.E. (1985). *Marketing ethics: Guidelines for managers.* Lexington, MA: Lexington Books.

Lohr, S. (1988, August 7). British health service faces a crisis in funds and delays. *The New York Times,* pp. 1, 12.

MacPherson, K.I. (1987) Health care policy, values, and nursing. *Advances in Nursing Science, 9*(3), 1–11.

Mayberry, M.A. (1986). Ethical decision making: A response of hospital nurses. *Nursing Administration Quarterly, 10*(3), 75–81.

McCoy, B.H. (1983). The parable of Sadhu. *Harvard Business Review, 61*(5), 103–108.

Murphy, C.P. (1976). *Levels of moral reasoning in a selected group of nursing practitioners.* Unpublished doctoral dissertation. New York: Teachers College, Columbia University.

Murphy, C.P. (1978). The moral situation in nursing. In E.L. Bandman & B. Bandman (Eds.), *Bioethics and human rights* (pp. 313–320). Boston, MA: Little, Brown.

Newton, L. (1982). Collective responsibility in health care. *Journal of Medical Philosophy, 7*, 11–21.

Packard, V. (1957). *The hidden persuaders.* New York: Pocket Books.

Robin, D.P., & Reidenbach, R.E. (1987). Social responsibility, ethics, and marketing strategy: Closing the gap between concept and application. *Journal of Marketing, 51*(1), 44–58.

Schmeisser, P. (1988, July 10). Pushing cigarettes overseas. *The New York Times Magazine,* pp. 16–22, 62.

Sethi, S.P., & Post, J.E. (1985). The marketing of infant formula in less developed countries. In G.R. Laczniak & P.E. Murphy (Eds.), *Marketing ethics* (pp. 165–177). Lexington, MA: Lexington Books.

Sietsema, M.R., & Spradley, B.W. (1987). Ethics and administrative decision making. *Journal of Nursing Administration, 17*(4), 28–32.

Silva, M. (1983). The American Nurses Association position statement on nursing and social policy: Philosophical and ethical dimensions. *Journal of Advanced Nursing, 8*, 147–151.

Tull, D.S., & Hawkins, D.I. (1985). Ethical issues in marketing research. In G.R. Laczniak & P.E. Murphy (Eds.), *Marketing ethics* (pp. 55–70). Lexington, MA: Lexington Books.

Turk, P. (1979). Children's television advertising: An ethical morass for business and government. *Journal of Advertising, 8*(1), 4–8.

PART II

Marketing in Practice

Marketing a Professional Nurses' Association*

Ruth R. Alward, EdD, RN
Caroline Camuñas, EdM, RN

THE MARKETING PROBLEM

Many professional associations are faced with a declining membership or one that is small in proportion to the potential membership. This is true of the American Nurses Association, the American Medical Association, and the American Bar Association, as well as other nonprofit membership organizations. Member recruitment and retention is crucial to these organizations if they are to remain viable. Membership dues are generally the primary source of revenue; funds from other sources are often minimal. Low membership rosters mean low income, which, in turn, constrains activities. Less activity leads to diminished interest, which further decreases ability to recruit new members and increases the difficulty of member retention. The downward spiral becomes difficult to stop.

In the late winter of 1986, the New York Counties Registered Nurses Association (NYCRNA), also called District 13 of the New York State Nurses Association (NYSNA), established a task force to develop a marketing plan to achieve a healthy membership. The task force was made up of six members; all had research experience and some also had a working knowledge of the marketing process.

Not since 1980 had the membership numbers approached 6,000, yet this was the number consistently quoted. Of the approximately 26,000 possible members, only 5,750 nurses actually belonged to the association in 1986. The low point occurred in 1983 with 5,208 members; 1987 ended with 5,298. For these eight years, the average number of members was 5,508 (see Figure 1.1). The board of directors felt that membership must be increased, and discussed strategies that might be useful. In 1984, the bylaws were changed to allow membership in the district association without belonging to NYSNA. This change resulted in only 25 district-only members in two years. Although gross membership figures were available, the number of new members, renewing members, and those who failed to renew were not available.

*The authors wish to acknowledge funding provided by the New York Counties Registered Nurses Association for this study. We also thank Elizabeth Vecchione, EdD, RN, for her contributions to the study.

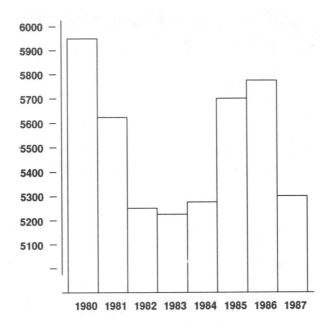

Figure 1.1.   NYCRNA Membership

It is not clear what brought about the dramatic decreases in 1982 or the large increase in 1985. The increase may have been related to the dissemination of a new, attractive brochure beginning in May 1985. These changes may also have been due to certification or decertification of bargaining units requiring NYSNA membership. The more recent decrease of 465 members may be attributed to changes in the tax law eliminating dues as a deduction. However, regardless of the causes, the fact remains that the association failed to retain members. It is reasonable to assume that needs and wants were not satisfied.

Another problem was that many members of NYSNA had joined for collective bargaining purposes and did not belong to the district association. Other problems of the association were too many inactive members and too many nonrenewing members. The demographic characteristics of members were unknown. The site of meetings was possibly a problem; meetings were held in one midtown location. No one knew if this caused mass transit, traffic, or parking problems for many members.

During 1986, the association had major financial problems. Expenses exceeded revenues. The financial objective was to correct the problem and create a cash flow situation that would allow for increased activities. Accomplishment of these objectives was essential to the life of the association.

MARKET RESEARCH

Internal Analysis

It was easy to see that the association was not market or customer oriented. Informal polling of active members and the leadership revealed that they had a product orientation (see Chapter 2). They ascribed nurses' failure to belong to the association to ignorance and lack of motivation rather than to a bad product. It was felt that if nonmembers only knew how important it was to support the association, they would join. Generally, members did not see the need for market research, and no market research had ever been done.

Most members defined *marketing* as selling. A sales orientation was identified in the solutions suggested to increase membership. Better salesmanship was encouraged. Included in this approach were a membership drive and other recruitment activities. Because we could not afford to advertise, there was an effort to increase publicity. Hence, public relations activities were enhanced.

Public relations was emphasized by increasing communications and developing a new image. The numbers of public service announcements and press releases sent to the media were increased. The attractive membership recruitment brochure had been developed with professional assistance in 1985. By 1986, the office was redecorated and a logo was in development. These activities were all centered on communication and the association itself. No effort had yet been made to identify and meet the needs and wants of members. It was believed that one "really good" strategy, such as a membership drive, was all that was needed. The leadership assumed that other nurses associations were our competition. They did not recognize that NYCRNA competed with work, family, and leisure activities for professional nurses' time and interest. Additionally, no attention was paid to retention of present members.

The marketing task force wanted to make the association into a customer- or member-focused organization with a marketing orientation. We wanted to know who and where the customer was, what the customer's characteristics were, what the customer's perceptions, needs, and wants were, and how they might change, and whether the customer was satisfied. In order to learn this, we had to do marketing research. We would then have to segment the broader market in a deep and sophisticated manner, identify a target market, reconceptualize the competition, and change products or services to meet customer needs and wants. We wanted to make the entire organization responsive to customers.

Initially, the task force planned to do focus group interviews to get an adequate sense of the direction quantitative studies should take and to identify questions to ask. Because of the weak financial situation of the association, it was not possible to hire focus group consultants (see Chapter 4). In fact, because of cash flow difficulties, the research was delayed for one year.

The Survey

Marketing research was undertaken to determine why nurses join professional organizations and what they want and expect from such groups. This information was important to meet the needs of present members and to attract new members. We decided to use survey research because of its flexibility and its capacity to meet our requirements, including budgetary constraints.

Members and nonmembers were surveyed. A total of 750 questionnaires were distributed to members of NYSNA who did not belong to the district association. Seven hundred of these were mailed. A random mailing of 300 questionnaires was sent in June 1987. In August 1987, a second random mailing of 400 was sent. The remaining 50 surveys were given to nonmembers at the September 1987 district meeting to which many nonmembers came because of an NYSNA presentation.

Three hundred questionnaires were distributed to NYCRNA members. At the September 1987 membership meeting 100 questionnaires were passed out. The names of all the members who had attended this meeting were removed from our mailing list. A random mailing of 200 was then sent to members.

Throughout the study, a similar cover letter was used. It was signed by the president of the district association, and was modified only to satisfy the requirements of the two groups in the study. Computer-generated mailing labels and first-class, colorful, commemorative stamps were used. Stamped (metered-mail), self-addressed envelopes were enclosed to facilitate and increase response rates.

Results and Discussion of Findings

Of the surveys returned, 208 (27.7%) from nonmembers and 121 (40.3%) from members were usable. When chi-square analysis was undertaken, there were some statistically significant ($p < .05$) differences in the demographic data between members and nonmembers. Members tended to be older than nonmembers. The largest segment of nonmembers (31.1%) was in the 31–36 age group, while the largest group (22.6%) of members was in the 37–42 age group. Of the members, 78.9% were 37 years of age or older; 38.8% of nonmembers were 37 years or older.

As could be expected from the age differences, members had more years of nursing experience than nonmembers. The largest group of nonmembers (75, or 36.2%) had 6–10 years of experience. While 66.7% of members had 11 or more years of experience, 46.4% of nonmembers had this amount of experience.

The United States was the country of origin for 74.2% of all respondents: 84.2% of members and 68.2% of nonmembers. The largest immigrant group was Filipino, representing 6.7% of the total members (8 respondents) and 18.2% of the nonmembers (36 respondents). Other Asians made up 3.0% of nonmembers and 1.7%

of members. Additional groups were about equal in percentage of members and nonmembers.

Educational levels for the two groups showed considerable variation. Diploma programs provided the basic education for 33.5% of respondents, but members had a highly significant difference in amount of additional nursing education. While 39.4% of members were diploma graduates, only 4.8% did not subsequently earn degrees. Of the 30% of nonmembers who were diploma graduates, over two-thirds did not earn degrees. The baccalaureate was the basic education for 37.7% of all respondents; 39.6% of nonmembers and 34.6% of members. The percentage of members having the baccalaureate as the highest degree was 30.2%; the percentage of nonmembers was 42.9%. Fifty-four percent of members had graduate degrees; 14.8% of nonmembers had graduate degrees. The doctorate was the highest degree for 11.1% of members; one nonmember (0.5%) had a doctorate.

The positions held by respondents reflected their education: 69.1% of nonmembers and 32.5% of members were staff nurses; 9.3% of nonmembers and 5.7% of members were head nurses; 2.9% of nonmembers and 18.7% of members were educators; 14.6% of members were administrators and 5.7% were supervisors; 1.5% of nonmembers were administrators and 3.4% were supervisors.

Members of NYCRNA were more involved in other nursing associations as well. Seventy-four percent of members and 27% of nonmembers belonged to other nursing organizations. Forty-eight percent of members and 12% of nonmembers participated in task forces or committees; 15.1% of members and 3.4% of nonmembers were officers in those organizations.

Marital status and number of dependents were not significantly different in members and nonmembers.

Preferences of Members

There were differences in the kinds of articles members wanted to see in the association newsletter, the kinds of programs they preferred, and the other kinds of benefits in which they were interested. Current issues, professional development, legal, and clinical articles were preferred by the majority (Table 1.1). Similar membership meeting program topics were selected (Table 1.2). Of the benefits suggested, none was preferred by a majority of respondents (Table 1.3).

Preferences of Nonmembers

Nonmembers were asked if they had ever heard of NYCRNA. The letterhead identified the organization as both NYCRNA and District 13 of NYSNA. Of the 208 respondents who answered the question, 169 or 81.6% *had not heard of the organization.* Only 37 or 17.9% indicated that they had heard of NYCRNA; two were unsure. When asked if they were interested in joining, 102 or 49.3% checked no; 69 (33.3%) answered yes, and 20 (9.7%) wrote in "maybe." Sixteen (7.7%) did not respond to the question.

TABLE 1.1   Kinds of Articles Members Would Like to See in *The Calendar*

	Meeting sample n=70		Mail sample n=58		Total N=128	
	#	%	#	%	#	%*
Current issues	44	62.8	39	67.2	83	64.8
Professional development	46	65.7	27	46.5	73	57.0
Legal	42	60.0	30	51.7	72	56.3
Clinical	37	52.8	29	50.0	66	51.6
Political	37	52.8	12	20.6	49	38.3
Women's issues/studies	26	37.1	17	29.3	43	33.6
Personal/financial	23	32.8	18	31.0	41	32.0
Advice/consultation	21	30.0	16	27.5	37	28.9
Research	20	28.5	15	25.8	35	27.3
Managerial	23	32.8	12	20.6	35	27.3
Theory	11	15.7	9	15.5	20	15.6
History	12	17.1	4	6.8	16	12.5
Other					8	6.3

*Percentages do not add up to 100%, as respondents could select more than one item.

The midtown location of membership meetings was convenient for 129 (61.8%) of respondents; 89 (43%) found the time convenient. One hundred and twelve (54.1%) responded that district dues ($45 per year) were reasonable; 60 (29%) responded that the dues were too high; 35 (16.9%) did not answer the question.

For responses to the question, "What would make you interested in joining?" see Tables 1.4 and 1.5.

TABLE 1.2   Kinds of Programs Preferred by Members

	Meeting sample		Mail sample		Total	
	# 70	% 100.0	# 58	% 100.0	# 12	%* 100.0
Current issues	42	60.0	25	43.0	67	52.3
Professional development	17	24.2	17	29.3	34	26.6
Clinical	10	14.2	15	25.8	25	19.5
Personal/financial	0	0.0	9	15.5	9	7.0
Managerial	1	1.4	7	12.0	8	6.3
Other					3	2.3

*Percentages do not add up to 100%, as respondent's could select more than one item.

TABLE 1.3   Interest in Benefits

	Members n=121		Nonmembers n=208	
	#	%	#	%
Malpractice insurance	60	46.9		
Travel programs	47	36.7		
Health insurance	40	31.3	78	37.7
Discount houses/programs	40	31.3		
Disability insurance	36	28.1		
Dental insurance	36	28.1		
Life insurance	24	18.8	46	22.8
Other	2	1.6	5	2.4

TABLE 1.4   Nonmember Interest in Programs

	Continuing education		Membership meetings	
	#	%	#	%
Professional development	109	52.7	69	33.3
Personal/financial	61	29.5	44	21.3
Clinical	55	26.6	34	16.4
Managerial	28	13.5	22	10.6

TABLE 1.5   Nonmember Interest in Professional Development Benefits

	#	%
Social and professional networking	77	37.2
Political voice	45	21.7
Helping others	39	18.8
Leadership opportunities	34	16.4
Committee membership	21	10.1
Other	4	1.9

MARKETING STRATEGIES

Not having an effective marketing plan for the association had resulted in slowly dwindling numbers of members. This started a cycle of shrinking resources, decreasing activities, minimal impact of the organization on the community and on nursing, and an increasing number of nonmembers in the district. It was the task force's responsibility to develop a marketing plan. In developing the marketing plan, the task force started by reviewing the association's mission and goal statements as well as the results of the survey. We then determined strategies to reach our marketing goals. These were presented to the board of directors. Subsequently the board, officers, and committee chairpersons participated in a retreat to select and set marketing priorities, as well as to plan for the achievement of other goals and objectives. Some elements of the marketing plan are presented below. Advantages and disadvantages of some strategies are included to assist the reader.

The Marketing Plan

I. *Member Recruitment*

Without continual recruiting efforts, membership in most associations tends to decline, while fixed costs tend to increase. Recently, many professionals have lost association dues as an income tax deduction.

Strategy 1: Mount a well-planned campaign to increase registered nurses' awareness of the association, evaluated by a follow-up survey.

Tactic A.   Direct mailing campaign.

1. Choose segments to target from
   a. Staten Island
   b. specific zip codes
   c. specialty association lists
2. Costs depend on weight, mailing class, and materials
   Advantages:
   (a) audience selectivity
   (b) flexibility
   (c) no other ad competition
   (d) personalization
   Disadvantage:
   junk mail problem

Tactic B.   Develop a slide show about the NYCRNA for use at meetings, talks, and lectures.

    Rationale: Eighty-two percent of nonmembers surveyed had not heard of the association.

Tactic C. Begin a support group for foreign nurses.

    Rationale: The survey showed a statistically significant number of foreign-born nurses (especially Filipino) who do not belong to the association.

Tactic D. Other awareness tactics considered but not recommended due to cost and inappropriateness.

1. Telemarketing sales (using the telephone to solicit sales or contributions)
2. Advertising
   a. Newspapers (1990 prices for one ad for one day in *The New York Times*):

full page ad, daily, national	$53,752
full page ad, daily, northeast	$39,803
full page ad, Sunday, national	$47,968

   b. Television: $1,500 for 30 seconds (Chicago, 1986).
   Advantages:
       (a) appealing
       (b) high attention
   Disadvantages:
       (a) high cost
       (b) high clutter
       (c) fleeting exposure
       (d) little audience selectivity
   c. Radio: $700 for one-minute promotional drive time (Chicago, 1986).
   Advantage:
       mass use
   Disadvantages:
       (a) fleeting exposure
       (b) attention lower than to television
       (c) little audience selectivity
   d. Periodicals:
       (1) popular press: $120,130 for one-page, four-color ad in *Time* (1990)
       (2) journals: $5,691 for one-page, one-time, black-and-white ad; $6,284 for one-page, one-time, two-color ad; $7,796 for

one-page, one-time four-color ad in the *American Journal of Nursing* in 1990 (circulation: 268,000 in 1990).

Advantages:

(a) credibility, prestige

(b) high-quality reproduction

(c) long life

Disadvantages:

(a) long ad purchase lead time

(b) selectivity a problem; question of how many nonmembers read any given periodical

e. Outdoor billboards.

Strategy 2:   Establish programs to take nursing students through the stages of buyer readiness: awareness, knowledge, interest, desire, intention, joining (see Chapter 5).

Tactic A.   Give priority to program for graduate nursing students and to registered nurses earning undergraduate degrees.

> *Rationale:* The survey showed that members had more education after entry into practice than did nonmembers. The survey results also demonstrated that nonmembers tended to be younger than members. By targeting this segment, the buyer readiness process could be sped up. The literature confirmed that nurses actively engaged in practice for less than five years are significantly lower in the use of professional organizations than nurses who have been in practice for more than five years (Monnig, 1978; Yeager & Kline, 1983).

Tactic B.   Share study findings with educators and request that graduate and undergraduate schools encourage membership in professional organizations by incorporating this expectation into curricula.

Tactic C.   Provide field experience for students in district office.

Tactic D.   Send newsletter to schools on a regular basis.

Tactic E.   Provide schools with *First Job Brochure.*

Tactic F.   Give talks at nursing schools on professional issues.

Tactic G.   Make joining the association convenient for graduating seniors.

Tactic H.   Invite students to programs by sending flyers to schools.

Tactic I.   Send letters of congratulations to new graduates.

Tactic J.   Send letters to parents of new graduates suggesting gift memberships.

Tactic K.   Have membership brochure available at graduate schools.

Tactic L. Eliminate or reduce dues for first year after graduation.

> *Advantages:*
> (a) ease of access
> (b) new graduates have their whole career ahead of them in which to be members, especially if they are socialized to expectation of membership
> (c) many students are already registered nurses and can join immediately

> *Disadvantages:*
> (a) possibly 1–10 years before this segment joins
> (b) limited and decreasing number of students

Strategy 3: Develop a recruitment campaign.

Tactic A. Have membership committee plan and implement a membership drive, appointing nurse captains in major health care institutions.

Tactic B. Publicize the campaign and document progress with visual aids.

II. *Member Retention*

Members are the life blood of any organization; they are forgotten to its detriment. Satisfied members are vital to recruitment efforts. To recruit without retaining members is costly and counterproductive.

Strategy 1: Develop editorial policy for the newsletter to better meet the wants and needs of members.

Tactic A. Define and develop short-term and long-term goals for the format and content of the newsletter.

Tactic B. Use marketing survey findings to plan content.

Tactic C. Solicit articles according to priorities identified in the survey.

Tactic D. Publish short version of the annual report.

Strategy 2: Development of "What NYCRNA Is Doing For You" campaign. (For other campaign ideas, see Lamb-Mechanik & Block, 1984.)

Tactic A. Continually publicize activities and benefits of the association in newsletter.

> *Advantage:*
> less cost
> *Disadvantage:*
> not always read

Tactic B. Annual report in abbreviated format.

1. Published in newsletter
2. Direct mailing to members

> *Advantage:*
> focused publication
> *Disadvantages:*
> (a) additional cost
> (b) work to prepare
> *Rationale:* publicizing district activities will increase awareness and knowledge about organization.

Strategy 3: Develop bimonthly membership programs that better meet the needs of members.

Tactic A. Use marketing findings to plan programs.

Tactic B. Publicize meetings by posting flyers in hospitals and making announcements in hospital newsletters.

Strategy 4: Investigate offering malpractice insurance and a travel program because these benefits were rated highest in the marketing survey.

Strategy 5: Establish a committee on retention or a retention task force.

Strategy 6: Remind nonrenewing members by mail and telephone of their lapsed membership.

Strategy 7: Communicate marketing task force findings.

Tactic A. Publish study.

1. In the newsletter
2. In other professional journals

Tactic B. Make study available on request as appropriate.

> *Rationale:* It is important to inform members about association activities and to emphasize that the association is interested in the needs

and wants of members. (See Bywaters [1987] for discussion.) In addition, communication of research is professionally responsible.

III.   *Nursing Profession Recruitment*

Recruitment to nursing is a responsibility of the professional organization. Competition for college students has increased. By 1991, American colleges will award approximately 14,500 BSN degrees, compared to approximately 16,000 MD degrees (Green, 1987).

Strategy 1:   Develop recruitment strategies for both traditional and nontraditional students, such as minorities, second-career people, men, and undergraduate students who wish to change majors.

Tactic A.   Develop methods and materials to increase students' awareness of the potential of nursing as a career.

1. Brochures
2. Popular magazine articles
3. Newspaper articles
4. Talks at local high school career days

IV.   *Improved Relationship with NYSNA*

The district needs access to nurses who are joining the bargaining units under NYSNA. Approximately 5,000-5,500 nurses belong to NYSNA without membership in the district association.

Strategy 1:   Negotiate with NYSNA so that they encourage members to join their district associations.

Strategy 2:   Request that NYSNA preprint "District ___" on membership cards.

V.   *Improved Relationships with Hospitals and Other Employers of Nurses*

The district needs access to students and nurses who work in local health care institutions.

Strategy: Negotiate improved relationships.

Tactic A.   Invite deans and nurse executives to an open house to discuss programs, issues, and concerns.

Tactic B.   Meet regularly with deans and nurse executives to continue dialogue.

VI.   *Management Information Systems Development*

NYCRNA needs current data in order to assess membership situation and to market the organization to new members, nonrenewing members, and nonmembers.

Strategy 1:   Streamline system for district-only renewals.

Tactic A.   Design an attractive renewal form that requests more information.

1. Age
2. Basic education
3. Highest education
4. Position
5. Employer category
6. Specialty

Tactic B.   Put information on computer to facilitate data access.

Strategy 2:   Develop a system to track other member renewals.

Strategy 3:   Do market research as necessary and appropriate.

Tactic A.   Ask carefully designed questions to get information needed.

Tactic B.   Pilot as necessary.

Tactic C.   Invest in franked envelopes (preferred over stamped envelopes).

Tactic D.   Send single-purpose mailings; combined mailings are *not* cost effective.

CONCLUSION

In June 1988, officers, board members, and chairpersons had a strategic planning session for the association. The direction for the next several years was set. Goals were identified and were subsequently brought to the committees to guide their work. The committees designed and implemented programs to achieve goals. Having the research-based marketing plan facilitated organizational work.

REFERENCES

Bywaters, D.R. (1987). Surveys: The smart manager's crystal ball. *Association & Society Manager, 19*(4), 8–13.

Green, K. (1987). What the freshmen tell us. *American Journal of Nursing, 87*, 1612–1615.

Lamb-Mechanik, D., & Block, D.E. (1984). Professional membership recruitment: A marketing approach. *Nursing Economic$, 2*, 398–402.

Monnig, Sr. G. (1978). Professionalism of nurses and physicians. In N.L. Chaska (Ed.), *The nursing profession: Views through the mist* (pp. 35–49). New York: McGraw-Hill.

Yeager, S.J., & Kline, M. (1983). Professional association membership of nurses: Factors affecting membership and the decision to join an association. *Research in Nursing and Health, 6*, 45–52.

Marketing Education Programs

Nancy Ann Sickles Corbett, EdM, RN
Susan J. Costello, BSN, RN
Maryanne P. Doran, BSN, RN
Carol Kronick-Mest, MSN, RN
Reba Stephan Scharf, BSN, RN
Lorraine C. Shoenly, MSN, RN, C, CCRN, CEN
Janet Gear-Wolfe, BSN, RN

THE MARKETING SITUATION

Zurbrugg Memorial Hospital is a 350-bed community hospital located in New Jersey close to Philadelphia. A range of health care services are provided: pediatrics, maternity, medicine, surgery, psychiatric services, and addiction treatment. The hospital also serves as a clinical site for two baccalaureate degree, one associate degree, one diploma, and one practical nurse program.

Patients who use the hospital tend to be drawn from three towns surrounding the hospital. These towns are middle-class communities in which home ownership is the norm. People work either in local industry or in Philadelphia, and hold a mixture of blue- and white-collar positions. There are still large farms in the area providing employment.

About one half of the patient population has Medicare coverage; the rest have Medicaid, commercial insurance, or no insurance. The county population is one of the fastest growing in the state. There is great diversity in patient age. Many of our patients are over 65 years of age and suffer from a variety of chronic illnesses, typically correlated with increasing age. At the other end of the age continuum, the obstetrical service delivers about 2,200 babies a year, a number that has remained stable for several years.

The Department of Education is responsible for coordination and planning of all education activities except continuing medical education. It has multiple publics whose needs must be considered in the planning and implementation of its various programs and activities. We felt the need for a good marketing program in order to promote high-quality health education to several publics.

243

MARKETING STRATEGIES

Segmentation and Targeting

A good marketing program was essential to accomplish the goals of an effective Department of Education. Because the department has multiple publics, we segmented our market into physician, nurse, community, and patient groups. We then targeted those who play roles in providing, promoting, and using services. This resulted in our targeting physicians and nurses along with the patient and the community. Marketing enabled us to be responsive to rapidly changing needs, and to maintain efficiency and effectiveness. Using the marketing process has helped us to meet consumer needs and wants both within the hospital and in the larger community. An example of how we met staff nurses' education needs was our "brown bag seminars," explained in Exhibit 2.1.

Marketing Patient Education Programs to Physicians

Physicians are an important targeted segment of our market. They refer patients to both inpatient and outpatient education programs, and thus must be familiar with the programs offered. We had to gain their acceptance of our role in patient education, especially in preparing the patient and family for discharge. Early discharge is a critical concern because of DRG reimbursement and the concomitant need of the hospital for financial success.

Patient education programs have to be acceptable to the physician, in that learning outcomes must be supportive of the goal of treatment. How do we define the product from the physician's perspective? It has been our experience that physicians do not respond to surveys dealing with patient education. Therefore, we have to use a less formal means to obtain the information we need. We find it helpful to spend as much time as possible with physicians in order to understand the product they require. Making rounds with physicians is an excellent way to observe the kinds of information they share with patients. Informal conversations in the cafeteria are also helpful. In our institution, the physicians tend to cluster together for lunch. At breakfast, however, they scatter at various tables. We make it our business to join them whenever possible to gather information.

Defining the product from the physician's perspective was only part of our marketing strategy. Many physicians did not perceive a need for patient education, so we had to create a demand for our product. Discharge planning rounds provide a mechanism to identify patients who have learning needs. We make it a point to approach physicians who rarely use education programs and request referrals for patients with obvious or complex needs. All physicians with admitting privileges receive written descriptions of new and revised programs so that they know what is available. Patient classes held in highly visible locations increase physician exposure to the programs. Therefore, the location of inpatient classes is used as a promotional strategy. While we still have physicians who are hesitant to refer their patients, we are seeing steady increases in referrals for the cardiac and diabetic classes.

EXHIBIT 2.1   Brown Bag Seminars

From an analysis of program evaluations and attendance patterns at staff development programs, we developed our "brown bag" seminars. Staff nurses found it difficult to complete their work and attend classes during the day. They did have an established regular pattern for covering one another so that they could leave the unit for their noon meal break. Plans were made to conduct informational discussions of clinical topics for staff nurses during lunch time.

The original plan was for nurses to bring their lunches to the conference area and eat during a 20-minute lecture and discussion. It was soon apparent that the nurses were unable to get their lunches and arrive at the conference room on time. Evaluations included requests that lunch be provided at these seminars. We attempted to solve this problem by asking the dietary department to prepare brown bag lunches and sell them at the seminar. This was beyond the resources of the cafeteria. Somewhat hesitantly, we approached a drug company representative and asked if the company would provide lunch. The representative was delighted to do so! Many other vendors have since provided lunch. From the vendors' point of view, this makes good public relations sense.

Lunch was added to the agenda and was advertised. Topics are advertised two weeks in advance using flyers and word of mouth with management. Staff nurses are personally contacted by staff development instructors during unit rounds on the day. Fifteen minutes before the presentation, overhead announcements are made to remind staff to prepare to leave the unit for the half hour. The 20-minute sessions are repeated twice, giving all staff an opportunity to attend.

Evaluations and attendance have improved. Attendance has gone from the original 5 hardy attendees to 25 nurses at each session. Interestingly, physicians are also beginning to attend and participate in the discussions.

Marketing Education Programs to Patients

Marketing health education to patients is accomplished in a number of ways. Patient education literature is available in waiting rooms, lounges, and other areas accessible to the public. We hold programs in visible areas and encourage patient attendance. Questionnaires and evaluation forms are mailed after discharge. Including a stamped, self-addressed envelope increases returns.

We know that patients who have a positive experience with education programs will "sell" the programs to other patients. They do this informally through casual conversations in the patient lounges. Some experienced patients become actively involved in the teaching process. An additional benefit is the support they give one another. When patients who have had a positive experience with our programs return to the community, they spread the good news about our services.

Marketing Patient Education Programs to the Community

The community is a very significant population to target. Because of the importance of the community, some of our educational programs are offered free of charge. We do this to promote the hospital as well as those education programs for which we do charge. We are increasing awareness of the hospital in the community by these activities. The hospital benefits by establishing a reputation for high-quality, patient-centered programs. Visibility and the perception of good care increase use of other hospital services.

Coverage in the print media is an excellent way to reach the general community. Positive news items are publicity for both the hospital and the specific education program. The public relations department helps us by sending press releases, but it is our responsibility to inform them of possible newsworthy activities. Another proven tactic has been to respond to requests from media personnel for interviews about specific programs. Our *Diabetes and You* program was recently featured in a prominent article, complete with photographs, by a large metropolitan newspaper. We also respond to requests for speakers on health-related topics. This is good public relations, and it gets us in the news. Local newspapers cover these events and publish reports about them.

Paid advertisements are used for specific programs. We carefully monitor the results of these advertisements to learn which newspapers provide us with the maximum return on our investment. The most expensive newspaper is not always the most effective. Matching the newspaper and the target audience is essential.

Brochures are used to reach segments of the community. For instance, we send brochures advertising health promotion programs to local businesses to interest them in providing health information to their employees. We emphasize that these programs can result in decreased ill and absent time and reduced injuries.

Specific Programs

Diabetes and You

One of our ongoing community education programs is *Diabetes and You,* a self-care seminar for Types I and II diabetic patients and their families. This is a series of classes scheduled once a week for four weeks. Patient evaluations are used to determine how well the program meets patients' needs. After analysis of the evaluation data, we make changes in the program to be more responsive to these needs. Based on the recent evaluations, we designed an advanced second series that will run for five weeks and for which we will charge a fee. The original program was offered at no charge, but after program evaluation, we decided to assess a $25 fee.

Diabetes and You is promoted throughout the community in a variety of ways. The program is listed in the public events column of local newspapers, and flyers are sent to past participants of programs. Physicians refer their patients for education. Word-of-mouth recommendations from patients who have gone through the program also helps to promote the program. We also received positive publicity when a nurse from our department gave a talk to teen diabetics at the local high school.

Since our Department of Education does inpatient as well as outpatient education, we establish contact with patients during their hospitalizations and inform them of the outpatient program. Staff nurses also refer patients and families to the program.

We have yet to establish a price for the new advanced series, *Diabetes and You, II*. Insurance carriers do not reimburse patients for outpatient education programs. It is important to remember that the price we set must not exceed what patients are willing and able to pay. On the other hand, it is a human tendency to devalue what is offered free or for a small fee. At this time, it is not necessary for the program to be self-supporting; Zurbrugg Memorial Hospital is willing to support the program as a means of maintaining positive relations with both physicians and the community.

There are indications that there may be changes in the reimbursement mechanism that will provide third-party payment for outpatient diabetes education. Our current program does not meet the proposed standards for reimbursement. The program as it is evolving allows us to maintain a presence in the community while making the necessary modifications. We are doing some market research to make the program meet the needs of patients and fulfill third-party payer requirements.

We have some concerns about the place and distribution aspects of our marketing strategies. There is some geographic restriction, due to minimal public transportation and no taxi service in the community. We are currently studying these factors to determine the size of the diabetic population without transportation and how we can provide services to it. These considerations will become more and more important to us as the program expands.

Smoking Cessation Program

When the state passed legislation restricting smoking in the workplace, we realized that a smoking cessation program would be in demand. We conducted a survey to validate our assumptions. It confirmed that there was a demand for this type of program. From this information, we developed and aggressively promoted the program to corporate clients.

Hospital employees were the first group targeted, because of their role in promoting healthy behavior by example and because of easy access. Having a president who is an adamant nonsmoker was helpful. Marketing the smoking cessation program to employees included offering the program at a reduced fee and giving a rebate upon successful completion of the program. Our in-house success with this program provided us with a valuable tool for selling the program to other employers in the area.

Corporate clients, including the hospital, share many similar needs. They desire more physically and mentally productive employees. Offering a smoking cessation program contributes to positive employee relationships, as it is a concrete expression of employer concern. Many employers also express a desire to decrease sick days and health insurance costs.

We have found that corporate clients also identify specific goals. A sportswear manufacturer expressed the need to reduce the risk of fire hazards on the job. He also saw a relationship between the quality of his product and whether the sewing machine operators smoked while working.

Direct mailings are used to interest our corporate customers. Potential benefits to the employer are described in the literature we send to businesspeople. We make it clear that we are willing to give the program at their place of business. A discount is offered. The discount seems to be a valuable strategy in selling the program to businesses, as the perception seems to be one of bargain. Increased volume offsets the cost of the discount for us.

Clients from the surrounding communities are solicited by direct mail, newspaper ads, public service announcements, and ads in the local shoppers' guides. Brochures and other literature are available in pamphlet racks in the hospital lobby and patient waiting areas. Graduates of the program also refer clients to us.

Physicians and dentists were targeted as potential consumers and as sources of referral. Health care providers recognize the need for patients to lower their risk factors for disease, and frequently advise patients to stop smoking. Since most people are unable to quit successfully by themselves, health care professionals need programs to which they can refer their patients. A hospital-based smoking cessation program can provide a valuable service. It provides tangible assistance and increases physicians' loyalty to the hospitals with which they are affiliated.

During the start-up phase of the program, physicians and dentists were sent personalized letters describing the program. Using a computer made personalization of the letters easy. Patients referred by physicians and dentists receive a 15% discount on the cost of the program. Each time we send a new schedule we remind them of the discount. We give feedback by sending a letter of thanks for the referral and by describing the patient's progress. This information is important to the physician or dentist, and helps us maintain the visibility of the program.

In developing the marketing plan for this program, we kept in mind the different needs of each targeted segment. For instance, we have targeted patients using the

Center for Women and Health. To this group, we emphasize the effects of smoking on the fetus and the effects of passive smoking on young children. Quality of life, health hazards associated with smoking, and the real savings of $400–$1,200 per year are stressed to all groups.

This program may be so effective that the need for it will be eliminated. However, that time is some years down the road, because 30–35% of Americans still smoke; also, there are difficulties in stopping and relapses due to nicotine addiction. We will monitor trends and make adjustments in the program as needed.

Basic Life Support Programs

Marketing the Basic Life Support (BLS) courses is directed toward two distinct populations: health care professionals (nurses and physicians), both on staff and in the community, and the lay public. The BLS Training Center offers three courses, developed by the American Heart Association, to meet the needs of the targeted groups.

In order to exist as an American Heart Association BLS Training Center, certification of specific numbers of the public is necessary. We must continually look for potential additional markets. The training center has developed several strategies to create consumer awareness and interest in the courses. Advertisements are placed in local newspapers, direct mailings are made to community members, and flyers are left in the hospital lobby and are enclosed with the quarterly hospital magazine that is sent to households in our service area. Word-of-mouth is also effective. For instance, the training center certified the entire recreational staff at a local lake on referral from one of their employees who had taken the course.

An idea for another potential market came from a small news item in a local paper. It stated that the state legislature was considering mandating certification in basic life support for workers in nursery schools and day care centers. Addresses were obtained from the telephone directory's yellow pages and a direct mailing was done to all such facilities in our area. Our letter described the courses and our willingness to go to the work site. Response to this focused mailing was very satisfactory. Direct mail also got us a contract to certify the managerial staff of the county Office of Aging, Nutrition Program. Staff in all five of their sites have been trained at our center. These two mailings generated enough clients to more than meet our quota of community members for the American Heart Association.

Nursing schools are another segment of our market. Because of frantic phone calls from students during the last week in August, we became aware that many of the nursing schools affiliating with Zurbrugg require BLS certification. To meet this need, we schedule extra courses just before the beginning of the fall term. The various nursing schools are informed. Both students and faculty have responded well to this plan.

Pricing this product was easy. We followed the American Heart Association guidelines, determined what our competition charges, and calculated the cost of transporting equipment to the work site. From these figures we came to an acceptable, reasonable price.

RESULTS AND EVALUATION

The common threads in all the programs described are commitment to high quality, ongoing evaluation, and sensitivity to market demands. This framework requires that Department of Education staff be flexible and innovative in meeting the needs and preferences of patients, nurses, physicians, and the community. We are pleased with the outcomes of our early marketing efforts and anticipate further developing our marketing perspective.

Marketing Nursing Products*

Mary Ann Crawford, MSN, RN
Vice-President for Patient Care Support Services
Akron General Medical Center
Akron, OH
Doctoral Candidate, Kent State Univeristy
Kent, OH

Mary L. Fisher, PhD, RN, CNAA
Associate Dean for Administration
Assistant Campus Dean, IUPUI
Indiana University
Indianapolis, IN

THE MARKETING SITUATION

As nurse executives at Akron General Medical Center, we planned for a Joint Commission on Accreditation of Hospitals (now named Joint Commission on Accreditation of Healthcare Organizations (JCAHO)) visit in 1984 with the goal of a perfect survey for nursing. One of the strategies we used to achieve our goal was to prepare a checklist audit tool developed to measure nursing's compliance with the JCAHO standards. Because a majority of hospitals seek Joint Commission accreditation, we believed that our checklist would have national marketing appeal. This belief and our success with the tool helped to launch a nationwide nursing marketing program that has now passed its sixth year.

Our marketing approach was defined as the promotion and sale of existing nursing products to other acute care institutions nationwide. This strategy evolved to include defining our target market, choosing competitive positioning, and developing an effective marketing mix to reach and serve our consumers (Kotler & Andreasen, 1987).

Marketing "relies heavily on designing the organization's offering in terms of the target market's needs and desires, and on using effective pricing, communication, and distribution to inform, motivate, and service the markets" (Kotler, 1982, p. 6). Our target market was other nurse executives facing circumstances similar to ours. Kotler and Clarke (1986) describe the responsive organization as one that

---

*Adapted with permission from Crawford, M.A., & Fisher, M.L. (1986). Marketing: The Creative Advantage. *Journal of Nursing Administration, 16*(12), 17–20.

makes every effort to determine and meet its consumers' needs. We designed our product offerings to respond to what we perceived were our consumers' needs.

External forces affecting the hospital business have resulted in numerous internal changes. Governmental and third-party payer reimbursement requirements changed the emphasis from inpatient to outpatient care, resulting in shortened length of stays, institutional downsizing, and rising acuity levels for hospitalized patients. Increased demand for high-technology approaches had escalated costs, while the operating margin was dwindling.

Many hospital administrators faced with these events called for cost containment measures such as eliminating or curtailing nursing staff support positions. At the same time, new technologies required accelerated staff education programs to meet the demands of a constantly changing care environment. Without qualified experts to serve as clinical staff resources, growing consumer needs were unlikely to be met.

Pointer (1985, p. 11) suggests the necessary survival requirements in an industry undergoing rapid and turbulent change: "Health service organizations must become far more creative and innovative if they are to thrive, let alone survive, in the new health care market-place." We believed that our products, nursing education curricula and policy and procedure manuals, offered a creative new approach to meeting some of the needs of our targeted consumer group. Our current catalogue demonstrates our approach to the target group:

> Whether you are initiating new programs, meeting standards, looking for convenient resources or updating current nursing practices—here are helpful policies, procedures, guidelines or content to expedite the process and save you developmental time and money!

The success of our marketing effort, measured by initial sales, repeat business, and requests for new products, affirms our belief.

Organizational Needs

Like other nursing executives, we were bombarded with data comparing our institution's productivity with local competitors and national averages such as Monitrend. Included in these comparisons were numbers of full-time equivalent staff per patient day and the number and cost of nursing staff support positions. These data exerted pressures on us to look creatively at methods of decreasing the expense associated with staff support positions. We also needed to find a way to continue staff education programs. Our response to these demands was a plan for nursing administration to become a revenue center.

For a number of years, the nursing staff development department had generated revenue through charging for educational services. We started to ask: How could the division of nursing develop new income sources? After exposure to the concepts and success of our hospital's general marketing efforts, our nurse managers decided that a marketing approach specific to the division of nursing was the option of choice. The identification of consumer and organizational needs provided the foundation for our marketing program. Product determination and evaluation involved more in-depth analysis.

MARKETING ANALYSIS

Reporting success offers credibility; our approach worked for us. We did not engage in a formal marketing research program as a part of planning for our first product. Instead, we relied on our understanding of nursing executives' needs and our knowledge of current products available in the industry. Our first product, the *JCAH Checklist*, was an attempt to share something that worked for us with others who had a common need.

When we expanded our product offerings, we became more involved in a process that Drucker (1986) describes as analysis of the result areas of a business, the products or services. Highly advanced tools or techniques, such as sophisticated computer systems, the use of advanced accounting methods, or market analysis may not be needed if the complexity of the business or product does not require it. Drucker promotes asking the right questions in the process of analysis. An important question is: "What is the simplest method that will give us adequate results?" (Drucker, 1986, p. 16).

Our initial marketing effort used simple methods. When they worked, we were motivated to expand our marketing program and product offerings through a more formalized analysis process. A specific blend of marketing strategies, known as the marketing mix, was used to achieve objectives in the target market. These variables are commonly grouped into four categories: product, place/distribution, price, and promotion. They are discussed in greater detail in Chapter 5. We considered all these in our internal and external analysis, and they became the basis for our marketing strategies.

We had a marketing orientation, with our major task being to put out a product that met our customers' needs. Considerable time was spent evaluating our products for their quality, features, and usefulness in meeting these needs. Our letters and flyers included suggestions on how the buyer might begin using our products immediately. The products were prepared so that the text was generic, without any reference to our institution. Permission was given for the purchaser to photocopy them. This proved to be an important feature that aided voluntary exchange with the customer. We received many requests for rush processing of orders, another indication of the appropriateness of our product.

A significant part of our internal analysis process involved determining what additional products were worth selling. To determine the kinds of requests nursing managers received from other hospitals for policies, clinical staff expertise, or educational programs, we logged inquiries requesting manuals not available on our product list. The areas with the most outside interest were evaluated as potential products.

Nominal group technique (see Case Study 8) was used to identify potential products from existing nursing manuals, current projects, and educational materials. Everything from computer-generated x-ray preparation instructions to educational curricula were considered, based on quality and potential for general appeal. We focused on existing materials to keep developmental costs low.

A marketing planning group was charged with the responsibility for selecting the products. It included the vice president for nursing, three directors of nursing, and a special projects coordinator. Some of the "place" marketing variables analyzed by this group included geographic coverage, distribution channels, and inventory control.

Any first-time venture has an element of risk associated with it. Risk can be reduced by the use of market research, targeted product development, and effective communication. To help offset the risk, funds were allocated in the nursing administration cost center budget to underwrite the expenses of the initial marketing project. The only requirement was that any new venture break even by meeting its *direct* expenses during the first project year.

Price and promotion were a consideration in our external analysis. Our pricing policy was both competitive and value-oriented. We wanted the price of each product to ensure our competitive position, yet we didn't want to give our products away! Our products and prices were compared with those in commercial catalogues advertising similar products. The cost of staff time needed to produce a similar product was estimated. This was done to ensure that buyers could quantify the value received for dollars invested. They could purchase our product for a fraction of what it would cost to produce it themselves. We used this analysis as a part of our promotion to those customers who inquired about products before purchase.

We believed that our products could be promoted nationally. For example, the *Checklist* would assist all JCAHO-accredited hospital nursing departments to measure standard compliance. Once we decided on a national promotional approach, we continued it for subsequent products.

Certainly, the assessment of consumer and organization needs and the marketing analysis process provided a strong base for our marketing strategies. We continued to use these analytic processes as we brought new products to the marketplace and evaluated the results of earlier marketing plans.

MARKETING STRATEGIES

Marketing strategies are every bit as important to the success of a sales campaign as analyzing the market. To succeed, an organization must develop a marketing strategy for each of its products. Product, price, promotion, and place or distribution all must be considered in any marketing strategy.

The Product

An organization's most basic marketing decision involves the selection of the products to offer the target market. We began our marketing efforts in 1984 with a single, unique product, the audit tool developed by our nursing staff to evaluate nursing department readiness for an accreditation visit. For our first manual, decisions regarding format, content, and style of the *Checklist* were made with the user in mind. One user-friendly approach was the double-column audit format that allowed staff to monitor compliance with standards by using the first column to identify deficiencies and the second column to reevaluate their unit's status after correction. The content was divided into nine sections, so that each specific nursing area would use only a single audit section. Because of the reference to standards, we sought JCAHO approval before publication.

In preparing manuals for publication, editing, copy, and design details were important. Copy was typed and printed in the hospital to keep production costs down. Manual covers and section dividers were typeset by a low-cost printing company, collated at the hospital, and spiral-bound by the printing company.

The success of the *Checklist* led to the decision to update it for 1985. Because of the success of our first product, we caught the ''marketing bug'' and began to look for additional products to sell. Other pertinent items in use within the nursing division that had marketing potential were identified by the marketing planning group. Each of these was reviewed by the special projects coordinator to determine its feasibility for marketing. Based on this review, final marketing decisions were made by the market planning group. The target market segment was identified for each approved project. For example, we targeted staff development directors for our *Nursing Management Core Curriculum*, and directors of psychiatric nursing for our multidisciplinary *Psychiatric Manual*. Following this step, possible completion dates for each phase of the marketing process were suggested with the use of a PERT (Program Evaluation Review Technique) chart.

Once the target market, project dates, responsibility lines, and manual developmental phases were determined, our marketing plan was ready to be implemented. Many aspects of this plan required simultaneous attention to assure that the manuals met market deadlines and that supplies were adequate for anticipated sales. Each marketing program then became the responsibility of the special projects coordinator. The PERT chart ensured that important details were completed on time.

Price

For the *Checklist*, we projected expenses per manual based on printing, typing, mailing, and developmental cost estimates for 50, 100, 150, and 200 manuals. Our final decision to proceed with marketing plans, the charge per manual, and a break-even point were based on these projections. The break-even target number was posted and watched for eagerly once orders started arriving.

Promotion

Promotional efforts centered on identifying the target market for the *Checklist*. Undoubtedly, it had national appeal, because all JCAHO-accredited hospitals must meet the same standards. We determined that the vice president for nursing at each hospital would have primary interest in our product. The hospital marketing department assisted the project by providing a national mailing list of more than 5,000 hospitals. Using a computer allowed us to do bulk mailings to generic "vice president for nursing" positions or any other category of nurse manager, depending on the nature of the product.

We then considered alternative sales approaches that included action cards, letters, flyers, and journal advertisements. Because vice presidents for nursing were the target group, we developed a one-page letter from our vice president. Our intent was to decrease marketing costs, speak to the audience on its level, and minimize the financial risk for our first project.

Hospital volunteers provided the hands needed for collating, labeling, envelope stuffing, and sorting. By using volunteer labor, promotion costs were kept to a minimum so that profits could be realized in a shorter time. Our second-generation products were promoted by the use of self-mail flyers. This process had the benefit of enhanced visual appeal, elimination of envelopes, and a savings in mailing costs. The use of a standard format for the flyers resulted in an additional benefit: instant visual recognition of a Akron General promotional piece. Our hospital logo became visible across the country, and soon was associated with a progressive and dynamic nursing division.

Distribution

Once the marketing letter was mailed, a system designed to process orders and to maintain records was established. Initially this function was performed manually, but it has since been automated. We set up notebooks in which completed orders were filed alphabetically, first by state, and then by institution name. Order date, purchase order number, payment status, and shipment date were kept on file. The staff development secretary assumed responsibility for distribution of products and recordkeeping. We assisted her in her new role by consulting the finance department on proper procedures and providing continuing education on bookkeeping. Functions included in the distribution process were inventory control, recordkeeping, packaging, mailing, processing funds, and evaluation. Orders were processed the same day they were received, since many customers stated an urgent need for our products. Requests for overnight delivery were specially processed for express mail.

Because of our marketing orientation, we wanted to know that our customers were satisfied with their purchases, so we devised an evaluation postcard to include with each order. The feedback we received assured us of the quality of our product.

Mail delivery time was eagerly anticipated. We measured our success by the number of orders received in comparison to the break-even point. Inventory was monitored closely. Subsequent printings of our manuals were anticipated and ordered in a timely manner so that customers would not experience delivery delays. Our next task was to decide on future marketing efforts.

RESULTS AND EVALUATION

Nursing executives at Akron General Medical Center began marketing nursing products in 1984 with the goal of generating revenue to partially offset salary costs for clinical specialists and staff development faculty. Four years later, we are still in the business, and have earned a profit of more than $122,900 for the institution.

The marketing operation expanded to six projects scheduled for distribution in 1985. They included: *1985 Checklist; Position Descriptions and Performance Evaluations, Volumes I and II; Nursing Management Core Curriculum; Psychiatric Manual;* and *Family Centered Maternity Care Manual.* Management of the program became more complex. We assigned each project to a specific work group comprised of nursing management staff in the specialty area where the product had originated. Continued use of a PERT chart kept the program moving forward; everyone was informed as to their role and deadlines.

For 1986, we added *Diabetes Patient Education Manual, Oncology Manual, Rad-Prep Protocols,* and *Nursing Grand Rounds.* Many customers took advantage of a special 15% discount offered when three or more manuals were purchased at one time.

Our sales promotion strategy was altered to take advantage of the larger number of products. We modified our brochure to list all 10 products so that all could be promoted in one mailing. This resulted in additional savings on the promotional end. Only one additional manual was prepared for sale in 1987: *Emergency Care Nursing Manual.* Product development continues. Anticipated for 1988 were *Critical Care Policies and Procedures* and a certification curriculum.

After only five months of selling our first product, we had a net profit (in 1984) of $14,000 from the *Checklist.* The year-end evaluation for 1985 indicated that each of our six products was profitable. Our total net gain for 1985 was approximately $40,000. With the addition of four more products in 1986, we netted $31,500. Likewise, 1987 yielded a profit of $27,400. Best sellers in 1987 included *Nursing Grand Rounds, Psychiatric Manual, Nursing Management Core Curriculum, Oncology Manual,* and the *Emergency Care Nursing Manual.*

These marketing efforts have generated pride in our nurse managers and staff. They were surprised and pleased that their work had general appeal on a national level. Hospital administration has acknowledged our efforts as being a valuable contribution to the hospital's prestige. The reputation for excellence that we already enjoyed was enhanced by the increased visibility for nursing and the entire hospital.

Now that we have set the expectation for revenue generation, there are future goals to meet. In light of leadership changes, this takes renewed effort, growth, and creativity on behalf of our nurse managers. The dynamic nature of human resource development is visible in the growth that accompanies success. As managers are empowered by their involvement in the process of change, the process becomes self-generating.

Marketing has helped to achieve national recognition for our nursing department and medical center. We presented a poster display about the marketing program for the Ohio Hospital Association and the American Organization of Nurse Executives (AONE) conventions in 1985. Participants were very interested in the marketing process, because few nursing organizations were actively marketing their products at that time. This experience with marketing has also helped us to grow professionally through publications in the *Journal of Nursing Administration* and the *Journal of Nursing Staff Development,* in addition to this case study.

REFERENCES

Crawford, M.A., & Fisher, M.L. (1986). Marketing: The creative advantage. *The Journal of Nursing Administration, 16*(12), 17–20.

Drucker, P. (1986). *Managing for results* (2nd ed.). New York: Harper & Row.

Kotler, P. (1982). *Marketing for nonprofit organizations* (2nd ed.). Englewood Cliffs, NJ: Prentice-Hall.

Kotler, P., & Andreasen, A.R. (1987). *Strategic marketing for nonprofit organizations* (3rd ed.). Englewood Cliffs, NJ: Prentice-Hall.

Kotler, P., & Clarke, R. (1986). Creating the responsive organization. *Healthcare Forum, 29*(3), 26–32.

Pointer, D. (1985). Responding to the challenges of the new health care marketplace: Organizing for creativity and innovation. *Hospital & Health Services Administration, 30*(6), 10–25.

Social Marketing: A Transplant Program

Faye D. Davis, MSN, RN
Executive Director
New York Regional Transplant Program
New York, NY

THE MARKETING PROBLEM

Public relations and public education have been integral parts of every organ transplantation and procurement program, but it was only five years ago that the label "marketing" was openly attached to these activities (Prottas, 1983). Fox and Kotler (1980) stated that when the product is an idea, it involves social marketing (see Chapter 2).

Prottas (1983) described how the concept of organ donation was sold, and offered suggestions for marketing strategies. In his framework, the product is the donation of organs, and the price is what one has to pay to donate. He also noted that, on a superficial level, it would appear that the product is very cheap, since it can be donated only after death. However, given the American attitude toward death, the product is difficult to sell.

Other issues complicate this marketplace: the next of kin must give permission, and the family often does not know of the deceased's wish to donate organs. Even when a person has made it known in life that donation of organs after death is wanted, the final decision must be made by the next of kin. The difficulty is compounded by laws that most states have, stating that families should be given the option to donate organs of a loved one after death. This final decision must be made after the potential donor is declared brain-dead and is on a respirator to keep the heart beating, the circulation intact, and the organs viable.

Physicians have been labeled the gatekeepers of organ donation, because the potential donor must be referred to the organ procurement agency by a physician. Stark, Reiley, Osiecki, & Cook (1984) and Davis (1981) suggest that attitudes of nurses also play an important role in the outcome of a potential donation. The National Task Force on Organ Transplantation clearly takes the position that organs are donated in a spirit of altruism and volunteerism, and constitute a resource to be used for the public good.

Manninen and Evans (1985) established that the need for cadaveric organs for transplantation far exceeds the supply. In 1986, the American Council on Transplantation (ACT) reported that, on any given day, a minimum of 300 patients await hearts, 300 await livers, and more than 9,000 wait for kidneys. The paradox of this shortage is that thousands of undonated organs are wasted annually.

To procure these organs, agencies must rely on health professionals who are willing to refer potential donors, assist in obtaining permission from the next of kin, and provide medical care for the potential donor until the organs are surgically removed. Health care professionals and the next of kin constitute the market segments that must be reached.

MARKETING STRATEGIES

Similar, but nevertheless different, marketing strategies are necessary for health professionals and next of kin. Marketing plans for both groups must take into account attitudes about altruism and death. While marketing to health care professionals involves straightforward marketing, selling an idea to the public requires a social marketing approach. Both methods are used daily by organ procurement agencies. Three programs are presented here to demonstrate how we used social and societal marketing concepts to develop strategies for a transplant program.

Program I: Centers for Disease Control, Kidney Activity Program

A pilot project in three cities was developed by the Centers for Disease Control in the late 1970s. The goal was to increase the number of cadaveric kidneys available for transplantation. The method for developing a procurement program is found in Exhibit 4.1. Components of the program included assessment (research), planning, implementation, evaluation, and modification (see Exhibit 4.2). Great detail in strategic planning, tactics, and logistics was emphasized in these activities.

Nursing personnel were hired by procurement agencies as transplant coordinators to carry out the program. The transplant coordinators' first task was to conduct a careful analysis of each *catchment* or service area, the hospitals within the area, and their interaction with one another, and to develop an awareness and respect for local sensitivities and procedures in each community.

Internally, our procurement organization laid out a plan for the roles of all personnel, the steps the organization should take, and how the steps would be implemented. Technical functions of the procurement program were defined in great detail (see Exhibit 4.3). The focus was to implement a formal, systematic, organ procurement program in all hospitals where donors might be found. A formal approach would allow for consistency and clear delineation of roles by all personnel involved in the partnership between the hospitals and the organ procurement agency.

EXHIBIT 4.1   Method for Developing a Kidney Procurement Program

Phase I: Retrospective record review

Records of intensive care unit and emergency center deaths that occurred in selected hospitals were reviewed retrospectively. This review assisted in focusing procurement efforts by enabling us to assess the number of potential organ donors and to describe the characteristics of those potential donors.

Phase II: Program development

Professional education

Professional education was conducted to inform hospital personnel about the need for procuring organs and tissue for transplantation. This education was continuous and repetitive to sustain interest and to develop resource people to help in all phases of donation and procurement. Continuity of education is essential in light of the constant rotation of hospital personnel.

For physicians, professional education was given by transplant coordinators and physicians from the New York Regional Transplant Program. Education for nursing and hospital administrators, paramedical, and medical support personnel was tailored to meet each group's special requirements and expectations. Seminars were held to train personnel for compliance with required requests and in approaching families for organ donation.

Policies and procedures

Specific policies and procedures were developed with each institution's staff, allowing for the unique features of each hospital's program and defining appropriate personnel roles and relationships. Policies and procedures were also established to ensure that all appropriate charges were sent to the Procurement Program.

High visibility

High visibility in all potential donor areas developed an effective relationship between the New York Regional Transplant Program and hospital personnel. Our presence also facilitated the establishment of procedures for the continual process of identifying and reporting potential donors so that donation and procurement takes place.

Current medical record review

A periodic sequential record review of all deaths occurring in critical care units and emergency rooms permitted identification of discrepancies between numbers of potential donors and actual donors.

Process analysis

Analysis of unsuccessful referral or procurement efforts contributed to the progressive development of a smoother and more effective donation program.

Phase III: Active participation in the donor process

Donor identification and management

The organ procurement staff was available 24 hours a day to respond to each referral of a donor. The potential donor was evaluated by a transplant coordinator to decide if the potential donor met medical and legal criteria. Under the attending and procurement physicians' guidance, and adhering to each individual hospital's policy, the coordinator expedited the donation process.

Specific tasks included assisting in or taking primary responsibility for explaining the critical need for organs, requesting permission for donation from the next of kin, and advising on the clinical support of the potential donor to ensure optimal physiologic status of the organs to be donated.

Coordination of surgical procedures

The organ procurement staff, working with the hospital staff and procurement physicians, was responsible for alerting and scheduling the surgical teams and any other persons involved in the removal of organs. The organ procurement staff was also responsible for the preservation and transplantation of all organs after surgical removal. When multiple organs were removed, and more than one surgical team was involved, the organ procurement staff coordinated the entire surgical process, assuring that the hospital's policies were properly observed.

Phase IV: Follow-up after donation

Transplantation

The transplant coordinator maintained a close relationship with the donor hospital by visiting the hospital to exchange information on the entire donation procedure, and by sending administrators a follow-up form and a letter describing the disposition of the organs and tissues. Similar follow-up was also provided to the attending and consulting physicians.

A letter of acknowledgment and appreciation was sent to the donating family. Any other follow-up with the family was carried out as appropriate. A survey requesting suggestions about the organ donation process was sent to each family.

Charges related to organ and tissue donation

The transplant coordinator and the billing department reviewed all charges related to organ and tissue donation. This ensured reimbursement to the donating hospital from the organ procurement program, and avoided any extra costs to the donor family.

Medical support for the program was obtained from nephrology services, where patients were being dialyzed and awaiting transplants, and through surgical services, where physicians performed nephrectomies or sought educational experiences for resident physician training. This support also created bonding between physicians in the transplant centers and the community hospitals.

Formal appointments were made with hospital administrators. Again, exchange theory worked. Administrators realized that organ donation should be a service available to hospital patients, and that the hospital would have more control over organ donation. Many also saw public relations benefits in promoting the hospital's support of transplantation.

The program was presented not only to administrators, but to other key personnel, including chiefs of staff, medical directors, nursing directors, and, frequently, a staff person from risk management or the legal department. Initially, a "soft" approach was made by asking for a retrospective record review to establish the potential donor pool. Once that was established, another meeting would take place to share the findings and to put the rest of the program in place.

Organ procurement coordinators soon began to realize that approval for record reviews could take weeks or months, during which time no progress for the program would be made. As their confidence and skills increased, coordinators began to be more aggressive, and tried to close the deal in one meeting. They would often get approval to begin a portion of the work in the plan, such as working with designated hospital employees to develop policies and procedures, working with medical staff to revise or develop brain-death criteria, or conducting inservice or surveillance rounds. Constant assessment and modification took place.

Results and Evaluation

Ongoing medical record review identifying missed donors provided the quality control for and evaluation of the program. Policies were also reviewed and revised when they were found to be inaccurate or insufficient. Solicitation of feedback from administration, physicians, and nurses was a major responsibility of the transplant coordinator, and helped to evaluate each program's success. However, the bottom-line evaluation was the increase in organs procured. There was a nine-fold increase in the number of kidneys retrieved during the first year of the program compared to the preceding year. This program was deemed very successful. Indeed, it has subsequently become the prototype for many other transplant programs. Only minor additions and revisions have been made.

Second only in importance to the increase in number of donated kidneys was knowledge that would make the program even more successful. Follow-up with donor families provided an enormous amount of information. Organ procurement personnel began to realize that grieving families benefited from the donation. According to the New England Organ Bank, 59% of families who donated felt the donation made something positive come out of the death. The two most frequent reasons for donation were to help others and to make a memorial to the deceased.

Once transplant coordinators realized that donation could help donor families, their own jobs were easier. This knowledge gave them a new tool with which to market the idea of organ donation. It is the foundation for marketing the donation concept to both health care professionals and the public.

EXHIBIT 4.2   Procedures and Logistics of Kidney Procurement Program

  I. Assessment and planning
        Define donor criteria
        Devise screening format
        Define program plan
        Develop record review protocol
        Define charges and billing procedures
        Develop and print educational material
        Define area and select hospitals
        Gain permission and do retrospective study and analysis
        Secure endorsement with contract or memo of agreement
 II. Implementation
        Obtain support of key personnel and establish surveillance system
        Define hospital-specific procurement retrieval process, with policies
            and procedures
        Conduct inservice programs
        Establish frequent rounds to key services
        Proceed with procurement process when potential donor is found
III. Evaluation
        Conduct ongoing prospective record review
        Compare review results with actual referrals
        Determine reasons for failure to get referral
IV. Modification
        Refine or reinforce system when needed
        Provide feedback to key hospital staff

Reprinted with permission: Davis, F.D., Lucier, J.S., & Logerfo, F.W. (1986). Organization of an organ donation network. *Surgical Clinics of North America, 66*(3), 641–52.

EXHIBIT 4.3   Technical Functions of Kidney Procurement Program

Business and administrative aspects, including policies and procedures

Professional and public education programs

Public relations, including interpersonal skills

Surveillance of areas where donors may be found

Donor evaluation criteria

Obtaining family consent

Donor maintenance

Donor nephrectomy

Organ preservation

Tissue typing

Recipient identification

Organ disposition and transportation

Data analysis or record review

Ability to train retrieval teams within the hospital

The Need for Social Marketing

Unfortunately, the Centers for Disease Control model for promoting organ procurement and transplant programs made no provision for the need of the public to know about organ donation. Procurement programs were federally funded through the End Stage Renal Disease Program. Federal emphasis was on educating professionals in the institutions where the donation would occur. Programs were discouraged from spending money on public education, as it was believed that it was better to reach the next of kin at the time of the donation. There was also no demonstrated effectiveness of public education programs. Gradually, organ procurement personnel began to document that obtaining permission was easier when families had knowledge of organ donation before being asked for consent. As a result, by the early 1980s, more emphasis was placed on developing public awareness and support for the public good in donating organs after death.

Several organizations, as well as organ procurement agencies and transplant programs, have developed their social marketing efforts to emphasize the good in organ donation, and to heighten public awareness that transplantation of livers, hearts, kidneys, bone, corneas, and skin are highly successful treatment modalities. Today organ procurement agencies are benefiting from using sophisticated marketing research and strategies that target specific population groups. Minority groups are frequently targeted because studies have shown that organ donation rates are lower in these populations (Callender, Bayton, Yeager, & Clark, 1982; Perez, 1988).

Problems of Evaluation

Proper evaluation of the social marketing effort is complex. Since one must die before donating, the concept could have been sold but the product not obtained. Still, the bottom line is the number of organs donated. Additionally, because the donor must be brain-dead, and this criterion excludes most potential donors, only a small fraction of those who sign and carry donor cards actually become organ donors. Thus, once again, the idea could have been sold but the organ not obtained.

Another way to evaluate the effectiveness of the organ donation program is to look strictly at the behavior of the targeted segment. This involves counting the number of people who want to donate, who tell a family their wishes, who sign a donor card or driver's license, and perhaps those who become advocates of the program. As you can imagine, this approach also is difficult and has many problems.

Program II: Donor Awareness

A public awareness campaign with the goal of fostering family discussions on organ donation was launched by the Boy Scouts of America. The target groups were the public at large and the families in communities where the Boy Scouts lived. Dow Chemical, USA, designed a program that involved more than two million Scouts, plus organ procurement agencies, the American Council on Transplantation, the White House, the American Red Cross, and some medical organizations. An executive from Dow Chemical was loaned to the Scouts as program coordinator. See Exhibit 4.4 for assessment, planning, and start-up phase activities.

Once Boy Scouts and their leaders were trained, the program went into full swing. Scouts went door to door, convincing families to discuss organ donation, responding to public education requests, and carrying out their other designated activities. The campaign lasted four months. It was deemed a huge success. Success was evaluated in part, by the following:

- 597,823 Scouts across the United States participated and handed out 14 million public education brochures
- 125 public service institutions, such as electric companies and banks, participated in the programs
- 346 newspapers carried the message to 21 million readers
- 628 television and 1,102 radio stations participated through talk shows and public service announcements.

EXHIBIT 4.4   Boy Scouts of America Donor Awareness Program

Assessment and Planning

Identify Scout groups and local liaisons throughout the United States

Design and print a public education brochure

Solicit funding and donations*

Design slide presentations to train Scouts

Prepare trainer's kit for Scout leaders

Identify support groups

Develop public service announcements

Design artwork for milk cartons

Prepare news releases

Decide on activities in which the Scouts could participate: write letters to editors, hand out literature, appear on radio and television talk shows, make posters, volunteer at member agencies of the ACT

Start-up Activities

Visiting organizations to present program and solicit help

Distributing speaker kits and slide presentations to all volunteers who assist in training Scout leaders

Mailing public service announcements and press releases

Distributing brochures to all regional and local Scout groups

---

*Dow Chemical, USA and the W.K. Kellogg Foundation funded the program; International Paper provided donor awareness information on milk cartons; Eastman Kodak provided a slide presentation to train Scouts.

As planned, Scouts who participated in the program received an honorary card signed by President Reagan and the president of the Boy Scouts of America. In fact, the program was so successful that the organ donor program was made a permanent part of the Boy Scouts Merit Badge Program. Scouts continue to work on promoting organ donation in the United States.

Program III: KDKA Second Chance Project

KDKA television station in Pittsburgh, Pennsylvania, a member of the Group W Broadcast Division of Westinghouse Electric, conducted an organ donation awareness project. The project had two goals: to increase the number of donor cards signed, and to stimulate family discussion about organ donation. Corporate sponsorship helped to defray the cost of the Second Chance Project. It consisted of the following:

- A one-hour special on transplantation and organ donation, hosted by a star of the *Knots Landing* television show
- A three-part news series which aired locally
- Three *PM Magazine* segments
- Twelve public service announcements featuring well-known personalities such as President Reagan, Bob Hope, and Ed McMahon
- A toll-free telephone number given each time the project aired.

At the annual convention of the National Association of Television Program Executives, the project was sold to other television stations. During the first hour it was on sale, 40 stations purchased the program. A total of 113 stations bought the program, giving it access to 85% of the national viewing audience.

KDKA produced a public education brochure with an attached donor card to help promote the organ donation idea. A toll-free telephone hotline was set up to answer questions. Members of the Junior League were trained to staff the hotline.

This project was aired over six weeks. KDKA's evaluation showed that the hot line received 2 million requests for donor cards. All the requests were filled. There were other positive outcomes. The one of which the station is most proud is that a family called to say that they had seen the show and wanted to donate the organs of their brain-dead child.

Program IV: Oregon Drivers' License Program

In conjunction with the Motor Vehicle Department (DMV), the Portland Donor Program obtained a federal grant to promote organ donation throughout the state of Oregon. The goal of this program was to increase the number of people who mark "D" for donation on their driver's licenses. Promotional strategies consisted of educating the employees at the 50 DMVs to enable them to answer questions about donation, and educating the public about the need for donors. An eight-minute film was developed for employee training, to be used at staff meetings and employee orientation.

All persons visiting the Motor Vehicle Department during a three-month period were targeted. A two-minute film was produced for the targeted public, and was played every 13 minutes during hours the DMV was open. The project was six weeks long.

Evaluation was made by the numbers of donors signed up in each of the 50 offices. Numbers varied by location, the workload in a department at any given time, and the size of the department. The evaluation showed that the busier the office, the less impact the film made. Overall, the increase in the number of donors was 6% to 12%.

After the initial evaluation, it was determined that a person from the donor program should remain on site to train DMV employees. Because DMV employees complained of sensory overload due to the added noise of the tape, it was decided to play the tape less frequently. In addition, a new group was targeted. To reach this market, donor information was inserted in all license renewal letters.

FOR THE FUTURE

As more marketing strategies are implemented, achieve success, and become models for emulation, we will see more segmented social marketing focusing on organ donation for target groups such as African-Americans, Hispanics, the clergy, lawyers, and so forth. New ways individuals can incorporate the concept of organ donation into their value system will be ripe for marketing strategies. Donor and recipient families will take their rightful places as educators and advocates. Topics such as death and brain death will be addressed along with the advances in transplantation technology. As more people are educated about, and became advocates of, organ donation, the need for organs will continue to increase. New marketing strategies will be needed and will be developed. Social and societal marketing are integral parts of every transplant and procurement program.

REFERENCES

Callender, C.O., Bayton, J.A., Yeager, C., & Clark, J.E. (1982). Attitudes among Blacks toward donating kidneys for transplantation: A pilot project. *Journal of the National Medical Association, 74,* 807–809.

Davis, F.D. (1981). Current strategies in the procurement of cadaveric kidneys for transplantation. *Nursing Clinics of North America, 16*(3), 565–571.

Davis, F.D., Lucier, J.S., & Logerfo, F.W. (1986). Organization of an organ donation network. *Surgical Clinics of North America, 66*(3), 641–652.

Fox, K.A., & Kotler, P. (1980). The marketing of social causes: The first 10 years. *Journal of Marketing, 44*(4), 24-33.

Manninen, D.L., & Evans, R.W. (1985). Public attitudes and behavior regarding organ donation. *Journal of the American Medical Association, 253,* 3111–3115.

Perez, L. (1988, January). *Organ donation in three major American cities with large Latino and Black populations.* Paper presented at the meeting of the New York Transplantation Society, New York, NY.

Prottas, J.M. (1983). Encouraging altruism: Public attitudes and the marketing of organ donation. *Milbank Memorial Quarterly, 61*(2), 278–306.

Stark, J.L., Reiley, P., Osiecki, A., & Cook, L. (1984). Attitudes affecting organ donation in the intensive care unit. *Heart & Lung, 13*(4), 400–404.

Marketing a Clinical Nurse Specialist

Marsha E. Fonteyn, MSN, RN, CCRN
Doctoral Student
The University of Texas at Austin
School of Nursing
Austin, TX

Sharon E. Hoffman, PhD, MBA, RN
Dean and Professor, College of Nursing
Medical University of South Carolina
Charleston, SC

THE MARKETING SITUATION

Strategies used for marketing services in a nonprofit organization such as a hospital are not very different from those used in for-profit organizations. Indeed, whether or not a health agency is for-profit, services are sold to generate revenue. Services such as health care are considered "public goods" that are augmented by community assistance through tax-exempt bonds, community donations, and volunteer labor. Thus, marketing of professional services such as those of a clinical nurse specialist (CNS) are subject to public scrutiny. Part of the scrutiny that CNSs face involves concern over the impact of their services on other professionals, particularly physicians. Strategies must be developed to assure nonnurse colleagues that services provided by the CNS add to patients' well-being, but do not compete with medical and other professional care. The employing organization needs to be assured that the CNS's services are unique and worth the cost, both to the employer and to the patient.

There is clearly an exchange transaction between CNSs and their target markets. The nurses exchange their skills as practitioner, patient advocate, change agent, consultant, and clinical teacher for specific benefits, which include salary, fringe benefits, job security, and respect. According to Kotler and Andreasen (1987), the customer or constituent is asked to pay or make some sacrifices in return for a benefit. The customer provides or sacrifices one or more of the following:

1. Economic costs. Administration provides the CNS's salary as well as fringe benefits and overhead, but ultimately the consumer pays this.

Adapted with permission from Hoffman, S., & Fonteyn, M. (1986). Marketing the Clinical Nurse Specialist. *Nursing Economic$, 4*(3), 140–144.

2. Sacrifice of old ideas and values. Physicians, patients, and third-party payers give up the belief that advanced clinical nurses are no more autonomous than staff nurses.

3. Sacrifice of old patterns of behavior. Patients give up unhealthy habits for a more healthy lifestyle. Families may have to give up free time to assist the client in this process.

4. Sacrifice of time and energy. Administrators, physicians, and nursing staff work on a patient care committee with CNSs or assist the accounting department and third-party payers to develop a method for obtaining reimbursement for the CNS's services. Staff nurses and physicians assist the CNS's efforts to provide a service to a patient.

In return for these payments, the consumers of CNS services receive economic, social, or psychological benefits. Administration can offer high-quality patient care and also receive reimbursement from insurers for the CNS's consultation services. Clients and their families receive additional knowledge and skills that should result in improved health. Physicians have more satisfied, self-sufficient patients. Nursing staff and members of the community receive the assurance that high-quality nursing care will be provided to patients.

Because so little is known about the market for CNS services, it is difficult to assess consumer needs for them. Lack of information and precedent makes it difficult to reach marketing decisions for planning and implementing strategies. Consumers, such as administrators, physicians, clients, nurses, and third-party payers, need to make major shifts in attitudes and behaviors in order to accept the value in, or recognize the need for, CNS services. A group that may be difficult to convince is hospital administrators, who do not always see the benefit of hiring a CNS. Another marketing problem is that many of the benefits of CNS consultation, such as health and increased knowledge, are intangible and difficult concepts to measure. Unlike a tangible product, which has properties that can be clearly delineated, services of a CNS are often difficult to separate from those of other health care providers. Despite this, there are ways to identify and market the advanced skills of the CNS. An initial step in this process is identification and analysis of the CNS's marketing environment.

INTERNAL AND EXTERNAL ANALYSIS

Because marketing is concerned with gaining and retaining customers, they must first be identified and segmented. Customers of CNS services consist of various constituents, both internal and external to the health care setting. These include administration, patients, physicians, nursing staff, the community, and third-party payers. The successful CNS will define the services needed by each of these groups and market services to each segment.

Internal markets include patients, physicians, administrators, and nursing staff. External markets include patients' families, community members, and third-party payers. After segmenting consumers into these groups, the CNS can develop services tailored to meet specific groups' needs and proceed to implement them, while being alert to possible changes in market conditions.

Services provided by the CNS must be substantially different from those already provided by unit nursing staff. The various customers must be able to identify these services as either higher in quality, more complex, or unique in some way. To potential customers, the value of these services is based on their perceived benefits. For example, if the CNS helps a physician solve a difficult patient care problem, such as failure to understand or to follow a treatment regimen, then the physician is relieved of a patient management problem and will likely seek the CNS's services again. Nurse executives and hospital administrators perceive high-quality patient care, specialized patient services, and the possibility of obtaining third-party reimbursement for CNS services as very strong benefits to their organization. Once CNSs have defined their unique exchange relationships and segmented their markets, their challenge is to promote their inherent capabilities and positive economic effects. The following experience of Marsha Fonteyn's success in marketing her CNS services at a small nonprofit hospital demonstrates the diverse marketing strategies that were necessary to establish the credibility of these services.

CNS in Patient Education

When I assumed the position of CNS in charge of patient education, it was a new role at our hospital. Marketing strategies became very important in establishing credibility as a CNS and in promoting the importance of patient education. My selection of strategies was based on the following questions suggested by Taylor (1985, pp. 7, 8): Who are the customers? What products (services) will be made (provided)? How will the products (services) be made (provided)? Who will be the competition? What will be the cost?

Who Are the Customers?

I determined that my customers would include medical staff, nursing staff, key hospital administrators, patients and their families, the community, and third-party payers. I selected, planned for, and implemented different strategies for each consumer group.

What Services Will Be Provided?

The services I would provide centered around patient education, but the meaning of these services differs depending on the consumer group's perspective and needs. I had certain expectations of what each target group wanted. The medical staff would want me to provide education for their patients that would improve outcomes and result in more knowledgeable individuals, thus making the future care of their patients easier. They also would want me to save them time that they would otherwise have to spend teaching patients and family about medications and treatments. Nursing staff would want me to provide the patient education services that they either were not qualified to provide or for which they did not have time. Key hospital administrators would want my patient education services to increase customer satisfaction, and to provide another means of increasing revenue. Patients and their families would want me to provide them with information about their health problems and to assist them in taking better care of themselves in order to avoid future illness. The community would want the best possible care to be provided to patients, and would see my patient education services as contributing to high-quality care. I hoped that people in the community would also want to learn more about maintaining and improving their health, even if they were not hospitalized. Third-party payers would want my patient education services to promote early discharges and decrease the number of readmissions for previously treated conditions.

How Will the Services Be Provided?

When I assumed the role of a CNS in charge of patient education, I realized that the services I provide to patients were specialized and consultative in nature. One way to make this position cost-efficient was to develop a means for the hospital to receive reimbursement for my services. The rationale for this strategy was based on a medical model of consultation services (Stevens, 1978). In this model, consultation is seen as an interactional process that occurs between health professionals: the consultant, who is a specialist in a particular area, and the client, who lacks expertise in that area. In my case, I was a medical-surgical CNS with a master's degree in nursing, who was asked to provide specialized nursing expertise to the client, a physician, who has requested my expertise. This expertise provided coordination of complex nursing and medical care to prevent complications and avoid prolonging the patient's hospital stay. Hospitals operating on the DRG payment system that rewards short patient stays would also directly benefit.

Who Will Be the Competition?

I did not have any specific competition for my services, but I realized that physicians might feel threatened if they saw my consultative services as competing with, rather than augmenting, the care they were providing for their patients. Therefore, I established a policy of not charging a fee for service unless the physician had requested a consultation in writing. I recognized the importance of marketing my services to both physicians and the nursing staff to effect a steady increase in referrals.

MARKETING STRATEGIES

Marketing to Physicians

The initial step in marketing my services to physicians was to write an informative announcement letter discussing my role as a CNS at our hospital. It also told them that third-party payers would be billed for my services. My letter emphasized the benefits of CNS consultation to both the patient and the physician. It was sent out, on hospital stationery, to all area physicians, after this procedure had been sanctioned by the hospital administrator. Following the initial mailing, all physicians new to the medical staff were sent letters as soon as possible.

Additional strategies for gaining physician support included sending a follow-up letter to physicians thanking them for referrals and providing them with specific information regarding what I had done for the patient and what results were obtained. Chart dividers labeled "Patient Education" were placed in all charts, and CNS consultation activities were documented in this area on specified forms: CNS consultation record, history and physical, and CNS progress notes.

Soon after assuming my position in patient education, I conducted a survey of the physicians to identify the educational needs of their patients and the methods of education the physicians preferred. I also asked them to identify patient education programs they would like to see developed. Questionnaires were mailed to all 44 members of the medical staff: 50% returned completed questionnaires. The results indicated that all the physicians recognized a need for an increase in both the quantity and quality of patient education. Specific educational needs seemed to be related to the health problems of their patients. From a list of 10 possible patient education programs that might be developed, the majority chose all 10 as important and desirable.

Appropriate dress was a factor in gaining professional recognition and respect from the physicians. I found it helpful to wear a lab coat over a dress or skirt and blouse, rather than the traditional white nurses' uniform. My name tag identified me as "CNS, Patient Education." It was important that the physicians view me as a specialist apart from the general nursing staff, even though I realized this might be a controversial issue with the nursing staff. Another means that I used to establish a collegial relationship with the staff physicians was to serve on committees that brought about hospital changes important to the physicians. For example, I assisted a surgeon in implementing a hospital policy that would improve the quality of care for burn patients. I also served on the discharge planning committee, a multidisciplinary team dedicated to making the patient's transition from hospital to home as smooth as possible.

Marketing to the Nursing Staff

Gaining the support of the nursing staff was also important in establishing the validity of CNS consultation. One method for accomplishing this was my high visibility in the various nursing units. Since part of my role as a CNS was that of expert practitioner and role model, I regularly scheduled time to provide direct patient care on a nursing unit. When doing this, I wore a uniform like the other nurses.

I distributed a questionnaire to the nursing staff to assess how they felt about patient education and what help they needed to educate their patients. Of the 100 questionnaires distributed, only 25 were completed and returned to me. Several factors that would have an impact on my marketing strategies, such as apathy and disinterest regarding patient education, or a perceived sense of nursing's inability to improve the current status of patient education at the hospital, may have contributed to the low response rate. The most common needs identified by respondents were formal programs of cardiac rehabilitation, diabetic, and postnatal education.

Another method I used to gain the support of the nursing staff was to seek their assistance in devising a plan of care for the patients that I saw in consultation. I also frequently praised and encouraged the nurses for carrying out care plans, and, based on their input, I revised the plans periodically. When individual head nurses approached me with patient education program needs for their unit (e.g., a more standardized pre-op teaching program for the surgical unit or an OB discharge class), I tried to make these needs a priority in program development, and I kept the head nurses informed of my progress.

Maintaining credibility as a CNS is important when dealing with a nursing staff that is composed of a variety of highly qualified members. This was done by keeping up to date through continuing education, seminars, and current nursing literature. New information was shared with staff members so that nursing procedures and policies would be current. Staff development activities, obtaining certification in my specialty, and publishing in nursing literature also helped me maintain credibility.

Marketing to Patients and Family

I found that patients were generally very receptive to me, and seemed pleased to have someone to talk with about their concerns and to answer their questions about their health problems and the treatment they were receiving. To be available for clients when they needed me, I was willing to accept calls at home in the evenings and on weekends. The need for education or explanation can occur any time during hospitalization, and is often accompanied by a sense of urgency. Newly diagnosed diabetics, for example, cannot wait until Monday if they need to learn to administer insulin injections on Saturday. Likewise, myocardial infarction patients, who suddenly find they will be discharged the next morning, may feel the need to talk about their concerns or to have their questions answered that evening. I left business cards with my home phone number for all patients and their families, and encouraged them to call me whenever questions arose.

Marketing to Third-Party Payers

The practice of nurse specialists charging patients (and thus third-party payers) for their services is relatively new, and insurance companies are initially suspect when such charges appear on the bill. They do not necessarily refuse to pay this charge, but usually they require further explanation prior to payment. I wrote letters describing the nature and specifics of CNS consultations. Because I maintained thorough documentation on all patients I saw in consultation, our accounting department was able to justify such charges.

Marketing to the Community

A final target group for marketing was the community. Exposure in the local newspaper provided good publicity. I frequently wrote health education articles for a "Focus on Health" column in the local newspaper. I also offered my expertise whenever requested by community groups. Teaching CPR at an elementary school provided an opportunity to explain my position at the hospital, and provided additional publicity when the local newspaper published a story on the event. Serving as a volunteer for health organizations, such as the American Heart Association and the American Cancer Society, gave me the opportunity to keep up to date on the associated health problems, and also provided me with a wealth of excellent patient education literature.

RESULTS AND EVALUATION

When the results of marketing strategies are measured in terms of goal attainment, it is possible to reach tenable conclusions regarding whether a venture is successful. My main goal was twofold: to provide high-quality patient education, and to demonstrate the cost-effectiveness of my CNS position so that I would be allowed to continue providing educational services to the patients at our hospital. I believed that obtaining reimbursement for my consultative services was one, but not the only, means of demonstrating cost-effectiveness. The total charges for my consultative services for the first year as CNS was about $5,000; but, because most third-party payers were not accustomed to this type of charge, only about 20% of this amount was actually collected. Since the practice of charging for CNS consultation was so highly innovative, I felt this amount of reimbursement was a very successful sign. As the year progressed, a slow but steady increase in reimbursement developed.

Another goal I achieved was a steady increase in the number of consultation referrals. Not only did physicians independently request my services, but greater numbers of the nursing staff solicited referrals for me. Physicians frequently told administration members how useful they found my services.

Additionally, I was able to document instances in which my efforts in teaching patients and their families resulted in earlier discharge than would have otherwise occurred. Numerous patients singled me out when providing feedback to the hospital regarding the positive aspects of their hospitalization.

As a result of this nursing venture, the hospital received a considerable amount of publicity from my publications and speaking engagements. Other CNSs were extremely interested in this method of increasing their cost-effectiveness. Our public relations director estimated that about $20,000 worth of publicity was generated for the hospital that first year through my speaking engagements and publications.

Problems Encountered

The process of developing and implementing marketing strategies must include a means of identifying and resolving problems and failures. Some of the problems I encountered while marketing my position included the following.

1. Little actual revenue from CNS consultation was generated during the first year. Because of the new, almost radical, nature of the concept of CNS consultation charges, I did not see the paucity of revenue generation as a problem. I believe the amount of revenue would have increased slowly, but steadily. Some members of administration, however, did begin to question the value of the position when revenue was not immediately forthcoming.

2. Some physicians did not consistently request my services despite obvious educational needs in their patients. Since the reasons for their reluctance were not readily apparent, I would have needed to expend more time and effort to identify their needs and those of the patients in order to determine appropriate marketing strategies to meet those needs.

3. Other equally important patient education needs seemed to have to take second place to my consultative efforts. As the director of the patient education department, I identified many needs and concerns regarding patient education at our hospital that did not require CNS consultation and yet seemed to be of equal importance. These included getting the nursing staff to see patient education as an integral component of the care they provided patients; finding the time, money, and administrative support for program development in patient education; identifying and using educational resources outside the hospital; and conducting research in patient education (an essential part of the CNS role). I soon realized that I would need to market these aspects of my patient education position with the same vigor as that used to market my consultative services.

Conclusions

Efforts of CNSs to establish the credibility of their position in a hospital are amenable to a marketing approach. The idea of marketing one's services may at first seem foreign, and perhaps even offensive to highly qualified CNSs who believe the value of their services should be readily apparent to all constituents. Unfortunately, the roles, performance expectations, and organizational fit of CNSs continue to cause confusion and force restraint in fully using the CNS in many hospitals (Wyers, Grove, & Pastorino, 1985). The success of this position may well depend on the use of a marketing approach, whereby the needs of the various consumers of CNS services are identified, and strategies are then planned and implemented to meet these needs. This case study has demonstrated how one CNS used such an approach in a small community hospital to solidify a CNS position and accomplish the goal of providing high-quality, cost-effective patient education.

REFERENCES

Kotler, P., & Andreasen, A.R. (1987). *Marketing for nonprofit organizations* (3rd ed.). Englewood Cliffs, NJ: Prentice Hall.

Stevens, B. (1978). The use of consultants in nursing service. *Journal of Nursing Administration, 8*(8), 7–15.

Taylor, J.W. (1985). *Competitive marketing strategies.* Radner, PA: Chilton.

Wyers, M.E., Grove, S., & Pastorino, C. (1985). Clinical nurse specialist: In search of the right role. *Nursing & Health Care, 6*(4), 202–207.

Social Marketing in the Community

Anne DuVal Frost, PhD, RN
Co-Founder of the Nurses Network of Pelham
Project CHILD Director and Principal Investigator
Associate Professor, Graduate Nursing Program Director
College of New Rochelle
New Rochelle, NY

THE MARKETING SITUATION

The development of a grass-roots organization, named the Nurses Network of Pelham (NNP), was based on the need of a group of nurses who came together and wanted to share their nursing skills with the community. NNP's goals were to develop programs to improve community health and to highlight the value of nursing's scientific knowledge, essential expertise, and professional independence. The goals led to a marketing strategy designed to improve society's understanding of nursing by demonstration of professional capabilities through community activities.

To realize these goals, the organization needed a marketing plan. The first step was to identify the needs of the population of Pelham, New York. Part of the needs assessment was to evaluate demographic characteristics, attitudes, and values (Frost, 1985). The town of Pelham is a commuter suburb of New York City and has a population of 15,000. Most of the residents are in the upper socioeconomic bracket, and have at least an undergraduate degree. There is an unspoken, but clearly felt, emphasis on success in the community, be it business, professional, civic, or academic. Kudos are given for innovation and being first. A winning attitude extends to sports, where competition and fair play are emphasized for both adults and children. With more equitable recognition of the community's professional women, there is concomitant recognition and equality for girls on town soccer and baseball teams. While the rate of divorce reflects the national trend, there is an emphasis on the value of the family and its role in healthy child rearing. The quality of the environment is promoted through an active volunteer, as well as professional, fire department, a large police force, and clean, well-paved and well-lit streets and sidewalks. Emphasis is given to ongoing maintenance of homes and grooming of property. Community spirit is applauded and involvement with a variety of clubs, agencies, and religious affiliations encouraged.

279

Most community projects are directed to children or the elderly. In summary, key community values include learning, innovation, competition, equality, family stability, environmental safety and beauty, and sharing.

ANALYSES

Internal Analysis

The resources of the Nurses Network of Pelham included 20 nurses who were practicing as administrators, educators, and clinicians, as well as real estate brokers and a town clerk. Several members were not employed. Areas of nursing specialty ranged from pediatrics to geriatrics, from acute to chronic care, with a variety of work settings such as emergency departments, home care, nursing homes, and private practice. Affiliations within the community spanned all socioeconomic levels, religious and ethnic groups, and all major organizations. There were strong connections to local government, the school system, businesses, social agencies, and the media.

Reactions within the organization to the idea of developing a successful marketing plan ranged from enthusiastic to skeptical. Enthusiasm was generated by recognition of the lack of bureaucratic restraints so often present in larger organizations and agencies. Members felt that there was opportunity for innovation and impact. This had special appeal for those not in nursing practice but who wished to revive or maintain a nursing identity. However, NNP's small numbers created skepticism about the ability to develop and implement a marketing plan for a successful health promotion program. Besides "person power," there was also a need for financial backing.

Projections for the size and scope of a potential program ranged from run-of-the-mill proposals to grandiose. We concluded that something practical but more toward grand was necessary to stimulate interest in the community. Anything less would fail to reach a population composed primarily of professional and corporate executives. These practical considerations, in addition to nursing's holistic and systems orientation (Riehl & Roy, 1980), suggested that the NNP develop collaborative partners for any program.

External Analysis

Our project began with a nursing colleague contact at The Fresh Air Fund. She and the director of The National Down Syndrome Society (NDSS) were interested in developing a community respite program for children with Down Syndrome. The need for the NDSS was to broaden the focus of their organization from genetic research to support services. Their motivation for working with The

Fresh Air Fund was to have the respite program come under the insurance umbrella of the organization's Friendly Town Program, a program which sends innercity children to suburban and country settings during the summer. The benefit to The Fresh Air Fund was to broaden their offerings without incurring great expense. While they would supply transportation for the children to and from the community site, the NDSS would pay the greater expense of hiring a part-time project director.

In order for the NNP to join as a collaborative partner, it was important to continue this market exchange analysis and identify the appropriateness of the program for the children and for the residents of Pelham. The identified benefits were as follows:

1. The child with Down Syndrome (guest child) would gain growth opportunities and the support of new relationships.

2. The parents of the child with Down Syndrome would gain freedom to attend to their own needs and those of other family members.

3. The children of the host parents (host children) would learn about interacting and sharing with a handicapped child.

4. The host parents would develop an understanding of the strengths of handicapped children, as well as of their needs.

5. The community would develop a greater unity by merging ethnic, religious, and socioeconomic values for a common goal.

It was immediately evident that the value of learning through discarding old myths for new insights was a strong component of the program. The fact that this would be the first program of its kind in the nation fulfilled the community's need for innovation and competition. Because the primary focus was on helping other families reduce their stress and increase family stability, potential host families were attracted to the program. Equality between sexes expands to equal opportunity for handicapped children. That most of the guest children were living in inner-city housing also was a motivating factor in recruiting community members to share their safe, pleasant, nurturing environment. The goals and values were clearly compatible.

The Nurses Network of Pelham, The Fresh Air Fund, and The National Down Syndrome Society had needs that had to be satisfied for the success of the program. Exploration of these needs as well as strengths led to the delineation of expected contributions from each group. (See Table 6.1.)

In addition to satisfying overt needs of the community and participants, NNP felt that sponsorship by two national organizations would add an image of significance to the program. The Fresh Air Fund is well-known for providing equal opportunity for children compromised by inner-city and lower socioeconomic neighborhoods. Although the organization is over 100 years old and is a stable New York institution, it has been recognized as an innovator since its beginning.

TABLE 6.1   Contributions of Organizations Involved in Project CHILD

Nurses Network of Pelham	National Down Syndrome Society	Fresh Air Fund
Project Director (unpaid)	Project Director (paid)	Liaison (paid)
Interview/select host families	Interview/select host families	
	Interview/select guest children	Interview/select guest children
Provide escorts		Provide transportation to and from Pelham
		Provide insurance

PROMOTION

Community Outreach

While respite care was clearly the goal of the three organizations, each had priorities for promotion of their own organization. Neither The Fresh Air Fund nor the NDSS volunteered funds for advertising the program in Pelham. The NNP also obviously needed a source of start-up funds. In addition, NNP felt that involving another organization from the community would strengthen community interest and ownership. The Junior League of Pelham was selected as an organization that represented influence in the community and had a successful track record for developing programs. Negotiations resulted in this new team member agreeing to assume the major role in community outreach. This would include promoting the program and soliciting host families. The Junior League also provided $1,500 for initial expenses. Coincidentally and fortunately, the brother-in-law of the league's liaison for the program worked in advertising and designed a logo and flyers for the program.

Again, to promote community interest and ownership, the Girl Scouts were asked to provide escort service for the guest children to and from New York City. This subprogram was called "Child to Child." Not only would the Scouts learn about children with Down Syndrome, but they could use this opportunity to earn badges and teach others at Scout functions. In addition, the Scouts are an important pool of future nurses. Both their age and involvement in the program provided a superb opportunity to promote nursing as an interesting career choice.

With the help of these agencies, the first respite program for children with Down Syndrome began. Guest children from New York City spent Saturday (overnight) and Sunday with host families in Pelham every six weeks for a year. Our plan served as a model for national implementation.

Naming the Program

A key element in our corporate identity strategy was selecting a name and logo for our respite program. The involved organizations met to brainstorm and reach consensus on these important aspects of our corporate identity. The Fresh Air Fund and The National Down Syndrome Society suggested "The Friends Program" or "Reach Out to Friends." Using the values assessment of the Pelham population as a basis, NNP suggested that gaining new friends was not as powerful an appeal as that of learning. Pelham residents often complain that there are too many social demands; offering more friends might be counterproductive. On the other hand, the emphasis on learning, which is a strong value in this community, would spark interest. With the help of the son of a NNP member who works in advertising, the acronym CHILD (Community Help in Learning About Down Syndrome) was developed. The program became known as Project CHILD. Besides being an effective mechanism to help remember a goal of the program, the acronym highlights the focus of the program—the children.

Logo

The next step was the development of a logo. Our logo depicts the outline of a home and family with their visiting child. Its stark lines and dark and light contrasts were used for a poignant impact. See Figure 6-1.

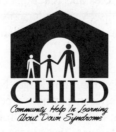

Figure 6.1.   Logo of Project CHILD.

Recruitment of Host Families

The NNP and the Junior League felt that sending a flyer home with every school child would be the most expedient way to reach the largest number of Pelham residents. In the interest of saving time and money, a photo and copy that the NDSS had used in a print ad was selected for the flyer. Contact names were given and the logo was placed in the center of the copy.

The superintendent of schools, a friend of a NNP member, was contacted for official approval and distribution of the flyer. The flyer was sent home with 1,500 Pelham school children. Calls from potential host families began to come in after a few days.

On-Call Service

To help recruit host families and to emphasize nursing's expertise, the NNP developed a weekend "on-call" service. During each weekend that children were visiting, a member of the NNP was available for consultation about any physical or emotional need. During our initial planning, a member of the NDSS questioned nursing knowledge of psychosocial care. We know this knowledge has often been associated with social workers, not nurses. The on-call service was an effective way to help to recruit families and to promote the broad scope of nursing expertise.

Graduate Nursing Students

Project CHILD provided academic and professional socialization for graduate nursing students from the nearby College of New Rochelle. One student became an investigator for the research, and two students interned as acting project directors for NNP. Their involvement provided the opportunity to highlight graduate nursing education, knowledge, and professional independence. Both of the acting directors wrote letters of introduction to the host families emphasizing nursing's role in prevention and the community as a primary site for independent nursing practice.

Involvement of the graduate students in the project proved to be more valuable than we had anticipated. Community knowledge about levels and requirements of nursing education, as well as roles and functions of nurses, was far more outdated than we had imagined. This discovery underscored the necessity and urgency of developing effective marketing programs for nursing.

Research Program

To emphasize nursing's scientific knowledge, NNP developed a research study entitled "The relationship between periodic weekend respite care and parental stress in families of children with Down Syndrome." Informal market research suggested that very few people knew that nurses possess research knowledge and skills. This was also true of our NDSS colleagues, who were very resistent to the study and whom we had to convince of nursing's scientific base. We began with a well-documented proposal and underscored the research experience of the five doctorally prepared nurse members.

Publicity

Newspaper Articles

From the inception of the program, stories accompanied by pictures regularly appeared in the Pelham newspaper. Emphasis was given to the Project CHILD's research study and to the on-call service. Several articles emphasized the independent role of nurses in health promotion and in the development of community programs. The articles also highlighted the relationship between the community's values and Project CHILD.

Radio

A member of NNP, who was also a host parent, and the liaison from The Fresh Air Fund were interviewed by the author on a New York City radio station. Project CHILD was discussed for an hour. Myths associated with Down Syndrome were eroded. Nursing's knowledge, expertise, and professional independence were demonstrated.

Events

Junior League—Nursing Network Dance

The Junior League holds an annual black-tie dinner dance and fund raiser. The NNP suggested that the Junior League emphasize its involvement with Project CHILD by allowing the NNP to co-sponsor the event, and splitting the proceeds between the organizations. This was a wonderful opportunity for the newly established NNP to ride on the coattails of a key community event. Needless to say, it would have been impossible for the NNP, with its limited membership, to plan an evening of dinner, dancing, and raffles for over 200 people. By soliciting the major raffle prizes, the NNP established a power base. The highlight of the evening was a sensitive slide presentation of Project CHILD weekend visits. It was shown on a giant screen and was accompanied by an audiotape of "Reach Out and Touch Someone." As one guest commented, "There wasn't a dry eye in the place." More money was raised than at any previous Pelham Junior League dance. The program was described as "the most dramatic in the community's recent history."

Contributor's Cocktail Party

The success of the dinner dance was repeated several months later when NNP held a cocktail party for its major financial contributors and key members of the Junior League. All community members who had contributed to NNP for the raffle or after the dance were also invited. A private showing at a college art gallery was the focus of the event. The reception that followed was held in a beautifully restored Victorian building called The Castle. Generous servings of jumbo shrimp and other hors d'oeuvres gave an aura of elegance and graciousness. In short, the cocktail party projected an image of style and power. After expenses we had raised $18,000 in just three hours!

NNP Awards

The Nursing Network of Pelham decided to give annual awards to highlight professional independence and to recognize contributions to the community. A member was presented with a Leadership Award for knowledge, expertise, and innovation. The person from the Junior League who had worked with us on Project CHILD was given a Community Liaison Award for sharing and community spirit. The awards presentation ended with a proclamation from the town council applauding the contributions of NNP to the community.

Host Family Dinners

Periodic dinners were held for host families by the NNP representatives of Project CHILD. This was a way to support the families, evaluate the program, and promote a positive image of nursing. The dinners achieved these goals.

Children's Parties

Picnics and pool parties were held for the guest children, their host parents, host children, members of NNP, and affiliating groups. The festive atmosphere and camaraderie were always enhanced by good weather and a bounty of food and games. The pictures of the smiling faces of guest and host children were published, along with a story, in the local newspaper.

Special Olympics

Collaboration with the Pelham Civic Association resulted in Project CHILD guest children participating in the annual Special Olympics. Besides the obvious benefits for the guest children, community ownership of Project CHILD was strengthened.

Project CHILD Video

Networking by the NNP director at a local dinner party resulted in a substantial contribution from another guest for development of a video telling about Project CHILD. A later chance meeting worked to get the video produced, when the director, while at a McDonald's with her family and guest child, met a neighbor who was an executive at MTV. She introduced the executive and his family to her guest child. Later she followed up with a phone call to the executive, asking for help in producing the video. Not only did he provide script consultation, but he also amplified the first contribution by providing a high-budget video for a low fee!

The 14-minute MTV production is a sensitive portrayal of the needs of children with Down Syndrome and their families. Interviews with family members attest to the relief the program has given them. It also provides documentation of the learning and personal growth experienced by the host parents and children. The unity of the community is reflected through the involvement of the various organizations and special events. A theme woven throughout the video is the knowledge, expertise, and professionalism of nurses. In recognition of its merit, the *American Journal of Nursing* gave the video an award.

Because the Project CHILD video delivers a powerful message about nursing, it has been shown at a variety of community and professional meetings. A recent presentation at the Pelham Rotary Club resulted in a lively question-and-answer period and a generous contribution to NNP. The video was the focus of a spring fund raiser given by the Pelham Civic Association for Project CHILD. Features of "The Pitch In For Children" included an auction and sports celebrities. Significant contributions were received.

The video was an effective adjunct to a presentation on the Project CHILD research that was given at a large research conference in New York. It was also shown at a conference on marketing for nurses in Texas. Several schools of nursing have used it to demonstrate to students the impact nurses can have on their communities. Praise for the video and strong endorsement for nursing's leadership came from the New York State Department of Mental Retardation. The assistant commissioner encouraged NNP to apply for funding to extend the respite program to other communities in New York State. We applied for, and received, a $62,000 grant from the state. In addition, we received $2,000 from the state for development of a brochure.

This video has enabled us to become independent of the Fresh Air Fund. We are able to expand our project to include children with developmental disabilities. Our name, therefore, has been changed to include this segment. The program is now called Project CHILDD. It includes in-house respite for medically dependent children at Blythdale Children's Hospital in Valhalla, New York.

EVALUATION

There is no question that the program has been highly successful in meeting all its goals. It has provided a needed service to children with Down Syndrome and their families. The host families of Pelham and the community at large have gained knowledge, insight, and the added benefit of providing a needed service.

In just three years, a more accurate image of nursing exists in Pelham and in other communities touched by Project CHILD. The financial contributions, professional assistance, and camaraderie with other community organizations are only part of the evidence of the success of the program. An expressed willingness to endorse nursing legislation and to contribute to future nursing research is also evidence of a greater value given to nursing. The effects of the program are just now being seen, but its potential influence can be estimated by a member of the Girl Scout Escort Service who announced: "Because of Project CHILD, I want to study to be a pediatric nurse!"

REFERENCES

Frost, A.D.V. (1985). Working together: Local community action. In D.J. Mason & S.W. Talbott (Eds.), Political action handbook for nurses (pp. 509–524). Menlo Park, CA: Addison-Wesley.

Riehl, J.P., & Roy, C. (1980). *Conceptual models for nursing practice* (2nd ed.). New York: Appleton-Century-Crofts.

The Model Marketing Plan

Christine M. Galante, MA, MSN, RN
Lieutenant Colonel, Army Nurse Corps
Doctoral Student, School of Nursing
George Mason University
Fairfax, VA

MARKETING PLAN FORMATS

Successful marketing programs are most often based on explicit marketing plans. These plans guide an organization's actions toward achievement of its goals. Management planning is difficult in any organization, and especially so in the face of ongoing operational responsibilities and turbulent, complex environments. Lovelock and Weinberg (1984) note that managers of public and nonprofit organizations face additional difficulties in planning when compared to their private sector counterparts. First, they often must develop and implement plans where the primary emphasis is on nonfinancial objectives for which outcomes are difficult to quantify. Second, they frequently must develop plans for benefactors or donors as well as clients or users. This complexity supports the adoption of an organizing framework, a formal marketing plan, as the primary means to achieve organizational goals and objectives.

Lovelock and Weinberg (1984, p. 255) define a *marketing plan* as "a systematic way of organizing an analysis of a market, of the organization's position in it, and of the direction of the marketing effort." They maintain that a marketing plan provides benefits such as:

- Coordination of activities of interdependent parties
- Establishment of a timetable
- Nurturing of improved communications
- Identification of expected developments
- Supportive preparation for meeting change
- Systematic focusing of efforts
- Serving as the basis for a control system
- Supporting the maintenance of organizational integrity.

The opinions or assertions contained herein are the private views of the author and are not to be construed as official or as reflecting the views of the Army or the Department of Defense.

Hillestad and Berkowitz (1984) note that in health care, organizations have tended to consider their internal needs first, and the needs of the marketplace second. Figure 7.1 details their model comparing internal planning versus market-based planning. The issue here is not to show a right or wrong planning approach,

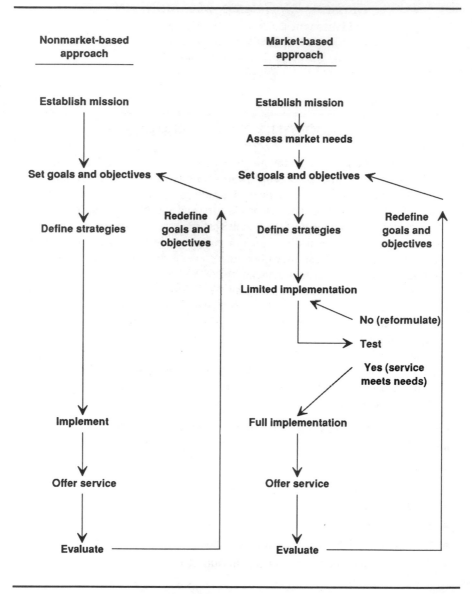

Figure 7.1. Internal planning versus marketing planning.

Reprinted from *Health Care Marketing Plans: From Strategy to Action* by S.G. Hillestad and E.N. Berkowitz, p. 32 , with permission of Aspen Publishers, Inc., © 1984.

but rather that, as human, material, and fiscal resources become more limited, the cost of mistakes increases. A market-based planning approach improves the chances for success.

Marketing plans vary according to scope (organization, division, department, unit) and focus (product- versus service-oriented, or by target markets). Numerous authors offer topologies detailing the market planning sequence and plan format. Strasen (1987), for example, defines a marketing plan as having five main elements:

1. Situation analysis: examination of the weaknesses, opportunities, threats, and strengths (WOTS) in the internal and external environments.
2. Identification of marketing goals and objectives.
3. Identification of marketing strategy, that is, the methods to be used to achieve the goals and objectives.
4. Establishment of the marketing action plan: a document that describes actions, responsibilities, accountabilities, and time frames for the marketing effort.
5. Ongoing review, evaluation, feedback, and revision (the control function of the plan).

The Hillestad and Berkowitz (1984, pp. 32, 33) model, detailed in Figure 7.2, has six basic steps for establishing effective marketing plans. These steps are: (1) setting the mission, (2) performing internal and external analyses; (3) determining the strategy action match and marketing objectives; (4) developing the action strategies; (5) integrating the plan and making revisions; and (6) providing appropriate control procedures, feedback, and integration of all plans into a unified effort. At each step of this model, three types of activities are necessary for success: performance of staff work to support decisions, actual making of decisions, and integration with other organization elements to support coordination of efforts.

Lovelock and Weinberg's (1984) marketing plan format, seen in Exhibit 7.1, is similar to the preceding two. It is enhanced by a detailing of the components of each step and by the use of four focusing questions. Regardless of the marketing planning model you use, these four questions must be answered:

- Where are we now?
- Where do we want to go?
- How do we get there?
- What is our budget and how shall we spend it?

Increasingly, nurses are adopting a marketing orientation and developing and implementing marketing plans. Benedict, Gemmell, and Anderson (1988) define a *marketing plan* as the organization's set of service strategies that addresses the specific needs of all patients, visitors, physicians, and employees. They

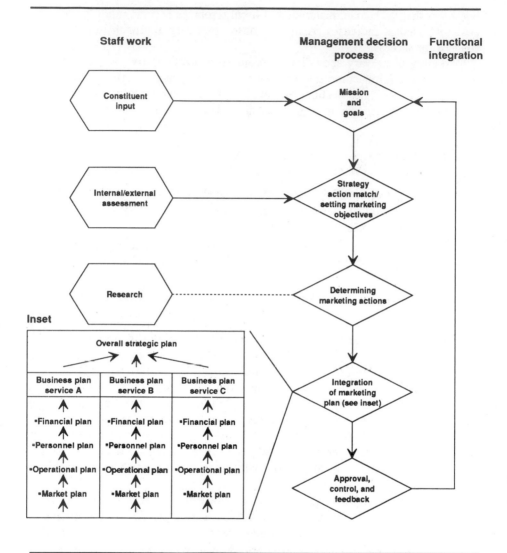

Figure 7.2.   The marketing planning model.

Reprinted from *Health Care Marketing Plans: From Strategy to Action* by S.G. Hillestad and E.N. Berkowitz, p. 35, with permission of Aspen Publishers, Inc., © 1984.

note that as the need to fulfill customer expectations grows in priority, nurse administrators must implement their marketing plans from the dual perspective of the organization and the nursing division. Patient and nurse satisfaction are the cornerstones of their model, as seen in Figure 7.3.

EXHIBIT 7.1   Marketing Plan Format

Executive Summary

Situational Analysis (Where are we now?)

External: environment, consumers, employees, funders, distributors, competition

Internal: objectives, strengths, and weaknesses

Problems and Opportunities: momentum forecast, identify gaps

Marketing Program (Where do we want to go?)

Characteristics: specific, realistic, important, prioritized

Marketing Strategies (How do we get where we're going?)

Positioning: target segments, competitive stance, usage

Marketing mix: product, price, distribution, communication

Contingency strategies

Marketing Budget (How much and where?)

Resources: money, people, time

Amount and allocation

Marketing Action Plan

Detailed breakdown of activities for each goal or strategy

Responsibility by name

Activity schedule in milestone format

Tangible and intangible results expected from each activity

Monitoring System

Source: *Marketing for Public and Nonprofit Managers* (p. 256) by C.H. Lovelock and C.B. Weinberg. Copyright © 1984, New York: John Wiley & Sons, Inc. Reprinted by permission of John Wiley & Sons, Inc.

While their degrees of detail and specificity vary, an analysis of these models finds seven consistent key elements in a marketing plan:

1. Mission statement.
2. Situational analysis.
3. Establishment of program goals.
4. Identification and selection of marketing strategies.
5. Integration with other plans.
6. Establishment of action plans.
7. Monitoring system.

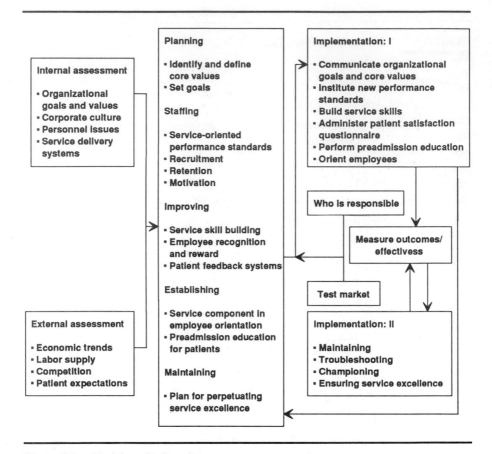

Figure 7.3.   Model marketing plan.

Reprinted from *Nursing Administration Quarterly*, Vol. 12, No. 4, p. 45, with permission of Aspen Publishers, Inc., © Summer, 1988.

DEVELOPING A MARKETING PLAN

Application of the marketing plan process in a health care setting is demonstrated in the following scenario. The seven common elements of marketing plan models are used to organize the plan. This discussion centers on both the organizational and nursing division applications of the process.

Metropolitan Hospital, a 660-bed acute care hospital, is experiencing a significant revenue loss related to a pattern of decline in the use of inpatient, outpatient, and ancillary services. A comparison of the previous and current fiscal years' marketing audits provides the following information.

External Analysis

A significant finding in the broad external analysis is major patient demographic changes. The community population shows a 20% increase in the number of Afro-Americans, Asians, and Hispanics and a 25% increase in the population that is over 60 years of age. The increase in the aging population is related to the establishment of three new retirement developments within the community. Market research undertaken to learn customer health care preferences included telephone and mail surveys, as well as clinic patient interviews. Findings indicated that younger minority clients desire well-baby and pediatric health services. This group tends to favor bilingual providers. Elderly clients are interested in home care support and in assistance with the purchase of medical equipment and medications. Both groups believe they are underrepresented in health services planning. Competition among health care providers has increased with the opening of a for-profit acute care facility across town. This new facility is targeting two large direct mail campaigns at physicians and senior citizens. Ethnic groups are actively working to identify and support high-quality, low-cost care services, concentrating their efforts on chronic illness support and improved social service programs.

Current client satisfaction evaluations show all services, especially nursing, enjoying a strongly positive evaluation. Additionally, the hospital's longstanding reputation for high-quality care was recently bolstered in feature stories broadcast by a local television station.

Internal Analysis

A task force from the executive committee contracted for the services of a marketing consultant, who completed a marketing audit. This involved an independent analysis of the hospital's entire marketing effort. It began with an assessment of the mission and goals. The mission statement and objectives of the organization had undergone no major revisions since the facility opened 10 years ago. Organizational strengths include a positive public image, above-average workforce stability, and a mature, cohesive top management team. Primary weaknesses include a pattern of decline in physician referrals for inpatient and ancillary services, decreased physician status, a weak organizational marketing orientation, and decreasing fiscal surplus. Opportunities identified include building on the current positive public image, targeting services to the ethnic groups, and expanding the nursing care delivery role by use of a managed care model.

Establishment of Program Goals and Strategies

Organizational Goal 1

Top management will initiate an internal marketing program focusing on meeting the specific needs of patients, visitors, physicians, employees, and the community.

Division of Nursing Goal 1a

Nursing will demonstrate understanding of, and support for, the mission, values, culture, and business direction of the organization and the division of nursing.

Divisional Strategies: Goal 1a

1. Develop a quarterly inservice education program that fosters a marketing orientation.
2. Schedule the programs for day, evening, and night shifts.
3. Publicize time, date, and location via flyers and memos to nurse managers.
4. Evaluate learning with a pre-test and a post-test. Seek to obtain a score of at least 85% on the post-test.

Division of Nursing Goal 1b

All levels of nursing employees will indicate they are satisfied or highly satisfied with their work environment and its components.

Divisional Strategies: Goal 1b

1. Develop a valid and reliable employee satisfaction questionnaire.
2. Request annual completion of the questionnaire on a voluntary and confidential basis.
3. Publish aggregate findings in the nursing newsletter.

Division of Nursing Goal 1c

Employees will be acknowledged for excellence in clinical, administrative, research, or educational job performance through a system of monetary and non-monetary recognition programs.

Divisional Strategies: Goal 1c

1. Appoint a committee to develop, pilot, implement, and maintain an employee excellence recognition program.
2. Achieve a 10% increase in monetary awards and a 25% increase in non-monetary awards within two years.

Division of Nursing Goal 1d

Patients (or significant others) will indicate satisfaction with the quality and quantity of services delivered.

Divisional Strategy: Goal 1d

1. Distribute a facility-wide patient satisfaction questionnaire to a random sample of 10% of discharged patients and 10% of ambulatory clients.
2. Achieve a satisfactory rating from at least 85% of those surveyed.

3. Report findings to the executive committee and to the consumer and employee councils.

Division of Nursing Goal 1e

Patients (or significant others) will indicate that they would return for health care and would recommend the facility to others.

Divisional Strategy: Goal 1e

1. Include on the patient satisfaction questionnaire an item that asks if the patient would return for care or recommend the facility to others.
2. Obtain an indication that at least 90% of patients (or significant others) would return for future care or would recommend the facility to others.
3. Report findings to the executive committee and to the consumer and employee councils.

Organizational Goal 2

The entire organization will market the facility as a "Center for Excellence" that is continually identifying and responding to the needs of its patients.

Division of Nursing Goal 2a

The nursing division will coordinate the establishment of a consumer council made up of seven former clients.

Divisional Strategies: Goal 2a

1. Ask nursing personnel to respond to questions from the consumer council.
2. Encourage all patients to participate in consumer council surveys.
3. Provide a senior nurse manager to serve a two-year term as organization liaison to the group.

Division of Nursing Goal 2b

The division will implement a case management project to support client needs for continuity and coordination of care and to provide a proactive response to the continued shortage of professional nurses.

Divisional Strategies: Goal 2b

1. Seek a grant from the National Center for Nursing Research to fund the first two years of a case management project.
2. Pilot case management on one medical and two surgical units.
3. During the third through the fifth year, fund the project from revenues generated by returning and referred clients.

Organizational Goal 3

Existing programs and services will be expanded or repackaged to concentrate on the Asian, Black, Hispanic, and elderly target markets.

Division of Nursing Goal 3a

The division will begin redesigning services with the pediatric acute care, ambulatory care, and well-baby programs, as well as the geriatric ambulatory clinic, to better meet the needs of the targeted markets.

Divisional Strategies: Goal 3a

1. Change divisional mission statements, organizational charts, and staffing to support expansion of ambulatory and inpatient pediatric nursing services as well as geriatric ambulatory care.
2. Advertise service changes by targeted mailings, posters, and a videotape.
3. Support a twice-weekly mobile community health teaching program.
4. Teach targeted populations preventive health strategies during ambulatory and inpatient visits.
5. Provide courses in needed foreign languages for health care personnel.
6. Make maximum use of bilingual personnel.
7. Achieve a 90% satisfaction rate from surveyed clients.

Division of Nursing Goal 3b

The division will support by referrals a social services project aimed at providing financial assistance to patients in need of medical and pharmaceutical supplies.

Divisional Strategies: Goal 3b

1. Appoint an interdisciplinary task force to develop the project.
2. Incorporate relevant questions into discharge plan and ambulatory care nursing assessment form.
3. Design a social service referral form.
4. Refer clients in need of supplies to the designated social service caseworker.
5. Conduct patient and provider surveys at 6 and 12 months after implementation of program to identify economic outcomes, satisfaction levels, and recommendations for change.

Organizational Goal 4

Compatible with the mission and available resources, top management will initiate new programs and services having above-average expectations of social and commercial success, based on market research. An innovative care and services committee will be established to review and manage proposals.

Division of Nursing Goal 4a

Encourage and support intrapreneurial and entrepreneurial efforts of staff.

Divisional Strategies: Goal 4a

1. Encourage all nursing staff, managers, patients, and visitors to submit written nursing care and system improvement recommendations to the vice president of nursing as a member of the innovative care and services committee.
2. Support selected ideas with research, information, technology, seed money, and extramural funding information.
3. Measure effectiveness of improvement to program by responses on patient satisfaction surveys and other system audits.

Integration with Other Plans

The key to success of the overall marketing effort lay in coordinating activities of the various divisional committees with the department heads and the executive committee's marketing subcommittee. This subcommittee served a monitoring and controlling function for the chief executive officer (CEO). It was composed of the associate administrator, the chief financial officer, the directors of human resources and marketing, the vice president of nursing, and employee, union, and consumer representatives. Their tasks involved evaluating the total marketing management effort for congruity with mission, resources, and goals, as well as coordinating changes with the respective departments. In the case of disputes, the CEO served as the final authority.

Establishment of Action Plans

The organization and the nursing division used the following format in the development of their marketing action plan document. They identified: (1) specific action steps; (2) responsibility points; and (3) a time frame for completion. This document brings together the strategies and outcomes described earlier with assignment of accountability and a timetable for action. It proved to be one of the most valuable and important parts of the marketing plan.

Monitoring System

A monitoring system used by our facility linked six major implementation processes:

1. An approval mechanism.
2. Feedback loops.
3. Review cycles.
4. Evaluation points.

5. Communication systems.

6. Revision procedures.

Approval of the formal marketing plan begins its implementation. Throughout implementation, however, approval continues to be an important part of the monitoring process. The monitoring system exists to support evaluation of the effectiveness of the plan and, as necessary, provide a mechanism to make changes in it. Feedback loops and communication systems move information on the progress of the plan. Review cycles and specific evaluation points provide opportunities to assemble and examine this information. Finally, a clear set of revision procedures provide for the approval and implementation of changes to the plan.

While there is general agreement that much more needs to be done to maintain our competitive advantage and to respond more quickly to opportunities, some achievements are apparent. Evaluations of the results at 6 and 12 months of the marketing plan were positive. See Exhibit 7.2 for some examples.

EXHIBIT 7.2   Marketing Plan Outcomes

Six-Month Evaluation Examples

1. A halt in the pattern of revenue decline.
2. Establishment of marketing orientation programs in all major clinical and support services.

Twelve-Month Evaluation Examples

1. Regained lost market share and 10% in revenues for the year.
2. Seventy percent of employees attended a marketing orientation program; 80% of these successfully completed the post-test.
3. Achieved a 25% increase in nonmonetary awards through implementing the employee excellence recognition program.
4. Achieved satisfactory ratings from 90% of surveyed patients.
5. Attained more than 50 new patient admissions a month.
6. Attained more than 50 new ambulatory patients a month.
7. Established the consumer council that is now making recommendations.
8. Implemented a managed nursing care delivery system with plans to double the case load in the coming year.
9. Measured increased satisfaction of targeted client groups with questionnaires.

Problems encountered in the marketing plan process involved organizational goals 3 and 4. The goal component addressing the elderly target market was implemented by the division of nursing as a project of financial support to assist the elderly with obtaining medical and pharmaceutical supplies. Members of the task force for this project were unable to reach consensus on issues such as size and source of the aid or screening criteria. Rather than cancel the project, a decision was made to scale back the size of the task force. They were then able to develop a pilot program to assist elderly clients with the lease or purchase of medical equipment and pharmaceuticals.

Organizational goal 4 addressed the management of initiatives for new programs and services. An innovative care and services committee was established as the mechanism for review and management of these initiatives. However, the number and skill levels of the committee members proved to be insufficient to handle the volume of care improvement proposals submitted. Additionally, conflict arose as a result of the absence of written guidance in areas such as the submission and evaluation process of initiatives. In an effort to improve timely response, the committee was disbanded. The responsibility for processing proposals was given to a project manager within the department of marketing. Written guidelines for initiatives and a proposal evaluation and tracking process will be developed and presented to the executive committee for review and approval.

Conclusions

The majority of the hospital's employees believes that the adoption of a marketing orientation was a wise choice. Inpatient, outpatient, and ancillary referrals and revenues have increased. Questionnaires show improved satisfaction on the part of patients, visitors, physicians, employees, and the community. It is apparent that further long-range (strategic) approaches to organizational planning and management will result in growth, efficiency, and effectiveness of the marketing program and the organization itself.

REFERENCES

Benedict, M.B., Gemmell, L.E., & Anderson, D.M. (1988). Achieving excellence through a superior service strategy. *Nursing Administration Quarterly, 12*(4), 39-51.

Hillestad, S.G., & Berkowitz, E.N. (1984). *Health care marketing plans: From strategy to action.* Homewood, IL: Dow Jones-Irwin.

Lovelock, C.H., & Weinberg, C.B. (1984). *Marketing for public and nonprofit managers.* New York: John Wiley.

Strasen, L. (1987). *Key business skills for nurse managers.* Philadelphia, PA: Lippincott.

Marketing Research Using the Nominal Group Process

Sharon E. Hoffman, MBA, PhD, RN
Dean and Professor, College of Nursing
Medical University of South Carolina
Charleston, SC

Sharon P. Aadalen, PhD, RN
Director of Nursing Education and Research
United Hospital
St. Paul, MN

THE MARKETING PROBLEM

Market measurement and forecasting is particularly difficult in the service sector where trends are complex, demand is not stable from year to year, and historical data are unavailable. All stages in new product development, from idea generation to launching an offering, depend upon market research. This is true in developing any new products, whether goods or services. Gathering data for idea generation is particularly difficult when the market is not well defined, and has diverse concerns and characteristics. Our marketing challenge arose when we designed a national institute for public health nurse leaders. The primary objective of the institute was to sponsor an annual continuing education conference. Many issues, such as geographical dispersion of our target audience, varying levels of education and experience, and diverse practice settings and concerns, made our task difficult. We used market surveys of national nurse leaders and the nominal group process to obtain the data that resulted in a new product, an institute for public health nurse leaders. Nominal group technique is a highly structured qualitative research method used to facilitate group interaction when consensus, creative, and evaluative decisions are needed.

Consumer Needs

In the 1970s, a significant increase in the number of nurses employed in outpatient settings such as community-based home health care and public health agencies, coupled with the increasing requirement of mandatory continuing education for relicensure, created a problem for public health nurses. During the early

1980s, little was available to meet their continuing education needs. As continuing education directors, we had a problem in programming for this diverse audience.

Public health nurses were a small percentage of the total registered nurse population. They seemed to function in relative isolation from one another. Their roles differed from agency to agency, and they practiced in a variety of settings and organizational structures, from private entrepreneurial organizations to county- and state-operated agencies. Concurrent use of both public health nurse and community health nurse titles is one clue to the diversity of this population. Both titles are used because of the continuing role controversy: Do these professionals provide nursing care to individuals in the community or to the aggregate of the community?

On first analysis, we seemed to be confronting a marketing nightmare. Several basic questions had to be answered. Who was the market? Which group was the potential market, the available market, the served market, and were there any penetrated markets? (See Chapter 2.) These questions were difficult to answer, particularly without any unified mailing lists or representatives of organizational bodies to serve as a consulting group. The opportunity to meet the continuing education needs of public health nurses was both intriguing and challenging. We decided to try to penetrate the larger market by providing continuing education for leaders in public and community health nursing, through a national institute. Our first step was to formulate a marketing research plan that included idea finding, idea screening, and evaluating stages of the new product development process (Kotler & Andreasen, 1987).

EXTERNAL MARKET ANALYSIS

Idea Finding

In this model, the idea finding stage included systematic searching for new ideas through reading, professional meetings, and consultation. We began the process by forming a local advisory committee of nine public health nursing leaders from the private, public, and academic sectors. After several brainstorming sessions, it was agreed that a national perspective was needed to identify the issues and challenges—present, emergent, and future—that faced public health nurses. An open-ended survey was developed querying national leaders as to the 10 most pressing issues facing public health practitioners. These leaders were used as intermediaries, assisting us in gathering data from an audience that we were unable to tap directly. Estimates of middlemen are often used in business when reaching the ultimate consumers is too expensive or difficult. These *middlemen*, individuals who are assumed to be close to the consumers and to know their needs and desires, are asked to forecast what the actual consumers are likely to be interested in, and thus estimate potential demand. Care must be taken to screen for middlemen bias. In our case, the next step of the process used another group of experts to act as a check-and-balance mechanism for the leaders' forecasts.

The decision to use a survey marketing research method to query national leaders posed a problem, for we were short of time and money. We decided to distribute the questionnaires at five national and regional meetings that the advisory council members would be attending over the next month. Advisory members agreed to seek acknowledged national leaders at these meetings, ask for their cooperation in filling out the instrument, collect the questionnaires before leaving the meeting, and return them to us. The advisory members collecting data would use their judgment in pursuing those informal and formal leaders they thought would provide grass-roots forecasting. This personalized, nonrandom approach worked surprisingly well; in one month's time we had accumulated completed surveys from 93 leaders. Our wide distribution, using professional networking, gave us data from 31 states.

Analysis of the survey completed the idea finding step of our marketing research plan. We now had a prioritized list of public health issues that were categorized according to primary, secondary, or tertiary interventions. Through the networking process, we also identified leaders in education and service from five contiguous states who were willing to come to a program planning session on our campus. From the names solicited by the initial advisory group, we selected public health nurses in leadership positions from Minnesota, North Dakota, South Dakota, Iowa, and Wisconsin. This group was carefully selected to be a mix of public health nursing educators, agency directors, and state consultants. A one-day program planning meeting to build consensus was the important next step in the market research plan. With the initial data in hand, we were able to persuade a group of rural banks interested in rural community health to underwrite the expenses for a one-day program planning session.

Idea Screening

The next phases of our marketing research plan consisted of idea screening and evaluating. Assessing new ideas and eliminating those without merit are the essence of idea screening and evaluating. An organized approach was required to develop consensus. After considering several options, we decided to use a nominal group method adapted from the Delbecq Van de Ven Program Planning Model (1971), a process used extensively in business and industry. *Nominal group* means a group in name only, formed for a specific decision-making task. In this case, the group established another list of prioritized continuing education issues. This method's advantage over the usual brainstorming planning sessions is that all individual ideas are solicited, recorded, grouped, and prioritized. Shy members' ideas are received and given the same consideration as ideas of more verbal group members; the group is never monopolized or sidetracked.

Nominal Group Process

After introductions and an orientation to the nominal group method, the group was divided into five round-table groups, each with five members and a facilitator. These work groups were mixed to include members from diverse geographic and practice settings. Each group was given written instructions to generate 10 conference themes reflecting public health nursing issues and concerns from the perspective of their own organization and region. Members independently and silently wrote down their 10 issues. The facilitator then asked each participant to present one idea from the list, moving around the circle until everyone participated. As they were given, the ideas were recorded by the facilitator on a large flip chart easily seen by all group members. No discussion took place during this recording session. Evaluation was not allowed, although other group members were encouraged to add to the suggestions or to consolidate them, if possible. This recording and round-robin exchange continued until all suggestions were exhausted. Next, the facilitator led a group discussion of each idea in sequence and recorded on the flip chart. Expressions of support, clarification, rationale, or nonsupport were elicited, and all members were encouraged to participate. Every item was thoroughly discussed. The person who gave the idea had no responsibility to defend, explain, or provide rationale for any suggestion. Following this, the group silently cast individual ballots to rank-order the items. These votes were summarized by the facilitator, accepted as the decision of the work group, and shared with the advisory group.

Nominal group process was also used to generate suggestions for session topics, speakers, and formats. Issues that evolved represented an excellent mix of rural and urban public health problems, perspectives from large and small public health nursing service agencies, concerns related to practice and education, and geographic diversity. The planning session provided participants with an opportunity to exchange ideas, share experiences, and link their organization's needs with others' continuing education needs.

Outcomes of these five groups were compared and contrasted with the lists generated by the national leaders. We had achieved a mechanism to unblock the system of idea generation. Ideas that might have been considered inappropriate or not relevant had as much chance to get on the list as others.

Advantages of the nominal group method include limited time involvement, low cost, reliability, and high-quality outcome. The time required for one prioritizing session was approximately two hours. This time commitment can be compared with the construction and analysis of several questionnaires, brainstorming meetings, and individual or group focus interviews. When compared to these alternatives, we felt it was well worth the effort. Reliability of the information gathered was increased because of the number of people involved. The process insured that a few participants could not dominate the discussion or force their ideas on others. It is clear that the selection of involved, enthusiastic, and creative participants affects the outcome. Quantifying the data by priority ranking increases group consensus. The cost of this method is often less than that of other group assessment strategies, such as paid focus groups or individual interview sessions. Using the survey from the 93 national leaders, we had generated a list of potential institute registrants who were already committed to the program and would be willing to advise co-workers of its worth. They all remained committed to the institute, and were used as session moderators and evaluators at the time of the program presentation.

If careful attention is devoted to the group formation, to the relevance of questions, and to feedback provided to group members, the nominal group method works well. Combining this method with survey research provided us with an effective check-and-balance system to test the middlemen's forecasting. In this way we generated overall goals and themes for a three-day national continuing education program.

SUMMARY

In this case study, we have described the successful use of the nominal group process as a qualitative marketing research method. As a result of our efforts, the first institute was held in 1981, and has become an annual event. The institute serves as an ever-increasing national and international forum for community health leaders. It has evolved as a recognized meeting place and as a prestigious annual conference for the profession.

REFERENCES

Aadalen, S., Hoffman, S., & Vegoe, S. (1984). Continuing education for public health nursing leaders. *International Nursing Review, 31*(3), 76–81.

Kotler, P., & Andreasen, A.R. (1987). *Strategic marketing for nonprofit organizations* (3rd ed.). Englewood Cliffs, NJ: Prentice-Hall.

Scott, D., & Deadrick, D. (1982). The nominal group technique: Applications for training needs assessment. *Training and Development Journal, 36*(6), 26–33.

Van de Ven, A.H., & Delbecq, A.L. (1971). Nominal versus interacting group processes for committee decision making effectiveness. *Academy of Management Journal, 14*(2), 203–212.

Marketing a Nursing Department to Physicians

Phillippa F. Johnston, MS, RN
Assistant Administrator
Capitol Hill Hospital
Washington, DC

THE MARKETING PROBLEM

Brian Hospital is a 350-bed, full-service, acute care community hospital in a metropolitan area. The nursing division is decentralized. First-line managers of each patient care unit report directly to the chief nurse executive (CNE), who is a vice president. The nurse managers have 24-hour accountability and responsibility for the management of patient care and the unit, and are called nurse directors (ND). In the hospital hierarchy, they are department heads. Budgeted positions are adequate. Organizational structures and systems for smooth, effective management of the nursing division are in place.

Like many other health care institutions, Brian Hospital is trying to survive in an economic environment with a reduced demand for inpatient services, and increased competition from managed care plans and other hospitals. In 1987, Brian Hospital made $3.5 million; 1988 projections were merely to break even. There are at least two factors aggravating this financial situation: (1) a rise in the number of indigent patients, and (2) an increase in budgeted nursing personnel costs because of the nursing shortage, with resulting use of agency nurses and increases in salaries.

Physicians were dissatisfied because they perceived the nursing care to be of lower quality at Brian Hospital than at other hospitals where they practiced. The physicians also complained that they received too many phone calls regarding their patients. As a result, many were admitting patients to other area hospitals.

Nurses were dissatisfied because they felt that physicians did not recognize and respect their contributions to patient care. The physicians did not seek out the nurses for information about their patients; they seemed to avoid direct, face-to-face discussion. They did not share the medical plans of care. Too often, medical orders were not clear, or a nurse's request for orders was ignored. A phone call to the physician was then necessary even though the physician had just left the hospital. This situation wasted valuable nursing time.

The CNE has a good working relationship with the medical director and other physician leaders. These physicians are comfortable discussing patient care issues

307

with the CNE. They know that the nursing division is focused on excellence and that their concerns will be followed up. After many discussions with the medical staff leadership, the CNE identified that a problem existed in daily communication between physicians and nurses, centered around quality of patient care. There were also other physicians who did not use established systems of communication to make their concerns, complaints, and dissatisfactions known.

The marketing goals identified were to increase physician and nurse satisfaction with work relationships, to increase patient and physician satisfaction with, and use of, services provided by Brian Hospital, and to facilitate physician and nurse recruitment and retention. Attaining these marketing goals would help the organization maintain financial stability and provide high-quality products.

MARKET RESEARCH

Sample Groups

Because the majority of physicians on staff are internists, we decided to first study them and the nurses on the two medical units. The Department of Medicine is headed by an elected chief and assistant chief. The department is divided into subspecialties such as endocrinology and oncology. Fifty internists have admitting privileges at Brian Hospital; however, only 25 are active. These 25 physicians are responsible for more than 80% of all admissions to medicine, so this active group was selected to participate in the study. The other 25 either admitted no patients or less than three during the last year.

Some important external factors have an impact on these physicians. Physicians are faced with increasing competition. They must compete for patients with other physicians, with managed care plans, and with alternative care delivery systems such as free-standing emergency care centers. In addition, in this era of prospective reimbursement, patients must be discharged earlier. This often causes interpersonal conflicts between patient and physician as well as intrapersonal conflicts for the physician making professional decisions.

All registered nurses on the two medical patient care units were invited to participate in the study. The two medical patient care units are staffed similarly. Each unit has its own ND and two assistants. Both NDs have masters degrees and head nurse experience at other hospitals; both have been at Brian for two years. Registered nurses, licensed practical nurses, and nursing assistants make up the staff; registered nurses account for 75% of the positions. Most have baccalaureate degrees in nursing. Turnover of RNs on each unit is 30%. Team nursing is the method of delivery of care.

Method

To obtain the information needed to develop a marketing plan, the CNE decided to use focus group interviews with the physicians and nurses rather than individual interviews or telephone or mail surveys. It was felt that group interviews allowed for greater flexibility and depth in those areas of greatest importance to physicians and nurses.

Small-group interviews with five to seven physicians or nurses were conducted. The groups were not mixed and not paid. They were encouraged to participate by the chief hospital and nursing executives. To increase participation, groups were convened at breakfast and lunch times; food was provided. We conducted four physician and six nurse group interviews.

Interviews were exploratory; we wanted to identify and define the problems. The following topics were discussed: perception of the medical and leadership staff (in nurse groups), perception of nursing and leadership staff (in physician groups), specific changes participants would like, specific preferences regarding nursing care, and values held by each group.

Results

Analysis of the interviews with the internists gave us the following information. These physicians perceive the nursing staff to be generally unfriendly, not interested, and unknowledgeable about their patients. They receive more telephone calls from nurses at Brian than from nurses at any other hospital. When the internists call the medical units, they are put on hold for a long time before a nurse answers. The nurses seem to provide good care because their patients are satisfied; they receive few patient complaints.

While the internists do not know the NDs very well, they perceive them as being competent and responsive. However, they find it frustrating to ask a ND a question about a patient only to be referred to the nurse caring for the patient. The physicians do not understand why the ND is not informed about all of the patients. "In other hospitals," they said, "head nurses know everything about the patients."

These physicians want few but vital changes. They want fewer phone calls, and more assistance from secretaries in getting needed information such as laboratory results. Space is a problem; there is no space to sit in the nurses' station and there is no place to talk privately with families.

Preferences regarding nursing activities vary widely. Some physicians want the nurse to call the house officer; others don't. Still others want the nurse to use professional judgment in calling the house officer. This difference in wants was also seen in relation to most nursing activities and doctors' orders. In general, what these physicians want is good nursing care and no errors. They want satisfied patients. Other wants are recognition and respect, patient information, and not being hassled. They want to use their time effectively.

The analysis of the nurse interviews also yielded useful information. Nurses perceived the physicians as not wanting to talk with their patients, as undervaluing the nurse's role, and as withholding pertinent patient information. They perceive the medical director and the chief of medicine to be very good physicians who are able to resolve patient care problems and conflicts with physicians. Both work well with nurses. The nurses do not have much interaction with the subspecialty chiefs.

These medical nurses want changes in the way nurses and physicians communicate. They see the need to streamline the system to facilitate communication. Implementation of joint rounds and review of current orders and patient needs would save time, wear, and tear on both the physicians and nurses. Similar to the internists, the medical nursing personnel want recognition and respect. They also want patient information, good communication with physicians, and to participate in patient management and decision-making. Their most important desire is to have time to give direct patient care.

MARKETING STRATEGIES

In order to achieve the marketing goals, the nursing division developed strategies to improve the nurse-physician relationship. We did this by sharing the results of the interviews with both groups. All agreed that they needed to look at how they were communicating and what values they were exchanging. Misconceptions had to be discussed and clarified. Solutions to identified problems needed to be negotiated. Both the physicians and the nurses had a great deal of skepticism as to whether the situation could be improved. Nevertheless, six physicians and six nurses volunteered to develop resolutions for these communication problems.

These 12 volunteers named themselves the Medical Division Collaborative Practice Group. They identified as their goals: (1) to clarify misconceptions; (2) to develop an effective communication process; and (3) to implement the process to improve patient care. The vice president for marketing was a consultant to the group, and the CNE was a facilitator. Six three-hour meetings led to the conceptualization of the marketing mix outlined in Exhibit 9.1, and to the development of the following tactics:

1. Delineate the nurse's role at Brian Hospital to the medical staff. This includes explaining the organizational structure, the system of care delivery, goals and objectives of the nursing division, and the roles of other care providers and employees.

2. Demonstrate excellence in nursing and medical practice as evidenced by patient satisfaction, reduced errors and incidents, JCAHO assessment, quality assurance programs, and the like.

3. Delineate the physician's role to the nursing staff. This includes discussing the highly political, competitive, cost-constrained environment inside and outside of Brian Hospital.

4. Implement a system that facilitates two-way communication. This includes:

   a. Nurse to physician

      (1) Post nurse assignments so that physicians know which nurse to look for, and where to find the nurse.

      (2) Orient physicians to the unit.

      (3) Make rounds with physicians.

      (4) Try to meet with physicians when they are on the unit.

      (5) Have all patients of a particular physician admitted to the same unit/area whenever possible.

   b. Physician to nurse

      (1) Make rounds with nurses.

      (2) Discuss patient needs with nurse caring for the patient.

      (3) Have all patients admitted to the same unit whenever possible.

RESULTS AND EVALUATION

The Medical Division Collaborative Practice Group set target dates for implementation and specific methods and criteria for evaluation. Evaluation would include feedback from all nurses and physicians involved. They ended the planning sessions optimistic that the goals would be accomplished. They believed the plan would take six months to show benefits. For members of the group, improved communication was immediately apparent.

Even though the nursing staff was able to implement all of the strategies, at this time only 20 of the 25 physicians consistently make rounds with nurses. For these 20, communication is more efficient and effective. The number of telephone calls they receive has diminished considerably. Nurses who work with these physicians have found that they are invited to participate in collegial patient care decisions, that they are helped to understand the medical care plan, and that physicians review orders with them. As a result, time is not wasted sorting out confused communication, and instead can be used for patient care. Both groups like the consistency gained by the assignment of all of a physicians' patients to the same unit.

We have found that patient care issues, expectations, and preferences of physicians and nurses are now easily discussed. This approach has been so successful that the CNE is going repeat this marketing process with the division of surgery.

EXHIBIT 9.1   Conceptualization of Marketing Mix

Product
High-quality patient or nursing care
Collegial communication
Hassle-free service

Place/Distribution
Patient care questions discussed face-to-face on the unit instead of over the telephone
Rounds and meetings conducted on units

Price
Physicians and nurses:
Provide care to patients admitted to Brian Hospital
Receive respect, recognition, goodwill, and payment

Promotion
Medical director and chief of medicine discuss plan at meetings with internists
Medical and nursing newsletters feature articles and provide updates
Nurses and physicians discuss nurse-physician relationships at respective staff meetings
Nursing's message to physicians: purchase nursing care here; admit your patients to Brian Hospital

Marketing a Nursing Education Service Line to Improve Image

Karen J. Kelly, MS, RN, CNAA
Associate Director of Nursing for Education and Research
Greater Southeast Community Hospital
Washington, DC

THE MARKETING PROBLEM

Greater Southeast Community Hospital (GSCH) is a 450-bed urban hospital located in southeast Washington, DC. It serves a very diverse service area population, with two-thirds of residents characterized as economically disadvantaged and one-third above the median income level for the area. In the early 1980s, the administration decided to dedicate significant resources to position the hospital as a premier health care provider for our community and to project a better image to the Washington metropolitan area. The new image would show that we were talented health care professionals interested in providing humanistic care to the residents of our community. While the communications department was busy with radio and print ads, slogan and jingle development, and other common image projection strategies, the staff of the Center for Nursing Education (CNE) was busy implementing its own marketing plan.

An opportunity that would contribute to the organizational goal of a new image was evident to the staff of the CNE. We had the service line, talent, and capability to help position the organization as a high-quality health care provider *and* a good place to practice professional nursing. CNE made a planned effort to position the department as a responsive, ''can-do'' service within the organization. Concurrently, this conscious effort contributed to the overall organizational goal to change our image in the community and helped recruit nurses to the hospital; thus, we were also playing with the team!

At that time, there was also a paucity of high-quality, reasonably priced continuing education programs for nurses in the Washington metropolitan area. While many national conventions and conferences were held in the nation's capital, this type of several-day, multitracked, and specialty focused program did not meet the need of professional nurses to update general knowledge and skills related to their specialty areas, such as medical-surgical, critical care, and oncology. In addition, these programs were very expensive for nurses who frequently had to pay for continuing education out of their own pockets.

313

Although continuing education is not required for relicensure in Washington, DC, or the surrounding states of Virginia and Maryland where many nurses also work and reside, hospitals often have an educational contact hour accrual requirement as a performance standard. Others may require contact hours for specialty nurses or those in clinical ladder programs. GSCH has a performance standard of 20 contact hours per year for all clinical nurses. Those in the clinical ladder program are required to accumulate more each year, depending upon their level. Thus, nursing administration of GSCH already had a history of supporting and valuing continuing education as one method of maintaining and developing professional competencies.

An internal image problem also existed in the CNE. The providers of educational services (CNE) were not perceived by nursing administration as the consumer of their service or as a responsive department that could contribute to organizational goals. New members of CNE felt that an internal marketing plan could be developed to address this issue as well. We also feared a lack of support on the part of nursing administration if we did not resolve this problem. Contributing to this difficult issue was the organizational structure, for at that time the CNE was located within the human resource development department, in the personnel division rather than the nursing division.

MARKETING RESEARCH

Method

In order to become a provider of high-quality, reasonably priced continuing education (CE) for nurses in the Washington community, we needed answers to the following questions:

How to get approved by the American Nurses' Association (ANA) as a CE provider;

How nurses make decisions about the continuing education in which they participate;

How to reach those nurses who participate in CE;

How to promote our CE programs so they were connected with the organization's efforts;

What the costs and potential revenues of these efforts would be;

What other benefits might be experienced as a result of a program like this.

To address the internal image problem that CNE was experiencing with nursing administration, we investigated the following:

What was the source of these perceptions?

What internal programming was needed by the CNE to help the nursing division reach specified goals?

What were the expectations of the key members of the organization?

Would nursing administration support the proposal to market selected CE offerings to the nursing community?

Three major marketing research techniques were chosen to collect the external and internal data we needed to develop a marketing plan.

Questionnaires were mailed to 800 registered nurses in the Washington area (not employed at GSCH) to develop a profile of decisions and preferences related to CE. A mailing list of 17,000 nurses in the metropolitan area was purchased from a professional nursing journal. Names were drawn from the mailing list using a systematic sampling technique. Each potential respondent received a packet that included a cover letter, the questionnaire, a stamped, addressed envelope, and a coupon for a $10 reduction in registration fees for one of our CE programs. The coupon said, "In appreciation for completing the survey," and was an incentive to increase returns. One week later, a postcard reminder was sent to all subjects. Three weeks later, subjects who had not returned the questionnaire received a letter requesting participation.

A self-mailer postcard questionnaire was sent to 17,000 nurses to determine their interests in becoming CE consumers and to develop our mailing list. We used the same purchased list for this survey. Each nurse was sent a double postcard. One part described the need of all professional nurses to participate in continuing education, briefly described our program, and asked the recipients if they would like to receive future announcements about our programs. The tear-off, postage-paid return card requested some limited demographic data and continuing education interests.

To collect internal data for the marketing plan, the CNE director and staff interviewed eight key organizational leaders, including the vice president for nursing, members of the nursing executive council, the director of human resources development, the hospital CEO, middle- and first-line managers, and staff nurse consumers.

Results

The mail survey to 800 nurses in the Washington metropolitan area yielded a 42% return rate and rich data that helped us target our marketing appropriately. For example, we learned that surveyed nurses prefer a great deal of descriptive information about conferences and seminars and prefer to receive their CE in a one- or two-day package. Nurses generally bought their CE from brochures and catalogs mailed to their homes. Location preferences generally excluded downtown locations; preferences were expressed for hotels with good (preferably free) parking, but churches and other sites were also acceptable. Prices nurses were willing to pay were unreasonably low, regardless of their annual income, although nurses with bachelors degrees or higher were willing to pay more. Accreditation of CE by the ANA was highly valued by most respondents.

The second market research strategy to determine actual interest also yielded a good return. From returns of the self-mailer postcard questionnaire, a mailing list of just over 2,000 potential participants was developed.

The costs of the continuing education proposal were also investigated and yielded the following estimates on an individual program basis:

2,500	professionally designed brochures	$400
100	folders, name tags, paper	$150
100	refreshments (coffee, donuts, soft drinks)	$200
100	handouts and support material	$ 50
	Total per program:	$800

CNE staff, faculty honorarium, and travel costs were already part of the CNE budget and were not expected to change significantly, since we would be using available resources.

To become an ANA-approved CE program provider required completion of an application. We already met most of the criteria specified to meet the standards.

Finally, the potential additional benefits of this proposal to the organization were elicited during the key interviews. The perceived benefits were:

Retention of nurses due to accessibility of on-site CE programs

Recruitment of new nurses

More competent and confident nursing staff

Opportunity to model a high-quality hospital-based CE program

Improving the image of the GSCH nursing department in the organization and the community

Opportunity to feature our own talented staff as faculty, when appropriate.

Of course, ultimately all these additional benefits would contribute to the quality of patient care delivered at GSCH.

The interviews with key organizational members yielded most valuable data that in turn contributed immensely to the outcome of this effort. Regarding the internal image of CNE, nursing administration cited many examples of CNE failing to respond to important learning needs of staff essential to achieve the nursing administration goals. High frustration was expressed about the lack of timeliness in delivery of requested programs. A lack of confidence was also expressed in the ability of the department to design good, sound programs for a busy and constantly developing nursing staff.

As a new member of the department, I was able to listen without becoming defensive, and began to develop new relationships and clarify mutual expectations that were reasonable and rational. Perhaps an indicator of success of this process was the consensus of nursing administration to support the proposal to provide CE to the nursing community.

MARKETING STRATEGIES

Analysis of the market research data led to the decision to implement the following strategies to market the continuing education programs:

Apply to the ANA for approval as a CE provider

Market approximately 12 CE programs over one year to our staff, the potential participant list of 2,000 nurses, and to area hospitals

Set a very reasonable price of $35 per program to attract nurses and help offset part of the direct costs

Maintain a no-charge policy for GSCH nurses

Develop, with the marketing department, a high-quality brochure that would appeal to nurse-buyers, as defined in the mail survey

Co-sponsor selected programs with specialty nursing divisions to gain support and commitment, and to feature talented staff

Use the well-designed GSCH conference facility for programs to attract nurses to this organization

Review results in one year to make decisions about continuing or expanding the program.

Strategies to address the internal image of CNE were identified as follows:

Use the CE program proposal to demonstrate program design capacity

Deliver within six months several internal programs that had been requested several times but never delivered

Respond to all requests for service by delivering a program, referring to other resources, suggesting alternate strategies, or negotiating other mutual agreements

Continue the key interview process biannually to define goals and determine educational programming needed to support those goals

Continue to clarify mutual expectations

Attend key meetings to determine and resolve issues.

RESULTS AND EVALUATION

The first program marketed externally was titled *Critical Care Highlights*, and featured a variety of GSCH and other local faculty. Program design included multiple tracks. While we anticipated 100 participants, 80 from GSCH and 20 from the community, we had an overwhelming response of 110 GSCH participants and 82 nurses from the community. Our conference facility could accommodate up to 200 and, with some program design modifications, we were able to provide a sound educational experience for the participants. What a positive first experience!

Our professional-looking brochures even caused our own nursing staff to view the CNE department differently. A note of pride was detected in many as they referred to our education department.

The first year's programming continued to yield an average of 125 participants. An average of 15 to 20 nurses from the community attended each program. We identified these nurses as our guests and requested our staff to assist them as needed. At each program, 1 or 2 nurses asked about our hospital, and it is estimated that about 12 nurses actually became employed at GSCH after they attended a CE activity, including one education specialist in the Center for Nursing Education.

Revenue generated from participant registration fees due to this effort was approximately $8,000 during the first year. When expenses were calculated, including the cost of outside speakers and CNE staff, there were no direct monetary profits. Benefits, in addition to those discussed above, came from our improved internal image.

The image of CNE with nursing administration was positively affected as a result of this program. Our efforts also yielded a good collaborative relationship. CNE was moved organizationally to the nursing division the next year.

Our success continues. We have maintained a solid program of CE that is ANA accredited. We market 10 to 15 programs each year to the community, to maintain our image of a high-quality care institution of professionals who care about our nurses and our patients. For a reasonably low cost, direct and indirect benefits have been experienced by the many participants in this concerted effort to improve the organization's image.

Marketing Home Health Care

Adina Kolatch, MBA
Director of Community Affairs
Visiting Nurse Service of New York
New York, NY

THE MARKETING SITUATION

Who is the customer in home care? Answers include:

Patient

Family

Caregiver

Nurse

Physician

Hospital

Social worker

Hospital discharge planner

Insurance company

Federal, state, and local government

Employers.

For many consumer products, the *customer* is the one who decides whether to purchase the product, who uses the product, and who pays for it. In home health care, however, the person who uses the service is the patient; the payer is usually the insurance company or other third party. The person who generally makes the decision whether to use the service is the physician, the patient, the social worker, the discharge planner, or a family member. This case study focuses on the physician as customer for home care services.

The Visiting Nurse Service of New York (VNS) developed a marketing plan to increase the number of referrals made by office-based physicians. We targeted physicians for three reasons. Physicians were a major referral source for the agency, second only to hospitals. The hospital market had received a lot of attention, while the physician market was relatively neglected. Physician referrals held steady from 1980 to 1986, representing only 3.5% of total referrals. Compared to physicians' referrals to other certified home health agencies, ours were a much smaller percentage of total referrals. As gatekeepers, physicians have the ultimate say about whether home care services will be provided. This is reinforced by most

319

insurance companies, as they require that the physician give written authorization for the plan of care in order for services to be covered. These factors led us to develop the goals to increase the medical community's awareness of VNS and to increase the number of physician referrals.

Marketing is a comprehensive process that culminates in an exchange of values between two parties. For example, two 6-year-olds, one with a vast supply of bubble gum and one with an extensive baseball card collection, will not trade unless the bubble gum magnate wants baseball cards and the baseball card mogul wants bubble gum. Each must value what the other has to offer. VNS engaged in the marketing process to increase the number of exchange partners.

MARKET ANALYSIS

To develop a customer (physician) profile, we did secondary market research. Data were collected on demographic aspects of physicians in the VNS service area, trends and changes in the industry, and patterns of use of home care service by physicians. For example, according to the American Medical Association Physician Masterfile for 1983, there were 27,336 physicians in New York City. Of these, 21,500 (80%) provided patient care, 11,912 (45%) had office-based practices, and 9,595 (35%) had hospital-based practices. Our secondary research confirmed our belief that physicians were indeed a worthwhile market to pursue. It expanded our knowledge about physicians, and it laid the groundwork for market analysis and subsequent plan development.

The role of the physician in the United States is changing. It was necessary for us to identify and understand these trends in order to understand physicians' needs regarding home care service. We found five important factors affecting the physician market: increased competition, increased number of group practices, increased marketing activities, new models of practice, and joint ventures with hospitals.

To deal with increased competition, physicians are providing outpatient surgery and home visits, setting up laboratories and radiology units, and purchasing imaging equipment. Patient demands for service have also increased competition. If the physician does not provide what the patient wants, the patient will go elsewhere for the desired service. In an effort to compete more effectively, physicians are forming group practices to develop larger referral bases. They are also using marketing to gain and maintain a competitive edge.

New models of practice are being developed. An increasing proportion of physicians are salaried rather than maintaining fee-for-service practices. Hospitals, PPOs, and HMOs are developing large staffs of salaried physicians. Hospitals are also strengthening ties with physicians through a variety of activities, such as joint ventures for professional office buildings, HMOs, PPOs, outpatient and diagnostic centers. A nationwide survey of 400 hospital executives conducted by Ernst and Whinney (1985) revealed that 50% of those surveyed were already involved in joint ventures. Of those so involved, 40% were with physician group practices. Of those not yet involved, 48% were interested in discussing possibilities with physician groups.

An important result of these trends is that many physicians are seeking competitive practice advantages. We felt that providing home care was one way physicians could seek and gain such advantages.

National studies on home care revealed that physicians generally have negative attitudes towards home care. The studies showed the following about attitude and usage of home care services:

1. Many physicians underuse home care because they are unaware of the range of services available (Baginski, 1985).

2. Many physicians see home care agencies as dominated by nurses (VNS informal staff interviews).

3. Many physicians shy away from home care because they have been trained to work in an institutional setting (Bernstein, 1987).

4. Many physicians are fearful of losing fees for office visits and tests that might come their way if the home care nurses were not out in the field (Baginski, 1985).

5. Many physicians resent not receiving case management fees for overseeing and coordinating home health care (Bernstein, 1985).

6. Many physicians do not know when a patient's insurance coverage includes a home care benefit (Bernstein, 1985).

We realized that our marketing campaign must take these factors into account in order to convert objections into positive attitudes.

Several studies indicated that some physicians do directly refer cases for home care. Frost and Sullivan (1983) conducted a national study of home care and found that 16% of all cases in certified home care agencies were referred by physicians. These findings actually understate physician referral activity because they failed to include hospital referrals initiated by physicians.

Although VNS had significant contact with physicians in New York City, physician referrals between 1982 and 1986 accounted for approximately 3.5% of total cases. This is significantly lower than the Frost and Sullivan findings. Clearly, there was potential for direct referrals that VNS was not capturing. VNS was underperforming in the physician market when compared with other home care agencies. We concluded that we had the potential not only to meet the current market norm, but to increase referrals beyond the 16% finding of Frost and Sullivan.

As the role of physicians changes, their negative attitudes about home care are softening. As more attention is given to the phenomenal growth of the home care industry, physicians are becoming more aware of the benefits of these services. In addition, the prospective payment system has forced the discharge of patients "quicker and sicker." Physicians must order early discharge. Consequently, physicians are becoming more knowledgeable about, and comfortable with, early discharge coupled with effective care at home.

MARKETING STRATEGIES

The changing role of physicians and their interests in home care gave VNS an opportunity to increase its market share and improve its competitive position. We did this by marketing to physicians in our area. A marketing plan was formulated based on the analysis of the secondary marketing research. See Figure 11.1 for services VNS could provide to physicians in exchange for patient referrals.

VNS found that various factors influence physician practice patterns and use of home care. Specialty, location of office, size of practice, hospital, HMO or PPO affiliation, past experience with home care, patient population, philosophy of care, medical education, age, and sex are important characteristics that must be considered when assessing the physician market for home care referral potential. We recognized the great diversity among physicians and decided to segment the market based on prior demonstrated usage of VNS (see Table 11.1). It was judged that it would be easier to increase referrals from existing customers rather than to cultivate new customers. Therefore, physicians who had previously used our services were targeted for this program.

TABLE 11.1   Physician Market Segments Based on Prior Usage

Segment	Referral Record
High potential	Refers 10 or more cases a year
Medium potential	Refers 3 to 9 cases a year
Low potential	Refers 1 to 2 cases a year
Unknown potential	Does not directly refer to VNS

The most effective way to promote VNS and expand physician referrals was through direct sales calls to physicians in their offices. A staff of six home care consultants was hired and trained to do this. VNS decided to use nurses and train them in sales rather than hire nonnurses and train them in home care. Five of the consultants were registered nurses; the sixth had a business background. Consultants received a two-part training program: training in basic selling skills, and learning about physicians and their usage of home care in New York City. Problems that might be encountered in working with these physicians were discussed.

Instruction in various approaches to increase referral frequency were given to the home care consultants, who used several marketing strategies. The first was *communicating the full range of services VNS provides.* Many physicians were

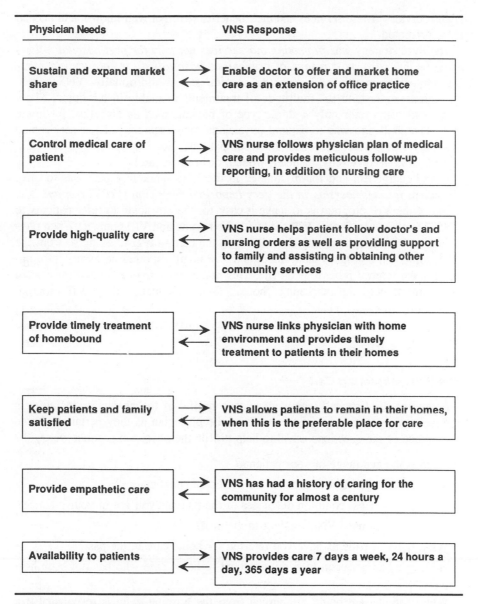

Physician Needs	VNS Response
Sustain and expand market share	Enable doctor to offer and market home care as an extension of office practice
Control medical care of patient	VNS nurse follows physician plan of medical care and provides meticulous follow-up reporting, in addition to nursing care
Provide high-quality care	VNS nurse helps patient follow doctor's and nursing orders as well as providing support to family and assisting in obtaining other community services
Provide timely treatment of homebound	VNS nurse links physician with home environment and provides timely treatment to patients in their homes
Keep patients and family satisfied	VNS allows patients to remain in their homes, when this is the preferable place for care
Provide empathetic care	VNS has had a history of caring for the community for almost a century
Availability to patients	VNS provides care 7 days a week, 24 hours a day, 365 days a year

Figure 11.1.   VNS response to physician needs.

underutilizing our services because they were unaware of what we could do. We explained our services and how the services could benefit patients.

Explaining the new services VNS had added was our second strategy. These services included providing oxygen for respiratory therapy, durable medical equipment, intravenous and antibiotic therapy, meals on wheels, AIDS care, and mental health services. These services and their benefits were not well-known, and needed to be promoted.

The third strategy was *promoting our services not only for post-hospital follow-up care, but also as a means of preventing hospitalization, preventing nursing home placement, and shortening hospital stays.* Additionally, VNS helped physicians understand the multitude of treatments available in the home. Many physicians often refer only a single type of patient, such as diabetics, for home care. The challenge was to expand physicians' understanding of our services so that they would refer a broader range of patients. For example, VNS can help patients who need ostomy, catheter, wound, or hospice care.

A key component and fourth strategy in the VNS marketing plan was to offer physicians *free membership in the Very Important Physician (VIP) Program.* The thrust of the VIP program is to make it easy for the physician to refer patients to VNS. Members are given a VIP card with their name and VIP number. When physicians call the telephone number printed on the card, a registered nurse from the VNS admission unit takes their names and VIP numbers; other necessary information for the referral process is on file. This makes referring easier and faster. We called this strategy our marketing "hook." Other advantages to the VIP program are outlined in Figure 11.2.

Personal Selling

The First Marketing Call

A goal of the first call was to develop a profile of the physician, including a comprehensive assessment of the needs of the physician as they pertain to home care. Some of the questions asked to help profile the physician account were:

What is the age range of your patients?

What percentage of your patients are Medicare beneficiaries?

What are the most common diagnoses of the patients you see in your practice?

How have you used VNS services in the past?

What types of patients have you referred for home care in the past?

Have you had occasion to admit a patient to home care who has not been hospitalized?

When patients are being discharged from the hospital, who is responsible for determining if home care is needed or desirable?

Which cases do you find most difficult to service?

Based on the answers to these questions, the home care consultants developed tactics for increasing referrals from each physician. The home care consultants saw the need to work with each physician in a very specific and different way. Some examples of the types of incentives offered to physicians are:

Welcome V.I.P.!

You have been selected to join our **V**ery **I**mportant **P**hysician program. As a VNS HOME CARE V.I.P., you can take advantage of a wide range of special programs designed to speed the referral process and help you ensure the highest level of professional care for your patients.

The V.I.P. Advantage:

• *Preferred access.* Your V.I.P. number is your key to expediting referral of your patients to VNS HOME CARE. Please be prepared to give your V.I.P. number, along with the information listed on your VNS HOME CARE CHECKLIST, when you call us to refer a patient.

• *Extend your reach.* Your private practice can offer a home care extension through your V.I.P. affiliation with VNS HOME CARE. Under your guidance, we can provide your patients with the continuity of care they need to achieve their highest level of health and independence.

• *Maximize your time.* The VNS HOME CARE V.I.P. program helps you use your time most efficiently, because total home care services are one call away.

• *Start-to-finish care.* We can provide, under your direction, in your patient's own home: professional nursing; physical, speech and occupational therapy; medical social work; medical equipment; nutritional counseling; mental health care; maternal/child health and pediatric care; hospice care for the dying; long term care; and personal care by certified home health aides. Each time you refer a patient, a nurse will visit the patient's home to design, in collaboration with you, a plan of care tailored to his or her specific physical, emotional and social needs.

• *Hands-on assistance.* As a V.I.P., you and your patients benefit from the constant administrative support of VNS HOME CARE personnel. A *Home Care Consultant* will routinely visit your practice and work with you to best meet your needs and those of your patients.

• *Maximize healing at home.* In some cases, our home care services may be able to reduce early re-admissions following a hospital stay by providing careful, professional post-hospital follow-up care.

• *Not just for hospitalized patients.* Keep in mind that VNS HOME CARE may benefit patients who don't require hospitalization. Patients suffering from an acute exacerbation of chronic problems or chronically ill patients with multiple diagnoses may be well served by VNS HOME CARE services.

• *Insurance analysis.* We will research your patients' insurance coverage to help them maximize available resources. And when needed, we will help your staff and patients with referrals to other community agencies for financial and social services.

• *REMEMBER:* In order to take advantage of your V.I.P. benefits, you must call VNS HOME CARE. Make sure to tell your discharge planner, social worker, or office manager to specify VNS HOME CARE when referring patients.

• *Finally, we are available 24 hours a day, 7 days a week, 365 days a year — whenever you need us!*

Call to refer a patient: **212-714-9250**

VNS

350 Fifth Avenue, New York, NY 10118

HOME CARE

A nonprofit subsidiary of the Visiting Nurse Service of New York

Figure 11.2.   The VIP program.

Reprinted with permission

1. Standing orders are developed so that the physician has only to reference the standing orders and specify modifications.
2. VNS admission nurses call the physician's office manager three times a week to pick up new referrals.
3. A VNS nurse goes to the physician's office once a week, confers with the physician regarding potential home care clients, and writes up each referral. The VNS nurse also provides the physician with clinical follow-up on all active cases.
4. VNS creates a home care extension for the physician's practice by dedicating a visiting nurse to that practice. The nurse would coordinate all home care services, including case finding and treatment.

Marketing Tools

Marketing tools were developed to structure and organize staff activities. Every home care consultant was given the following:

1. A physician audit file containing an alphabetical and geographical listing of physicians in their territory. This list contained the names, phone numbers, specialties, and hospital affiliations of all the physicians, plus the number of direct referrals to VNS each made in prior years.
2. A schedule delineating performance standards for each home care consultant. It specified how many physician sales calls were expected per day and per week during the first 12 months of the program. It also indicated how many new calls and repeat calls should be made each day, and the total number of sales calls for a given month.
3. Itinerary sheets that were used to plan each day and also served as route sheets.
4. Expense sheets to keep track of all expenses.
5. Phone logs to keep track of each telephone contact made and the result of the call. These logs enabled VNS to determine how many phone contacts were needed to make an appointment.
6. A physician call report containing a profile of the physician, call results, and a plan of action for the next sales call.
7. A week-in-review log providing a summary of all marketing activity for the week.

Monitoring the Activity

At the end of every week, the home care consultants submitted copies of the week-in-review log and physician call reports to their managers. This enabled the manager to keep a central master file on the physician-related marketing activities and to evaluate each consultant's activity. A listing of all physician referrals was generated at the end of every month. It was used to show the results of the sales activity as well as to identify new physicians on whom to call.

RESULTS AND EVALUATION

A key result was that the percentage of cases referred directly by physicians increased from approximately 3.5% between 1982 and 1986 to 6% in 1987. One hundred new referrals were generated in three months through the dedicated nurse incentive. Maintaining the physician contacts was critical to developing them as a referral source. Being visible, accessible, helpful, and following up inquiries was essential to keeping VNS home care on the physician's mind.

Office nurses and managers emerged as an important segment to target because physicians were often unavailable. By promoting VNS to managers and nurses, referrals were increased. In fact, these people seem to be the true gatekeepers to the physician practice. Good rapport must be established with them in order to obtain referrals from the physician.

Our results confirmed the market research findings that many physicians were unaware of the range of home care services and the reimbursement available. Many physicians viewed home care as nursing service only, and had not known of our other services. Many physicians had been unaware that home care services are covered by third-party payers other than Medicare and Medicaid. Many thought that Medicare still required a prior three-day hospitalization to qualify a patient for home care services; some physicians were under the impression that reimbursement for home care was limited to only those patients who had prior hospitalization. To dispel these reimbursement myths, VNS designed a Home Care Checklist providing physician reimbursement guidelines and the necessary information to make a referral.

Many physicians indicated that they did not handle referrals, and suggested that the home care consultant contact the hospital social worker or discharge planners. This inevitably expanded the sales promotion activity to include hospitals as well as physicians.

VNS is currently evaluating the costs and benefits of these marketing strategies. Preliminary data indicate that they are time-consuming and expensive, and that other activities, such as liaisons in hospitals, yield a greater return. We are investigating the cost per referral to reach other segments. New targeted segments could be the patient, social worker, or discharge planner.

Constant planning, flexibility, evaluation of current marketing activities, responding to opportunities, and setting priorities for effective use of resources are the keys to marketing success. Developing an agency-wide marketing orientation and strategic outlook that is market driven will position an agency for growth and development. This is the essence and goal of any marketing plan. It is the best recommendation we offer to other health care providers.

REFERENCES

American Medical Association MasterFile (1983). Department of Data Release Services and Data Resources.

Baginski, Y. (1985). Marketing home care to the doctors. *Caring, 4*(9), 34–40.

Bernstein, L.H. (1987). The physician as your second sales force: The role of the physician in home care marketing. *Caring, 6*(5), 40–46.

Ernst & Whinney (1985). *Health care joint ventures.* New York: Author.

Frost & Sullivan (1983). *Home care products, services, and markets.* New York: Author.

Marketing a Pediatric Private Doctors' Clinic*

Rebecca S. McAnnally, RN
Divisional Director of Nursing
Ambulatory Care Services
The Children's Hospital of Alabama
Birmingham, AL

THE MARKETING SITUATION

The Children's Hospital of Alabama (TCH) is a 160-bed private, nonprofit teaching institution. It is the only hospital in Alabama dedicated solely to pediatric care. Affiliated with the University of Alabama, Birmingham (UAB), the hospital serves as a referral center for the state, as well as for several surrounding southeastern states. Typically there are more than 10,000 admissions a year and over 100,000 annual outpatient visits.

In 1976, a private after-hours pediatric clinic was established at the hospital to provide an efficient system of outpatient care delivery for that patient population. No marketing survey was done; the clinic was the product of needs perceived by the medical director and the nursing director of ambulatory care services. There was a clear need for separation of private physicians' patients who were not critically ill from patients who required emergency care. Space in the emergency department (ED) was at a premium; there were only four rooms at that time. The new clinic was located in an adjacent specialty clinics area and answered the need for separation of patients and for more space.

During the next five years, visits to the ED and Private Doctor's Clinic (PDC) consistently increased annually. As space became more limited for both outpatient and inpatient services, a building program was undertaken to provide a relocated, enlarged ED. By this time, a moonlighting pediatric resident had been employed for several years to provide care to private inpatients and to outpatients in the PDC and ED.

Even with the improved physical plant, there were still only four exam rooms designated for the PDC. There was no separate waiting area, and staffing was shared with the ED. Patient flow became a problem during peak hours if more than four physicians arrived to see patients. Patients for the PDC were typically

---

*Adapted with permission from McAnnally, R.S. (1987). Marketing utilization for expanding an existing service. *Nursing Economics*, 5 (4), 186–188.

less acutely ill; therefore, they had to wait to register when seriously ill or injured patients took precedence.

In addition, the Medicaid program in Alabama had been severely restructured to decrease costs. This resulted in the limitation of payment to 12 inpatient days, regardless of diagnosis. Reimbursed outpatient visits were reduced to three a year. As a result of these limitations, the hospital's percentage of unfunded patients increased substantially, due to the influx of indigent patients referred from outlying and area hospitals. We received many transferred patients whose covered patient days and outpatient visits had been used. The referring institutions had managed in the past to deliver care until discharge to these same diagnosis groups. Consequently, families of private physicians' patients increasingly perceived our hospital as primarily an indigent care institution. This perception produced dissatisfaction among private patients, physicians, and nursing staff. Private admissions and outpatient visits declined in 1984, falling from 5,020 in 1983 to 4,616 in 1984.

Clearly, there was a need to upgrade the inpatient and outpatient services and to offer incentives to the pediatricians as a way to bond loyal users more firmly and form new bonds with practitioners not using TCH. We also recognized that if we could offer improved services to parents, we could successfully bond that market to our institution. The inpatient quality of care was satisfactory. Physical amenities were attractive; all rooms were private and units were newly renovated. Thus, it seemed reasonable to believe that we should concentrate our upgrading efforts on the PDC. To confirm this assumption and analyze the needs and wants of our primary markets, we studied first our physician market, using a qualitative research method, and later our parent market, using a quantitative method. Plans were developed and implemented to meet the identified needs and preferences of these targeted groups. Results of our marketing plans were evaluated.

MARKETING ANALYSIS

Qualitative Market Research—Physicians

In 1984, as part of a marketing plan developed by the divisional director of ambulatory nursing and the head nurse of the ED, a marketing research study of attending pediatricians was conducted. It focused on learning their perceptions of incentives and improvements needed in our inpatient and outpatient services. The study also explored external factors influencing private admissions and visits to the PDC. Sixteen private pediatricians who most frequently used our services were interviewed individually by two members of our hospital's marketing department. Physicians were not paid to participate in this qualitative research study. The questions we asked are found in Exhibit 12.1, and the following paragraphs refer to those questions by number.

EXHIBIT 12.1 Interviewing Questions for User Physician

1. Are you aware of the PDC and how it works?

2. Approximately how many times per month do you use the PDC?

3. If you do not use the PDC, what other arrangements do you make for after-hours patients?

4. What are your hours of practice?

5. What support staff do you keep after hours?

6. On which days is an after-hours clinic busiest?

7. Would or do you schedule visits for after hours?

8. Do any of your patients utilize emergency medical center, urgent care center, or other commercial family medical clinics? (List comments you have heard from them regarding these clinics.)

9. Name the strengths and weaknesses of the PDC.

10. How would you revamp the PDC?
    Location
    Number of exam rooms
    Ancillary services
    Telephones
    Waiting area
    Parking
    Staff
    Fees

11. How far would parents travel after hours before they would look for an alternative solution?

12. Scenarios:
    Your patient has arrived at TCH and a house officer has screened the patient. If the house officer considers it necessary, he/she notifies you. OK or not OK?
    Your patient has arrived at TCH and is screened by a paid TCH pediatrician. The physician then notifies you of his/her findings. OK or not OK?
    Your patient has arrived at TCH and is screened by a local private pediatrician who, on a voluntary basis, is staffing the clinic. The private physician notifies you, if necessary, post-screening. OK or not OK?
    Your patient has arrived at TCH and is screened by a local private pediatrician who receives a stipend from the PDC. The private pediatrician notifies you, if necessary, post-screening. OK or not OK?

Your patient arrives at TCH and waits until you arrive to see him/her. OK or not OK?

13. If local private pediatricians could develop an arrangement for staffing an afternoon clinic at TCH, how would this work? How would you want to participate?

14. What would be the best hours for an after-hours clinic?

15. If you met your patient at an after-hours clinic at TCH and your patient needed hospitalization, would you admit the child to TCH?

16. Would you ever have a circumstance where you would admit the child to another hospital?

17. What would be the advantages to you in having an after-hours clinic at TCH? Disadvantages?

18. If you could name the clinic, what would you call it?

19. Can you name the top five diagnoses seen after-hours?

20. If a new format for an after-hours clinic was developed, what promotional efforts should be undertaken?

21. Would you actively support such a clinic at TCH?

Results of the Interviews

All physicians interviewed were aware of the services provided by the PDC (Q1). Average utilization by each physician was 18 times per month (Q2). Most physicians were using the PDC, one competing outpatient clinic at a local hospital, or their own offices for after-hours care (Q3).

After-hours care was most commonly needed from 5:00 p.m. to 10:00 p.m. on weekdays, 8:00 a.m. to 1:00 p.m. on Saturdays, and 12:00 p.m. to 10:00 p.m. on Sundays (Q4). Pediatrician office staffing after hours usually included a registered nurse, aide, receptionist, and laboratory technician (Q5). All agreed that weekends were the busiest times (Q6). Most respondents stated that they would not electively schedule after-hours visits (Q7).

All respondents stated that their patients used all competing types of after-hours services. Negative comments regarding these other services included high prices and poor quality of medical care, including overtreating and mediocre diagnostic skills. Positive comments centered around convenience and fast service (Q8).

Identified strengths of the PDC were the personnel, equipment, efficient and accurate ancillary services, helpful moonlighters, and convenient location in the hospital with access to the admission office and tertiary care. The program was perceived as providing high-quality care. Weaknesses identified were expense, mixed registration with ED patients, inadequate waiting area, lack of sufficient space, lack of staff dedicated exclusively to PDC, and proximity to the indigent population (Q9).

Suggestions for revamping the PDC included locating the clinic away from the ED with independent registration, increasing the number of exam spaces, dedicating staff exclusively to the PDC (including a laboratory technician), providing sufficient telephone lines, providing a separate waiting area, improving parking facilities and access, and charging a flat fee for services (Q10). Most physicians felt their patients would travel as far as necessary for these services (Q11).

Of the scenarios listed, the responses indicated that the physicians would not object to the house officer or a paid TCH pediatrician seeing their patients, but they did not favor a voluntary basis physician or a local private pediatrician receiving a stipend. Most preferred to screen their patients on the telephone prior to bringing the patient in to be seen (Q12, Q13).

The suggested hours for the clinic were 5:00 p.m. to 11:00 p.m. weekdays and 8:00 a.m. to 11:00 p.m. weekends and holidays (Q14).

Sixty-three percent of the respondents stated that they would admit their patients to TCH; none stated they would not (Q15). Circumstances requiring admission to another hospital were: adamant parent preference, older teenaged patient, belonging to a preferred provider organization, a need for neurosurgery, and no beds available at TCH (Q16).

Advantages of the TCH after-hours clinic were competitive and high-quality care, convenience, cheaper supplies, more time off, and negotiating power. No disadvantages were identified (Q17). Most respondents preferred to keep the current name of the clinic (Q18).

The five most common diagnoses were otitis media, pulmonary problems, minor trauma, seizures, and pharyngitis/ tonsillitis (Q19).

Promotional efforts suggested were: aggressive courting of private pediatricians not using the service, advertising, and developing a brochure to parents for placement in private pediatrician offices (Q20). Some physicians stated that they would aid in the promotion. In response to the last question in the interview, 63% of the physicians stated they would actively support the clinic (Q21).

Quantitative Market Research—Parents

In March of 1986, a marketing survey was conducted by a group of graduate students at the Health Administration School at UAB under the direction of Dr. T. McIwain. The project was conceived by a registered nurse employed part-time in PDC and enrolled in the graduate program. Its purpose was to determine if there was a gap between the quality of care expected and perceived by parents and significant others who brought children to be treated in the PDC. A modified version of SERVQUAL (Parasuramen, Zeithaml, & Berry, 1986) was the instrument used in the study. In their work to further develop a scale to measure service quality, Parasuramen and others created a refined, 26-item instrument containing five dimensions of quality. The dimensions are:

1. *Tangibles*—Physical facilities, equipment, and appearance of personnel.

2. *Reliability*—Ability to perform the promised service dependably and accurately.

3. *Responsiveness*—Willingness to help clients and provide prompt service.

4. *Assurance*—Knowledge and courtesy of employees and their ability to convey trust and confidence (a combination of communication, credibility, security, and competence).

5. *Empathy*—Caring, individualized attention the organization provides to its clients (understanding, knowing customers, accessibility of staff).

Each of SERVQUAL's 26 scale items is comprised of a pair of identical statements: one assesses consumer service expectations, the other assesses their service perceptions. Respondents evaluate the items on a Likert-type scale that ranges from 7 (strongly agree) to 1 (strongly disagree). Measures of service quality are obtained by subtracting expectation scores from perception scores. The higher the resulting score, the higher the level of perceived service quality. Parasuraman and others (1986) found that, among service firms they studied, SERVQUAL scores averaged around -1. This negative score revealed that on the average, expectations were slightly higher than perceived quality. Thus, they surmised that this -1 score could serve as a benchmark against which quality scores of other service organizations could be compared.

One item on the questionnaire was deleted by the UAB graduate group. Expectation statements were changed to reflect health care services and perception statements to reflect TCH in particular. Demographic information questions were added at the end of the questionnaire. See Exhibit 12.2 for the questionnaire.

The modified questionnaires were administered over a two-week period. PDC had numerous repeat patients who could evaluate a past visit while waiting for their child to be seen during a current visit. A sample of 61 parents or significant others was obtained. The majority of the sample was female, between the ages of 16 and 45 years. Most had some college education.

Results of the Parent Survey

In our first analysis of the parent survey data, there were statistically nonsignificant gaps in all five dimensions. All five gaps were negative, meaning that the perceived quality of care was less than the expected quality of care in the PDC. No gap greater than -1.0 was found, but there was room for improvement in all areas, especially in the reliability, responsiveness, and assurance dimensions. We knew that the gaps could be reduced either by lowering the consumers' expectations or by raising their perceptions of the quality of the service provided. Since lowering expectations of service quality was deemed to be inappropriate at TCH, taking steps to raise the perceptions of high-quality service was the marketing strategy selected.

EXHIBIT 12.2   Parent Questionnaire—Expected and Perceived Quality of Care

1. A facility should have up-to-date equipment.
2. Its physical facility should be visually appealing.
3. Its employees should be well dressed and appear neat.
4. The appearance of the physical facilities should be in keeping with the type of services provided.
5. When a facility promises to do something by a certain time, it should do so.
6. When patients have problems, a facility should be sympathetic and reassuring.
7. The facility should be dependable.
8. It should provide services at the time it promises to do so.
9. It should keep its records accurately.
10. It should not be expected to tell patients when services will be performed.
11. It is not realistic for patients to expect prompt service from employees of the facility.
12. Its employees do not always have to be willing to help patients.
13. It is okay if they are too busy to respond to a patient's requests promptly.
14. Patients should be willing to wait a little while to get appointments with the facility.
15. Patients should feel secure in their dealings with a facility.
16. Patients should be able to trust employees of a facility.
17. Patients should be able to feel safe in their transactions with a facility's employees.
18. Patient's dealings with a facility should be very pleasant.
19. Its employees should be knowledgeable.
20. Its employees should be polite.
21. It is unrealistic to expect employees to know what the needs of their patients are.
22. It is unrealistic to expect a facility to have its client's best interest at heart.
23. It should not be expected to have operating hours convenient to all its clients.

24. It is okay if patients have to wait a long time to receive services.

25. Clients should not have to cut through a lot of red tape to talk to higher level officials.

MARKETING STRATEGIES

Physician Market

Based on findings of the research study of physicians, a marketing plan was submitted to TCH administration. Components of the plan included the following seven marketing strategies.

Relocate the PDC to an area used during the day by another clinical service.   The area chosen was one floor directly above the ED, with immediate stairwell and elevator access in case of emergency. This location was also one floor directly below laboratory and radiology services, and was immediately adjacent to medical records and admitting departments. It would have eight exam rooms, a large separate waiting area, easy access to the parking deck, and could be quickly supplied with additional equipment. A crash cart, oxygen, suction machine, stock supplies, and pharmaceuticals would be available. Permission to use the area was sought and gained from the adolescent service that occupied this space during the day.

Provide the equipment for separate registration.   The adolescent service did not register patients into our computer system. Purchase of a computer terminal and printer was projected in order to register patients efficiently.

Schedule clinic hours to meet patients' and physicians' needs.   Hours of current operation were 5:30 p.m. to 11:30 p.m. weekdays and 9:00 a.m. to 11:30 p.m. weekends and holidays. The adolescent clinic operated from 8:00 a.m. to 5:00 p.m. weekdays; therefore, PDC would not interfere with its schedule. A 30-minute interim between clinics would allow time for housekeeping to clean the area prior to PDC hours and allow PDC staff time to prepare to accept patients.

Develop a staffing plan and an alternative work schedule.   Staffing consisted of two full-time registered nurses, one part-time registered nurse, two nurse aides, and one and a half clerks. The two full-time nurses worked a seven day on—seven day off schedule. Salary projections were submitted in the plan.

Institute a more competitive pricing structure and a simplified billing procedure.   This strategy called for instituting a competitive pricing structure and a simplified billing procedure approved by the hospital financial department.

Form an administrative ad hoc committee. Formation of an ad hoc committee was suggested to work out the details for the relocated clinic. Specific managers, administrative representatives, and private and faculty physicians were suggested to comprise the membership.

Retain the present pediatric resident (paid service) in the ED. The physician's option of having private patients seen by the moonlighter in the ED was to continue. These visits would be identified separately in order to monitor admissions of private patients seen in either the ED or PDC.

Benefits of the expanded PDC were projected in the marketing plan. They included: increased private admissions, improved use of space, more efficient triage, decreased congestion in the ED, and improved public relations.

The proposal was accepted both by administration and by the board of trustees. It was presented to interested private pediatricians by the nursing divisional director and the head nurse, and met enthusiastic approval. An ad hoc committee was formed and met frequently to iron out details.

Changes in the original proposal were the addition of laboratory personnel, some minor renovations in the waiting area, and installation of a dictating machine. Fiscal administrators decided to completely revise charging mechanisms. Private physicians agreed to pay a set fee to the hospital for each patient seen; they in turn would bill the patient. Patients would not be billed by the hospital except for radiology services and for items and procedures excluded from the basic schedule. The basic schedule included:

1. Basic laboratory services: complete blood count, urinalysis, and screening throat and urine cultures.

2. Specific pharmaceutical supplies, including certain antibiotic injections.

3. Other basic supplies from the exchange cart necessary for a nonemergency visit.

A pamphlet describing the service was developed by the marketing department and was made available in the private physicians' offices when the clinic moved in February of 1985.

Parent Market

Aspects of reliability, responsiveness, and assurance were areas that we chose to address in an effort to improve the PDC service. For the most part, waiting time for service is dictated by the physicians; however, we could make this time more meaningful by supplying current reading materials and play activities for the patients. We also devised a preregistration form for use when there was a heavy patient load. This form provided enough information to allow the patient to be seen before full registration, which then could be done after the visit with the physician.

We continued to give the parent satisfaction questionnaire to all parents or significant others in the PDC, and intensified our efforts to encourage parents to return it. This was one way to let them know that we recognized and appreciated the family's patronage. We also encouraged personnel to speak to families at intervals and to offer explanation for long waiting times.

RESULTS AND EVALUATION

Statistical data from the first year of operation in the new location showed a 48% increase in visits and a 33% increase in private admissions to the pediatric service. Physicians who previously had extended office hours now used the PDC, thereby avoiding the additional expense of maintaining their own offices. The number of physicians using the clinic increased, and general satisfaction was expressed by all participants in the service.

Review and evaluation of the clinic was, and is, an ongoing process for clinic staff, nursing administration, physicians, and the parents of our patients. Annual formal update meetings for participating physicians and parents have been held every year since 1985. Financial, usage, and other significant information is shared. Suggestions for improvement and solutions to problems are solicited and discussed. We continually monitor the satisfaction of physicians, parents, patients, and staff by means of questionnaires, interviews, and formal and informal meetings. The parent survey described earlier is an example of one of our formal evaluation methods. We have continued to monitor the responses to the parent satisfaction questionnaire and receive scores near 100%.

During the summer of 1987, we experienced a drop in visits due to elimination of the services allowed by an HMO. However, in January of 1988, the hospital was approached by the same HMO to again contract for services at our institution. We learned that the reason for renewing the contract was that the HMO physicians demanded to be allowed to provide services at our institution and that the parents were adamant about not changing pediatricians. Thus, it seems that our original premise of the importance of bonding physicians and parents to our hospital was indeed correct.

REFERENCES

Parasuramen, A., Zeithaml, V., & Berry, L.L. (1986). *SERVQUAL: A multiple item scale for measuring customer perceptions of service quality*. Cambridge, MA: Marketing Science Institute.

Marketing Nursing in a Multihospital Corporation

Kathryn M. Mershon, MSN, RN, CNAA
Senior Vice President—Nursing
Humana Inc.
Louisville, KY

THE MARKETING SITUATION

It is no accident that marketing became a survival strategy in the health care industry during the 1980s. This was the decade in which consumers came into their own; and marketing, a consumer-focused process, serves their best interests. Marketing proposes to determine consumer's needs, wants, and values, and then to design and promote programs that satisfy them. This effort to satisfy consumers is founded on the premise that consumers have a right to ask for what they want and to negotiate with suppliers for favorable terms in return for their business.

Today's hospital executives rely upon marketing to insure institutional solvency and viability. Multihospital corporations have used the strategic planning and marketing process for the past 25 years. The current widespread use of this process by health care providers and administrators, however, bears witness to a major attitudinal shift that is occurring in the health care field. No health care agency would presume to develop a program and present it on a take-it-or-leave-it basis. Agencies today are sensitive to the demands of health consumers for high-quality health care that is affordable and convenient. The administrators of these agencies realize that not only do consumers know what they want, they are also willing to shop around until they find what they want. Administrators, therefore, look to marketing to provide strategies that will enable them to interact successfully with health care consumers.

Marketing techniques have also been widely used in the recruitment of nurses. The current shortage is forcing a vigorous use of these techniques as many providers compete for the same nurse. Despite the fact that more nurses are employed now than ever before, the supply is inadequate to meet the demand. In 1987, 1.5 million total nurses were employed in this country. This represents a 25% increase over the 1.2 million employed in 1980. The American Hospital Association reports that as of December 1, 1987, United States hospitals employed 817,952 registered nurses, up 30% from the 627,215 registered nurses employed in 1980.

It is important to note that this increase in hospital-employed registered nurses was reported at a time when the nation's hospital bed capacity significantly contracted as a result of medical technology and changes in practice patterns. The rising demand for nurses in hospitals exceeds the available supply, even though the nursing pool increased by 25% during the 1980s and 80% of all licensed nurses were practicing nursing.

According to the American Hospital Association, the vacancy rate for registered nurses in the nation's hospitals soared to 13.6% in late 1986, up from 6.5% in 1985. This alarming situation threatens to become worse. Enrollments in nursing programs have declined 20% since 1983. Declining enrollments led to the recent closing of some of the finest nursing education programs in the country, including those at The American University, Boston University, Duke University, and Skidmore College. In light of the sharply reduced enrollment in some nursing programs, analysts are predicting that the demand for nurses will exceed the supply by 1.2 million positions in the year 2000.

So serious is the nursing shortage that it has become the virtual preoccupation of health care managers. The most cursory review of the professional journals bears this out. During 1987, the *American Journal of Nursing* ran over 40 articles dealing with the nursing shortage and related problems, such as recruitment and the nurse's working environment.

In September of 1987, the Secretary of the United States Department of Health and Human Services established a special commission to study the magnitude of the nursing shortage problem and to determine the implications of the problem for national health policy. The report of the commission was published in December 1988. Among the issues that it addressed were increasing funding for the education of nurses; improving compensation programs, including higher pay for nurses, along with incentive bonuses and improved benefits; and finally, enhancing the image of nursing as a profession.

With the application of marketing techniques to the recruitment of nurses during this nursing shortage, nurses take on the privilege of the consumer to assert their needs, wants, and values. Nurses are concerned about pay and benefit packages, but they are concerned about a wide range of quality-of-care issues as well. Unfortunately, however, these issues are being raised at a time when the pressures of cost-containment policies limit the degree to which health care providers can respond. This limitation further complicates nurse recruitment.

The multihospital corporation has looked to marketing as the most promising strategy for dealing with the problem of nurse recruitment. To illustrate, I discuss here some of the approaches of one of the largest of the multihospital corporations.

The Multihospital Corporation

Humana is a 29-year-old, international, for-profit corporation that provides comprehensive health services. We have 85 hospitals distributed across 19 states, stretching from Alaska to Florida. In addition, there are two hospitals in England and one in Switzerland. This large system includes a wide range of facilities, differing according to size, location, and clinical specialty. For example, we operate a 545-bed, full-service facility in Dallas, and a 50-bed hospital in Destin, Florida. Within the system, we have specialty hospitals, such as women's hospitals, and within separate hospitals there are Centers of Excellence, which concentrate upon particular clinical specialties. The Humana Women's Hospital—Tampa, for example, is a regional referral center for obstetrics and gynecology. The Ophthalmology Institute is based at Humana Hospital St. Luke's—Bluefield, West Virginia; the Humana Heart Institute International—Audubon is in Louisville, and the Neurosciences Institute at Humana Hospital—Medical City in Dallas. Altogether, there are 28 Centers of Excellence in the Humana system.

Over 55,000 people, about one-quarter of whom are nurses, are employed by the corporation. There are opportunities for nurses in a wide variety of clinical settings and management roles. Nurses bring their professional experience and perspective to activities such as the recruitment of nurses and physicians, utilization management, education and training, development of new hospitals, and employee relations. Since 1985, nurses have also had the opportunity to assume any number of roles in the company's health insurance division. Opportunities seem to be virtually unlimited in a corporation prepared to offer its nurses coast-to-coast mobility and a practice setting that is not limited to a single facility, but dispersed over 85 facilities.

The large corporation also benefits from an economy of scale in its marketing activities, because it can build a marketing program around a cluster of hospitals. For example, we have 18 hospitals in Florida. When marketing costs are shared by this many facilities, expert marketing becomes a very cost-effective activity.

While the size of the multihospital corporation presents certain benefits, it creates certain problems as well. Staffing 85 hospitals is challenging in any day, but particularly during a nursing shortage. For us, as for all industry, the single greatest problem in recruitment is presented by location. It is always easier to attract persons to an urban center than to a rural community. Size presents the next greatest problem. Even within a desirable urban environment, the larger facility enjoys a recruitment advantage over the smaller one. Facilities having the least favorable prospects are those that are both small and rural. Some of these least-favored facilities, it must be remembered, are sole community hospitals that must be kept open in order to preserve access to health care for people living in isolated areas.

MARKETING TO NURSES

To illustrate the marketing of nursing at Humana, I discuss two separate programs. The first program relates to our marketing venture, begun in the early

1980s, for the purpose of creating a positive image of the organization within the nursing community. The second pertains to our efforts to capture the awareness of nursing educators, and through them, of nursing students across the country.

Program I: Creating an Image

The Corporate Nursing Department is responsible for developing a marketing program for nursing that will enable Humana to reach its goals. This responsibility begins with a careful study of the mission statement and then setting corporate nursing goals consistent with the mission of the company. The corporation defines its mission as achieving "an unequaled level of measurable quality and productivity in the delivery of health services that are responsive to the needs and values of patients, physicians, employers and employees." Briefly put, the company is committed to a goal of demonstrated high quality in the delivery of health services. It is also oriented toward productivity, and it strives to be responsive to the consumer in the delivery of care.

Consistent with the mission, the first corporate nursing goal is to "develop a corporate-wide nursing strategy conducive to acquiring and maintaining a productive workforce of competent nurses to meet the needs of Humana patients." The first marketing program for nursing was developed to support this goal. By that time, Humana had been in operation for 20 years. It was one of the largest companies in the health care industry and one of the largest employers of nurses, yet the compelling reason for developing a corporate recruitment program was to enhance and increase the image and awareness of Humana within nursing.

Ordinarily, the first stage of a marketing effort is research to provide precise and accurate information as a foundation for planning and action. In this instance, however, we were more empirical than scientific in our gathering of information. We relied upon the findings of our representatives at nursing conventions, career fairs, professional meetings, and the like. The findings of these representatives were consistent and startling: they indicated that the name "Humana" had very limited recognition among nurses and nursing students. No doubt this problem was in part attributable to the fact that hospitals within the corporation did not, at that time, carry the corporate name. Whatever the cause, it seemed certain that nurses could scarcely be attracted to practice in our hospitals if they knew little or nothing about the company.

The first objective of the corporate-level nursing marketing program was to create an image of the corporation that could be promoted throughout the nursing community. At that time, many health care professionals were opposed to image building, contending that the image did not matter as long as high-quality health care was being delivered. Our experience indicates that image does matter. It is a means of communication, allowing the public to relate to the organization both intellectually and emotionally. Health care facilities have to deliver good care, but they have to achieve credibility with the public as well, and this is a function of communication.

Marketing Strategies

One of the first strategies that we implemented was journal advertising. We chose the journals based on factors such as circulation levels and target markets. The overriding goal of our advertisements was to call attention to the human identity of this large, investor-owned company. Our advertisements were, therefore, designed to reflect at once the magnitude of the corporation, and the importance of individual hospitals within the corporation. For example, some advertisements featured a map of the United States and showed the location of each hospital across the country. Advertisements listed a toll-free telephone number, so that interested persons could call the corporate office for information on any of the facilities. The local facilities were then alerted to this interest so that they could follow through with an appropriate and a more personal response.

Another way we underscored the human dimension of our large corporation was in the theme adopted for our advertisements. All advertising carried the company name, logo, and the slogan, "Move up to Humana: there's more to move up to." Testimonials from nurses who had moved both laterally and vertically within the company were used to illustrate and personalize the theme.

The theme of moving toward and within Humana was readily accommodated to the promotional needs of the Mobile Nurse Corps, a group of professional nurses who are available to any hospital in the system for short-term staffing. This unit was initiated as a pilot program in the fall of 1980, with seven nurses on assignment in four south Florida hospitals. In the second year of its existence, the number of assignments jumped to 139 and the number of hospitals to 24. Currently, there are over 300 nurses on assignment with the Mobile Nurse Corps in 39 hospitals throughout the country.

The marketing effort to communicate a positive image to the nursing community was begun in 1980; but it has been, and will continue to be, an ongoing effort. More recently, the materials used in this effort have become more highly formalized, to enhance recognition. The focus of attention in the marketing effort has shifted somewhat. Advertisements, headlines, and even recruitment displays employ designs that are consistently used throughout the company. This consistency makes it possible to convey the image of a company that maintains broad corporate standards and at the same time provides varied and attractive sites for the practice of nursing. Mobility is possible within such a company; but stability, in the form of seniority and continuous benefits, is also a value.

We are currently conducting a campaign called "Move of a Lifetime," to convey just what it means to work for a multihospital corporation. It means, quite simply, that you can change career paths without changing companies.

Results and Evaluation

In the evaluation of our effort to promote a positive image within the nursing community, we are, again, more empirical than scientific. The experience that enables us to evaluate our success in reaching our goal includes our communication with nurses, both through professional meetings and through our toll-free telephone lines.

After a period of 12 to 18 months, our representatives noted that our corporate name was generally recognized by colleagues at regional and national meetings. In addition, calls on the toll-free lines, along with inquiries and referrals, steadily increased. The rapid growth of the Mobile Nurse Corps is one of the direct results of this enhanced name recognition.

Without a more precise evaluation tool, we are unable to distinguish between what has been accomplished on the corporate level, as opposed to the local level, in heightening awareness of our corporation within the nursing community. Other factors, no doubt, have played a part in making this objective a reality. For example, in 1983, every corporate hospital came to be designated first by the term "Humana Hospital" and then by the specific name of the facility; thus, Audubon Hospital in Louisville became Humana Hospital—Audubon.

Following this name change, our representatives at exhibit booths were approached by any number of persons who wanted to know when we had acquired a hospital that, in fact, had been owned or even built by the company years before the name change. Using our name consistently seems to have advanced the goals of the nursing marketing process quite effectively, by creating a higher profile for the company.

Program II: Recruitment Facilitated by Nurse Educators

In this program, our efforts focused on communicating with the nurse educators as a strategy for recruiting nurses. Nurse educators were targeted because of the substantial influence they exert upon the profession, through their opinions of what constitutes a congenial and progressive place in which to practice nursing. According to research conducted in the late 1970s, nearly 50% of job leads for newly registered nurses resulting in employment were generated by their classroom instructors.

We found it most disturbing to observe, as we frequently did, that many nursing educators simply did not know anything about us or about investor-owned health care corporations. It was clear to us that we needed to gain the attention of nursing educators. Our problem was to design a mode of communication suitable to our purposes and to our audience.

Marketing Strategies

Knowing that our identity was somewhat in eclipse with nurse educators, our first strategy was to enter into cooperative efforts with the most prestigious nursing organizations in the nation. Out of these associations, familiar to and respected by nursing educators, the identity of Humana would begin to take shape.

As an initial strategy, we created, in conjunction with the National League for Nursing (NLN), an Annual Award for Excellence in Writing. The competition was promoted in journals that appealed to nursing educators; the judges were well known to this audience. We offered substantial cash awards of $1,000, $500, and $300 to the authors of the top three manuscripts. These were published in *Nursing & Health Care,* the official publication of the NLN. After three years, the level of awareness of Humana had increased noticeably. When the numbers of manuscripts submitted began to decline, it was an easy decision to terminate this strategy.

The second strategy involved a cooperative effort with the American Journal of Nursing Publishing Company (AJN), which is a wholly owned subsidiary of the American Nurses Association. Humana contracted with the AJN to develop a three-part comprehensive study program designed to help students prepare for the National Licensure Examination (NCLEX). This package included a brochure with essays on "How to Prepare for the Licensure Examination" and "Test Taking Strategies." In addition, there was a cassette tape on "How to Relax for an Examination," and a pamphlet listing the specific test locations. Initially, these materials were made available to students through their faculty in schools of nursing within a 50-mile radius of Humana hospitals.

This program was a costly one. It was, however, successful, not only in creating an awareness among educators, but as an educational aid to student nurses. The program is still in use, although the original format has been modified to eliminate the cassette tape.

In a second cooperative effort with the AJN and the Kentucky Nurses Association, we co-sponsored a Nursing Boards Review that had a high level of success. The program included a 35-hour classroom course conducted by registered nurses holding graduate degrees. Participants received a free 400-page study guide presenting all clinical topics in which they were to be tested. This guide was made available only to participants in the Nursing Boards Review. Even though we were a co-sponsor of the program only in Kentucky, it was promoted in every school of nursing in the country because of the national advertising campaign implemented by the AJN.

Finally, our efforts to capture the favorable attention of nursing educators included participation with the NLN in programs offered around the country on effective student recruitment for schools of nursing. These programs were designed as intensive, one-day seminars for all personnel involved in recruiting efforts for LPN, RN, and graduate programs. All participants in the program received a copy of the *Reference Manual for Student Recruitment in Nursing,* developed specifically for this seminar.

In all of the strategies implemented to appeal to nursing educators, we made a conscientious effort to strengthen the image of nursing as a highly valued profession. The literature distributed to nursing students is career oriented, and is designed to promote professional development. We demonstrate continued interest in professional development through our interaction with nursing associations and our support programs for nursing excellence. In our effort to create a positive image both of Humana and of nursing, we establish a relationship between the two, with each influencing the perception and the reputation of the other. Humana is certainly aware that nurses are vital to its mission. The converse is also true, however. Our corporation is vital to the practice and the professional development of its nurses, and to some extent, of nursing generally.

Results and Evaluation

While we are confident of the professional value of our efforts, their evaluation as marketing strategies presents difficulties. When a nurse interviews for a position at one of our hospitals, we usually do not know whether the nurse was referred by an educator, nor do we usually know whether the interview resulted from a corporate or local recruiting initiative. It is, in fact, unrealistic to expect to be able to document the source of every interview or inquiry.

The most reliable indicators of our stature in the nursing market are our interaction with colleagues at regional and national meetings, telephone calls on our toll-free lines, and the volume of inquiries and referrals. While this kind of information does not lead to hard data, it has enabled us to identify our marketing needs, determine subjects for emphasis, and develop effective strategies.

CONCLUSION

The two marketing ventures just described were undertaken by a large multi-hospital corporation. Regardless of the size of the agency or company, however, today's hospital administrators and nurse managers are relying upon marketing techniques to help them determine the needs and wants of their customers so that they may respond to them appropriately. With the use of these techniques, managers are altering the manner in which they evaluate their activities. They know that their ultimate success depends upon their ability to plan and understand their respective markets. Failure in this will result in the loss of market share to another health care provider who does understand the market and competes accordingly. This sobering realization makes it clear just why marketing has become a survival strategy in the health care industry.

Marketing Nursing in an Academic Psychiatric Setting

Gail W. Stuart, PhD, RN, CS
Chief, Division of Psychiatric Nursing
Department of Psychiatry and Behavioral Sciences
Associate Professor, College of Nursing Graduate Program

Rebecca M. Reynolds, MSN, RN
Director of Marketing and Resource Development
Instructor, Department of Psychiatry and Behavioral Sciences

Mary F. Spencer, MN, RN
Program Nurse Specialist
Department of Psychiatry and Behavioral Sciences

Medical University of South Carolina
Charleston, SC

THE MARKETING SITUATION

In 1988, the Medical University of South Carolina (MUSC) opened a new Institute of Psychiatry as part of the Department of Psychiatry and Behavioral Sciences. The goals of the university in opening this new inpatient section of the institute were threefold: to provide the highest quality of patient care in the region, to become a premier training center for mental health professionals, and to become a renowned research center. Before the opening of the institute, MUSC had three psychiatric nursing units in the general hospital. These units provided adequate, if custodial, nursing care, minimal research, and a modest residency program. Occupancy rates were between 50% and 70%; generally they were closer to 50%. It was clear that there was a large gap between what existed in the old psychiatric services and the goals to be achieved by the new institute. Nursing saw this as a challenge to be innovative and to use the marketing process to improve our exchange relations with the institute's physicians and nurses.

347

MARKETING RESEARCH

Our first task was to do an internal organizational assessment with a particular focus on nursing. A nursing steering committee, consisting of eight nurses from management and staff, was formed to analyze the organization's goals, structure, processes, resources, and controls (see Exhibit 14.1).

In the process, it became clear that we had to make some drastic changes in what we did. It was decided that none of the problems were to be concealed to protect nursing; rather, all deficiencies in the system were to be used as an impetus for change and innovation. Our second task was to conduct an external community assessment that was an interdisciplinary effort to identify what the community needed and wanted in psychiatric services.

Primary and secondary market research were used for both types of assessments. Primary research methods were focus groups and surveys. Informal focus group interviews were held for physician and nurse participants, both together and separately. We seized the opportunity to interview in the cafeteria, at staff and management meetings, and at physicians' conferences throughout the state. A questionnaire was given to nursing staff to help us analyze the nursing organization and nurses' needs. Secondary sources were published epidemiological studies in the psychiatric literature, and data from the American Nurses' Association, the American Psychological Association, the South Carolina Department of Mental Health and Hygiene, and other regional and national sources.

Results

Analysis of the internal organizational and external community assessments identified that there was a need for: (1) psychiatric services for a large, underserved population at all levels of income and education; and (2) a psychiatric facility that was technologically advanced, research-oriented, and education-based, offering consultative and adjunctive therapy programs for use by referring mental health professionals.

The assessment also demonstrated that we had two physician target markets in mind. The faculty physicians wanted high-quality patient care and research conducted in the facility to benefit patients and enhance their own professional practices and careers. Community physicians wondered why they should refer patients to our facility as opposed to another facility in the area. Nurses were our third target market. The successful implementation of marketing nursing to physicians requires a concurrent effort to market nursing to nurses.

From this analysis, it became clear that we could capture faculty and community physician markets if we offered specialty treatment programs and were able to diagnose and provide care for patients with complex problems. To provide this

EXHIBIT 14.1   Nursing Organization Assessment

Environment
Demands
Opportunities
Constraints
Organizational culture
Organizational expectations

Goal Components
Nursing mission
Nursing philosophy
Policies and procedures
Standards of care

Structure
Staff characteristics
   Skills
   Education
   Work experience
   Certification
   Professional activities
Roles of nurse administrators
Table of organization
Position of nursing director
   Relationship to medical director
   Relationship to administrator
   Committee membership
   Faculty status
Committee composition and function
Nursing care delivery systems
   Primary nursing
   Modular nursing
   Team nursing
   Functional nursing
   Case management

Variables of size
 Beds
 Registered nurses
 Other employees
 Nurse administrators
 Physicians

Processes

Change
Conflict resolution
Communication patterns
Marketing
Strategic planning
Decision-making
Power and politics

Nursing Resources

Staffing patterns
Compensation
Career ladders
 Clinical, educational, administrative
Nursing research development
Staff development
Patient classification system

Control/Outcomes

Regulatory agency results (JCAHO, state)
Quality assurance program
Patient satisfaction surveys
Nurse job satisfaction surveys
Use of nursing research findings
Performance appraisal program

---

level of expertise, we needed a different mix of nursing staff, with more nurses than counselors, more than we needed an actual increase in the total number of staff (see Table 14.1).

TABLE 14.1   MUSC Psychiatric Nursing Staff

	1985	1986	1987	1988a*	1988b**
Total beds	38	38	38	38	47
Total nursing staff	62	71	70	70	70
Staff:patient ratio					
youth	2.0:1	2.1:1	2.0:1	1.8:1	1.6:1
adult	1.2:1	1.5:1	1.6:1	1.6:1	1.2:1
Percent RNs	53	54	66	74	74

* January through June
** July through September

In our internal organizational assessment, we analyzed the strengths and capabilities of nurses in general and the specific strengths and weaknesses of our nursing staff. For our institution, the most important strength needed was an ability by nurses to organize specialized treatment programs, to implement individualized patient treatment plans, and to assist in research studies. An analysis of our nursing staff indicated that most of the nurses on staff were graduates of diploma or associate degree programs; there were considerably fewer baccalaureate-prepared nurses. The staff generally lacked the knowledge and expertise required to function in a specialized and intensive psychiatric care setting.

It was clear that unless our nursing service was dramatically changed, we would be unable to provide an adequate level of nursing care to meet patient and physician needs, including those of research and education. A higher level of nursing expertise and a larger number of registered nurses were required. Nursing administration had to develop a marketing plan in order to fulfill its role in achieving the goals of the organization.

MARKETING STRATEGIES

The first step was to develop a model that would support an innovative approach to providing nursing care as well as assist in achieving the organization's goals, including high-quality patient care, research, and education as the commonplaces or topics (see Figure 14.1). Unique features of this model are identified

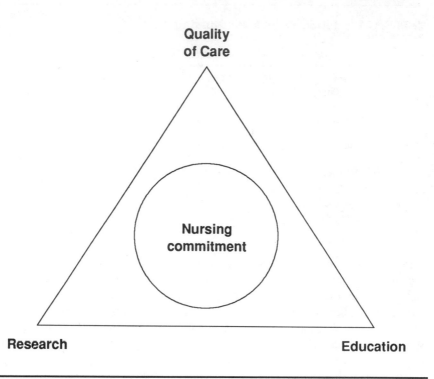

Figure 14.1.   Model psychiatric nursing service (MUSC).

Developed by Gail W. Stuart, NN, PhD., Michelle T. Laraia, RN, and James C. Ballenger, MD (copyright pending).

in Exhibit 14.2. Nursing commitment bridges the commonplaces and forms relationships among patient care, research, and education. It is nursing care that humanizes the environment, facilitating and enhancing the interaction among the components.

We then turned to developing roles to provide the advanced nursing care required to meet the needs of patients and physicians, as well as to achieve our identified goals. A new nursing organizational structure was necessary to implement this model of nursing practice (see Figure 14.2). One of the innovative roles we developed was that of the program nurse specialist. It was derived from our understanding of the clinical nurse specialist role, but would attempt to make the positive attributes of this role more accessible to nursing staff. In our search of the literature, we found that clinical nurse specialists typically hold staff rather than line positions, and act as consultants to nursing staff on a number of units.

EXHIBIT 14.2   Functions of Psychiatric Nursing Practice Model (MUSC)

- Moves clinical psychiatric nursing staff under an academic umbrella within the Department of Psychiatry and Behavioral Sciences.
- Establishes a Division of Psychiatric Nursing with a nursing chief whose role is comparable to other division heads in the department.
- Incorporates psychiatric nurses with graduate preparation as faculty members with joint appointments in the College of Medicine and College of Nursing.
- Utilizes a management triangle on each clinical unit that is led by faculty attending nurse with doctoral preparation.
- Divides traditional head nurse responsibilities between a clinical and an administrative nurse manager.
- Creates a new role of program nurse specialist to bring additional expertise and mentoring to nursing staff.

To meet our needs, we adapted this traditional position and created program nurse specialists who would be assigned to one unit, give direct patient care, and be immediately available to provide clinical expertise to staff nurses. Since the previous staff had not been exposed to a research environment, we identified this as an area for inservice education and training of the nursing staff by these specialists. To qualify for this position, a nurse had to demonstrate expertise in psychiatric nursing practice and have either a graduate nursing degree or years of experience.

As part of our marketing plan, we developed a new staffing proposal. For each 25-bed unit, we proposed that there be four to five program nurse specialists, in addition to the existing staff nurses and therapeutic assistants. In order to obtain approval for this significant expenditure, we had to present clearly the costs and benefits to administration.

The plan included extensive documentation of how the increase in numbers and expertise of nurses would be cost-effective. Nurses would be able to provide complex patient care. This would decrease the length of patient hospitalization. Third-party payers no longer provide coverage for unlimited or long-term stays; reimbursement for psychiatric care is generally for 10 to 14 days. Our services would help the patient attain more progress in less time, and would increase revenue for the hospital by minimizing unreimbursed days of care. High-quality patient care would be provided at decreased cost.

Ability to provide advanced nursing services would also enable the organization to implement plans for achieving goals related to research and education. These

354

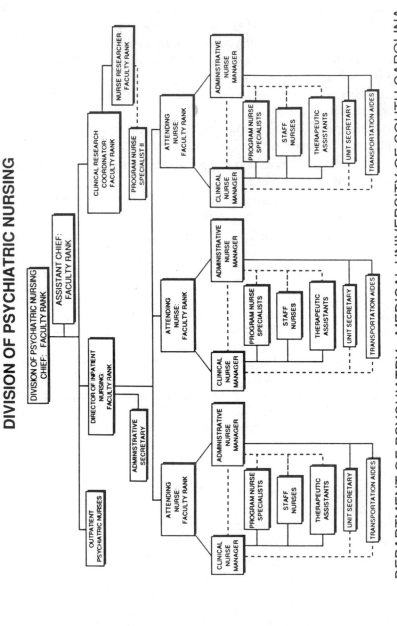

DIVISION OF PSYCHIATRIC NURSING

Figure 14.2. MUSC Division of Psychiatric Nursing table of organization.

DEPARTMENT OF PSYCHIATRY - MEDICAL UNIVERSITY OF SOUTH CAROLINA

goals were directly related to the faculty physicians' needs for ongoing research and training conducted on the inpatient units. We proposed that program nurse specialists were in the ideal position to teach nurses how to collect data, how to organize a research study, how to talk with families about informed consent, and how to be advocates for the rights of patients. This would result in increased use of facilities by faculty and increased referrals from community physicians. Care would be provided to more patients and more academic work would be accomplished. While the cost of salaries and benefits would increase, so would income. In addition to more revenue, the organization would benefit from enhanced stature because of the research and educational programs.

In order to implement the marketing plan, we had to recruit and retain nurses and provide a work environment that encouraged and supported professional practice. Our new organizational chart and job description for the program nurse specialist had been designed for these purposes (see Figure 14.2). The program nurse specialists were given line authority over staff nurses, but the basis of both their responsibility and their functions related to clinical care rather than to administration. Now we had to market the new role to nursing and medical staffs.

Implementation of the new job description and roles was not problem-free. Two critical elements contributed to the successful outcome of our marketing plan. The first was that the program nurse specialists had to be expert clinicians. Whenever a new role is instituted, a certain amount of confusion about the role, plus significant pressure to go back to the old system, is certain to be evident. This occurred in our institution. Staff nurses had a difficult time categorizing program nurse spe cialists. There was confusion about whether the specialists were nursing management or clinical nursing staff. Nursing staff also questioned the specialists' clinical competence. Only by demonstrating their expertise by working with the staff nurses every day were the program nurse specialists able to overcome these issues.

The second element necessary to the success of our marketing plan was making nurse-physician collaboration a reality. We wanted collaboration to be an expected norm of the institution. If we failed to implement this element successfully, the whole program could fail. A major problem was that nurses and physicians are not socialized, nor are they taught, to collaborate with each other. Neither group receives formal, academic preparation in this area. As a result, they are frequently at odds with one another in tense, stressful situations. Many physicians have not been exposed to nurses with masters and doctoral degrees, and may not know what to expect from them. Similarly, nurses traditionally have not been socialized to discuss their concerns with physicians directly. Too frequently, nurses have learned to accommodate and acquiesce instead of to articulate and assert. Therefore, nurses would have to be helped with collaboration, as would physicians, by means of ongoing education and support.

A final element related to this issue is the need for nurses to be mentors to other nurses. In order to grow and develop professionally, nurturing is required. Mentoring is encouraged for psychiatric nurses at the Institute of Psychiatry, and we believe it to be a driving element in the success of our model of nursing practice.

RESULTS AND EVALUATION

We evaluated the outcomes of the marketing plan based on the goals of the program. In relation to quality of patient care, the plan has been successful. Quality of patient care has dramatically improved. By virtue of our nursing capabilities, we offer the patient a chance to become more functional in a relatively shorter period of time. Nursing care hours have doubled. New nursing programs include the implementation of primary care as the method of delivery of care, the use of nursing diagnoses, and the revision of the method of nursing documentation. All of these programs have contributed to the improvement in quality of care.

Another positive result of these changes is that the Institute of Psychiatry is able to provide clinical educational experiences for nursing students. We now have nursing students from affiliated associate, baccalaureate, and masters degree programs. Program nurse specialists are preceptors for students and actively participate in their learning.

Our ability to articulate and demonstrate the value of nursing care is another important outcome. Nurses identify levels of nursing care intensity delivered to each patient. Those patients receiving the highest level of nursing care are assigned to more expensive intensive care beds. This directly reimburses the institute for the nursing care provided; thus, we are able to link the implementation of specific treatment programs with nursing care and ability. While we have not yet been able to implement a system of costing out nursing services, we have established the value and irreplaceability of nurses for the accomplishment of organization goals.

Increased satisfaction of staff nurses has also resulted from the plan. We have provided education and support for professional growth and development. In addition, the staff nurses have been exposed to more nursing expertise on a daily basis than is typical in many settings. These are important contributors to nurse satisfaction.

Among the outcomes that are directly measurable, many improvements have been made since the new institute opened. Nursing turnover has gone from 59% to approximately 17%; overtime costs have decreased from about $90,000 per unit per year to approximately $30,000; average use of sick days has decreased from approximately 11 days to 7 days a year. These are very positive outcomes. By using marketing strategies, we have successfully improved the quality of patient care, increased the level of professionalism, and helped to increase income for the organization. We have been able to achieve this while also keeping some costs down.

In relation to the organization's goals regarding education and research, advanced nursing care contributes to an increase in physician research, implementation of treatment programs, and an expanded residency program, thus increasing physician satisfaction. Occupancy rates have increased from an average of 50%–60% to 90%–100%. More community physicians are referring patients to the Institute of Psychiatry, and the number of regional referrals has also greatly increased.

By using the marketing process, we were able to develop and implement a plan that helped the organization achieve its goals of high-quality patient care, research, and education. Providing an advanced level of care helped the organization achieve the goals of professionalization and cost-effectiveness. We accomplished this by identifying what was needed and wanted and then by exchanging value for value.

Finally, we believe that these innovations have an impact on the future of nursing as a profession. For too long, nursing has continued to utilize traditional structures and functions for nursing staff, even though nursing qualifications and the organizational structures of our employment settings have changed. We believe our model establishes a high standard for nursing within an academic setting. This kind of innovation can help the profession, because it stimulates nurses to think in new ways; it suggests that nurses should challenge the institutions in which they work to create environments where nurses are best able to use a variety of skills. This would be to the complementary benefit of physicians, patients, and nurses alike.

Marketing to Recruit BSN Degree Completion Students

Nancie J. Thole, EdD, RN
Professor
Lewis University—College of Nursing
Romeoville, IL

THE MARKETING SITUATION

Schools, colleges, universities, and other educational institutions increasingly have marketing problems. All types of educational organizations are faced with declines in student enrollment and increased competition from neighboring institutions. These organizations can respond in many ways. One response is to do nothing and hope that the golden days of education, when the baby boom supplied ample numbers of students, will return. This is unlikely to happen.

A second response is to expand promotional efforts. The justification educators use is: "The reason for our reduced enrollments is that prospective applicants just don't know us. If they did, then they would actively seek us out. Consequently, we must vigorously promote ourselves." Promotion can be important in helping to boost enrollment, but it is doubtful whether, by itself, it serves as a long-term strategy for gaining competitive advantage in the marketplace.

Applying marketing principles to the situation is a third response. Central to marketing is the premise that the consumer is the focus of all organizational activity. Marketing is based on meeting consumer needs and wants.

In education, the competition is usually among institutions offering the same programs and the same terminal degrees. Yet, competition exists in other areas. We compete for people's time. This form of competition continually confronts educational marketers who target adult and life-long learners. Work, family, friends, and personal time demands also influence how, when, and what educational decisions are made.

Marketing turns around the traditional process of educational program planning and development. Instead of focusing on the needs of the institution, marketing places the needs of the consumers first and foremost. The marketing premises are simple: (1) when prospective applicants have choices, they will seek out and use those services, programs, and organizations that best meet their needs and wants; and (2) students are most likely to enroll in organizations that have minimized the real as well as the perceived barriers. This means that the easier it is to enroll, and the more convenient the educational offering, the more students the program attracts.

Prospective students face many barriers as they consider in which educational institution to enroll. It is not uncommon to find some, if not all, of the following pitfalls in the design and delivery of educational programs:

1. Failure to understand the wants and needs of enrollees so that the course offering or program is in synchrony with the needs and expectations of the user.

2. Failure to price tuition and related expenses so that they are perceived as affordable.

3. Failure to be sensitive to the fears students may have about going to school.

4. Failure to consider how choice is influenced by the distance traveled.

5. Failure to consider how the physical appearance of classrooms, buildings, and campus influences the perception of value.

6. Failure to communicate the benefits of a program or school correctly. Miscommunication can result because the message is faulty, the wrong medium is used, or the exposure is too infrequent to encourage the desired behavior.

In 1980, the college of nursing of a private, denominational university, in the far southwestern corner of metropolitan Chicago, sought and received a training grant from the Department of Health, Education, and Welfare to expand its degree completion program for registered nurses. We wanted to offer the four-year baccalaureate curriculum to a geographically dispersed group of students lacking easy access to the main campus. The BSN completion program provided university courses and support services at four off-campus sites in the metropolitan area.

By 1984, the program was considered to be successful. Approximately 250 students were enrolled at the main and off-campus sites. This program had earned the university a reputation for having the number one degree completion program in the area. However, the numbers were not all they seemed to be.

Program staff felt a growing concern over the uneven enrollment pattern of students from the designated service area. The pattern showed that the vast majority of enrolled students lived in the southern tip of one county. We did not know why we were not attracting significant numbers of students from other sections of the service area.

This could easily have been an academic question save for one important fact: competition. Since the beginning of the degree completion program, the number of schools competing had increased dramatically. In 1984, 11 schools were competing for students. It was clear that our long-term survival was linked to increasing our market share in the sections of the service area from which we recruited few students.

Out of the underrepresented areas, program administrators believed that one county represented a significant opportunity for further development. Four factors suggested that this county offered the most attractive possibilities:

1. The population was the second largest in the service area.

2. The average per capita income of the county was the second highest in the state, thereby making tuition costs less problematic.

3. The overall educational level of the residents was high, making the number predisposed to valuing degree completion higher than in other counties.

4. The students from this county had historically done well in our program, making them an attractive market.

Finally, one other factor was considered. According to the Illinois Department of Registration and Education, almost 9,000 registered nurses resided in this county. Of these, only 11 were enrolled in our program! There were large numbers of potential students in this county. We decided to target this segment.

MARKETING RESEARCH

Qualitative Method

In order to learn about the wants and needs of this target market, we decided to run two focus groups comprised of nurses living in the targeted county. Twenty-three nurses participated in the two groups. Their ages ranged between 24 and 65 years of age, with the majority between 35 and 39. All but one were female. A professor of marketing from the school of business moderated the focus group interviews, which lasted for $2\frac{1}{2}$ to 3 hours. We had four objectives for the focus groups:

1. To probe motivations for returning to school.

2. To explore the barriers that might prevent returning to school.

3. To evaluate competitor schools.

4. To assess recruitment literature from various schools.

Findings

Analysis of the focus group interview data gave us important information about barriers to enrollment. Key findings were:

1. Participants were confused about the value and purpose of the BSN degree for registered nurses.

2. Participants were frustrated because schools lacked uniform credit transfer policies.

3. Participants were influenced by convenience rather than tuition as a key determinant in school selection.

4. Participants were anxious about poor or dormant study skills.

5. Participants did not perceive any school in the area as the market leader in degree completion programs.

6. Participants saw the literature from local schools as impersonal, jargon-laden, repetitive, and undistinguished.

7. Participants found no school to have a distinctive image.

The finding that nurses were confused about the value of the BSN surprised program administrators. However, the nurses were being pressured by professional organizations, educators, and employers to earn the degree. In many cases, a BSN was mandated for entry-level positions. Practicing registered nurses who were no longer at the entry level had difficulty perceiving the relationship between these mandates and their nursing practice. They said, "Show me the relationship between required course work and the practice of nursing. How will this degree make me a better nurse?" Market efforts had to answer this question directly; the targeted population was clearly asking it.

Focus groups told us that convenience was more important than tuition in a student's choice of schools. In a very real sense, time *was* money. Thus, the site locations for courses, the travel time required, and the time of day courses are offered are critical elements in successful program design.

Credit transfer policies evoked strong negative comments. Focus group members felt frustrated because they perceived inconsistencies in schools' acceptance of credits earned elsewhere. Nurses often have course work evaluated by at least two schools. Prospective students found that credit transfer policies varied greatly. We needed to highlight credit transfer policies. Our promotional literature and student advisement should explain what credits are acceptable for transfer, and why added course work might be needed.

Participants wanted information presented to them in an objective, factual manner. They wanted to read, in easily understood terms, exactly what the school's course of study entailed. Vague, inconsistent, jargon-laden descriptions were not read by these individuals.

Returning adult students were concerned about their adequacy as participants in a class. They were anxious about competing with younger, academically savvy students. Lack of recent classroom experience and anxiety about having adequate study skills were commonly expressed fears. These perceived threats may be strong enough to keep students from entering, or remaining in, a program.

Finally, many adults attribute their achievements to their intrinsic motivation. Most significantly, focus group members said "The degree is important to how I feel about myself." Returning adult learners need to have personal clarity and motivation in order to sustain their efforts and achieve success. Faculty and staff should show appreciation of the knowledge acquired through life experience. As one participant said, "Pay attention to who I am, and respect what I've done."

MARKETING STRATEGIES

Since so many colleges and universities were competing for BSN students, we concluded that our program would be more successful if it had a unique identity and a carefully chosen market position. A marketing plan was developed for the BSN degree completion program. It included target groups and objectives, as well as the strategies, tactics, responsible persons, and communications support for each target group. We were guided by the focus group research. Emphasis was on three marketing strategies:

1. To position the program to better meet the needs of RNs.
2. To develop a media identity program.
3. To facilitate movement to buyer readiness.

Positioning the Program

To create our market niche, we made the necessary adjustments in the program. First, we carefully assessed the site locations of courses for ease of access from work or home, and the time of day the courses were offered. Locations were made as convenient as possible. Courses were slotted to allow sufficient time to travel to them after work. We had discovered that these considerations were more important than level of tuition. Most health care employers give some reimbursement for tuition, making our program affordable. In addition, the program was accredited; our degrees are highly valued by the nursing community.

Identity Program

Once we had adjusted our offering to meet our target markets' needs and wants, we designed the promotional activities. Our goal was to help our potential students understand what we provide in relation to what our competitors offer. We did this by carefully defining our image or identity. In this process, our discussion consistently returned to one theme: RNs feel frustrated and angry because no one sees them as individuals or acknowledges their professionalism. The question was whether a "we care about you" statement would convey our message. We determined that it was close, but not quite right. The "we care" theme was too close to popular jargon, and it sounded too much like what many health care organizations were saying. Many hospitals, a major pharmaceutical manufacturer, and charitable organizations were all using variations of the "I care" theme, so another variant of this theme was needed. "We treat you as an individual" was ultimately selected. Our message would be that the *individual* really does matter.

Identification of this theme gave us the center from which we could develop our marketing plan and position our program to reach our targeted segment. It helped us to dignify continuing education credits, personalize attention on the telephone and in admissions interviews, develop support groups, and make the whole process a partnership between the student and the program. Additional advantages were:

1. It facilitated quality control.
2. It clarified and anchored our identity, enabling us to identify innumerable ways to develop strategies.
3. It gave us a unique identity.

Style

A critical challenge was to replace the image of weak, ill-defined programs with a well-formed, distinctive, and bold identity. We needed to break through the perceptual defenses nurses used to screen out most promotional messages. The aim was to develop an image immediately identifiable with the program. A style that mirrored personality characteristics of the targeted nurse population was used. Because these nurses were unimpressed by extra frills, the program logo was a cross made up of small squares. Since nurses are serious-minded, we used a classic typeface on promotional materials. Ink color was bold and distinctive to differentiate our materials from eight competing schools. The layout was kept simple for these no-nonsense decision-makers.

Consumer-Oriented Language

Avoiding the impersonal, jargon-laden writing style of most recruitment literature was an important strategic decision. Program brochures were rewritten to allow readers to see themselves in the situations described. For example, in describing the registered nurses enrolled in the program, the brochure read:

> Our students have a strong desire to develop themselves personally and professionally. They want their education to broaden and challenge them.
> Our students value their technical skill and have demonstrated their competence in clinical situations. They want instructors who treat and respect them as professionals.
> Our students also value their time, since going to school still means finding time for work, for family and for themselves.

Buyer Readiness Program

We had to promote our program in ways that would achieve our strategy of bringing the target population to buyer readiness. Each target group needed a specific communication task (see Table 15.1). Key communication tasks were to:

1. Develop awareness that a new off-campus site was opening in the county.
2. Generate interest in this particular degree completion program.
3. Promote a compelling reason to enroll.
4. Reinforce the decision to enroll as an excellent choice.

TABLE 15.1   Communications Tasks for Specific Target Groups

Target Group	Communications Task
All nurses in county	Build awareness of program
Nurses interested in further education	Reinforce value of this educational program
Nurses interested in short courses	Refer to other schools who offer continuing education
Nurses interested in degree completion	Reinforce value of this degree
Nurses actively looking for a program	Promote interest in this program
Nurses interested in this program	Use one-on-one approach to convert interest into application
Nurses who apply for admission	Reinforce decision as the right choice

Marketing Plan

Target group: Nurses, health administrators, media.

Objective: Develop a positive image for the program.

Strategy: Differentiate all program print materials from standard university materials.

Tactics: Develop a logo for program.
Develop distinctive typeface.
Use a second, bold color to distinguish program.
Develop a tag line for program ("We treat you as an individual").
Use language of target market in all promotional activities.

Person responsible: Graphic designer (logo, type, layout).
Printer (stationery, brochures).
Consultant (copy for tag line, brochures).

Communications support: Stationery.
Brochures.
Mailers.
Specialty advertising items.

Target group: All RNs in designated county.

Objective: Generate awareness of BSN program.

Strategy I: Use public relations to gain publicity.

Tactics: Develop a press kit on program.
Send press releases to all county newspapers.
Send announcements to all county hospitals.

Person responsible: Public Relations (PR) Department (copy writing, placement, idea development).

Communications support: University press releases.
Program press kit.

Strategy II: Hold an open house to celebrate and show off educational facility.

Tactics: Invite all directors of nursing in county.
Invite all directors of continuing education in county.
Invite program alumni and their guests.
Send announcements to all county health care agencies.
Send press releases to all county newspapers.
Send public service announcements to radio stations.

Person responsible: PR Department.

Communications support: Invitations.
Press releases.
Public service announcements.

Target group: Working and professionally affiliated RNs.

Objective: Promote importance of baccalaureate degree.

Strategy: Work through districts of the Illinois State Nurses Association to develop awareness of program and value of degree.

Tactics: Call district presidents; set up speaking engagements with districts.

Develop chart comparing future potential earnings of RNs without degrees with BSNs.

Develop fact sheet showing future manpower need for BSNs.

Discuss how liberal arts studies relate to the nursing curriculum at the university.

Person responsible: Program administrators (contacting and speaking to professional groups).

PR Department (posters).

Consultant (copy).

Graphic designer (layout and paste-up of brochure).

Target group: RNs in county who are unaware of university and/or BSN program.

Objective: To make nurses aware of the university and the program.

Strategy: Use print media to reach group.

Tactics: Place ad in Illinois State Nurses Association publication.

Send direct mailings.

Develop brochure.

Develop "tickler" return postcard.

Obtain state registration list.

Target for a special promotion nurses in zip codes adjacent to site.

Submit articles about value of returning to school for spring and fall educational supplements of newspapers.

Person responsible: Graphic designer (layout, paste-up of ad and postcard tickler).
PR department (story placement).
Consultant (copy).
Students (preparation of direct mailings).

Communications support: Advertisement.
Program brochure.
Postcard tickler.
Article.

Target group: Any RN showing an interest in the BSN program.

Objective I: To demonstrate that at this university everyone is treated as an individual.

Strategy: Personalize each contact as much as possible.

Tactics: Develop a marketing information system (MIS) to track all contacts (part of this system should be a log of all incoming calls).

Send application packet in response to inquiries.

Use word processor to write personalized follow-up letters after each contact. For example, "Thank you for your inquiry" or "Thank you for your recent interview. Here's some additional information about the program we thought you might be interested in."

Personalize admissions interview. Use first minutes to gather personal and professional information that can be used later in the interview. Determine applicant's educational and career plans.

Tailor interview to fit the nurse's career objectives.

Individualize discussion of transfer credits.

Try to make each applicant feel good about previous course work.

If feasible, give an unofficial evaluation of transfer credits so that each applicant has something tangible from the interview. At the end of the interview, give each applicant a specialty item, such as a pen, pad, or key ring, with the program's name.

Person responsible: Admissions officer (MIS, follow-up letters).

Consultant (copy for applicant packet).

Graphic designer (layout and paste-up of applicant packet materials).

Communications support: Follow-up letters.
Applicant program packet.
Specialty advertising items.

Objective II: Reinforce credibility of program.

Strategy: Use alumni to confirm value of BSN from this program.

Tactics: Find alumni to be on call to answer applicants' questions.

Develop a list of alumni employed at all health agencies in target county. Give list to applicants.

Person responsible: Program administrators.

Communications support: Brochure.
Applicant packet.
Alumni list.

Target group: RNs working in health care agencies in target county who have been exposed to some message about the program.

Objective: Move them from awareness to interest in program.

Strategy: Do on-site recruitment sessions, prioritize the health agencies in rank order according to the amount of tuition reimbursement.

Tactics: Have admissions officer do on-site registration.

Present a brown-bag lunch and informal speech on the university and its new program.

Person responsible: Program administrators.
PR Department.
Admissions officer (on-site registration).

Communications support: Brochure.
Program packet.
Posters.

Target group: RNs who have shown interest by asking for an application.

Objective: To move this group from being interested to applying to the program.

Strategy: Reduce the perceived barriers to entry.

Tactic: Have interested RNs call a graduate for information.

Guarantee an evaluation of transfer credits and a proposed schedule within 48 hours of contact.

Include a franked envelope in every admissions packet. Mark envelope "Prompt attention; dated material."

Schedule courses to coincide with shift changes at health care agencies.

Have a 24-hour hotline that people can call for more information.

Establish a local telephone number in order to increase perception of being part of community.

Person responsible: Program administrators.

Communications support: Applicant packet.
Select list of graduates.

Target group: RNs who have requested information but who have not applied.

Objective: To find out why applicant has not applied.

Strategy: Use soft-sell approach.

Tactics: Conduct a follow-up telephone interview. Ask impressions of written materials and interview. Are they still actively considering the program? Why or why not? Have they enrolled somewhere else?

> Send a six-month, personalized, follow-up letter. "We haven't heard from you . . . can we still help you?"

Person responsible: Program administrators.

Communications support: Follow-up letter.
Telephone interview questionnaire.

Target group: RNs who have been accepted into program.

Objective: Reinforce that our program is right choice; reduce cognitive dissonance.

Strategy: Personalize response by using previously collected information.

Tactics: Send personalized letter welcoming applicant to the program.
Send specialty item to each admitted student.

Person responsible: Program administrators.

Communications support: Specialty items.
Follow-up letter.

Target group: Nurse recruiters.

Objective: Develop nurse recruiters as strong advocates of the program.

Strategy: Emphasize quality of education received.

Tactics: Get feedback from recruiters on their perceptions of the program and ask for improvement suggestions.
Give recruiters applicant packets.
Drop by every three to six months for feedback.
Send personalized letters thanking the recruiters for their support.
Send newsletter to keep them abreast of what is new and exciting in the program.
Take the recruiters to lunch.

Person responsible: Graphic designer (newsletter design).
Program administrators.

Communications support: Brochure.
Applicant packet.
Follow-up letter.
Portfolio.
Newsletter.

Target group: Directors of nursing (DON) in local health care agencies.

Objective: To gain support of directors for the program.

Strategy: Have an introduction meeting at the health care agency.

Hold a breakfast meeting for all DONs to give them first-hand information about program developments.

Invite DONs to an open house.

Send newsletter to all nursing administrators.

Person responsible: Program administrators.

Communications support: Brochure.
Applicant packet.
Follow-up letter.
Portfolio.
Newsletter.

RESULTS

Program staff successfully used a marketing approach to increase enrollment. Specific strategies and tactics were developed for each market segment. These strategies were successful in moving RNs from unawareness through the stages of buyer readiness to applying for admission and enrolling.

The cost of the focus groups was $5,000. Included in this cost was the consultant we hired to recruit participants, room rental, a buffet lunch for participants, taping the groups, and transcription of the tapes. Each participant was paid $40.

Promotional costs totaled $9,650. This included the design, development, and production of 10,000 direct mail brochures, for $3,000; 5,000 program brochures, for $2,250; 2,500 program packets, for $1,800; 5,000 newsletters for $1,500; and $500 each for posters and generic invitations. We also spent $2,100 for advertising. The HEW grant covered all these costs. In addition, the university paid for some advertising.

Our targeted promotional efforts paid off. Most of our new students resulted from these efforts. The unfocused advertising, which the university wanted and paid for, brought no students whose enrollment could be directly attributed to the advertising.

The results of the direct mail campaign, sent to 9,367 RNs in the targeted county, were 434 (4.5%) requests for program brochures; of those requesting brochures, 184 (42.4%) also requested applications. From this group, 24 new students enrolled in the program the following semester.

Marketing a Managed Care Addiction Program

Elizabeth L. Torresson, MSN, RN
Former President, Penn Recovery Systems, Inc.
Director of Medical Surgical Nursing
Rancocas Hospital and Zurbrugg Hospital
Willingboro and Riverside, NJ
Doctoral Candidate, Teachers College
New York, NY

THE MARKETING SITUATION

Penn Recovery Systems (PRS) is a small business owned and operated by three mental health professionals with expertise in addiction treatment. The three principals—a psychiatrist, a nurse manager, and a program director—came together as the management team of an inpatient detoxification and rehabilitation program in a 300-bed acute care hospital. We shared similar beliefs and values about addiction treatment. Our managerial and clinical expertise were complementary. Disturbed about the system as we saw it, we decided to do something about it.

Addiction is a chronic, progressive disease. It is a major health and social problem. Patients need treatment at various levels of intensity and frequency. Treatment needs range from inpatient hospitalization to weekly outpatient relapse prevention groups. At best, the health care delivery system provides fragmented addiction services. Some agencies offer only inpatient detoxification; others offer only outpatient services. Most insurance companies pay for a 28-day hospital stay and provide virtually no reimbursement for outpatient treatment.

After inpatient treatment, patients go from the safe, therapeutic hospital environment to their neighborhoods, where drugs, alcohol, and stressors surround them. Then they must wait several days for their first outpatient appointment. Without support, relapses are frequent. In the first two weeks after discharge, the major self-help support groups (Alcoholics Anonymous, Narcotics Anonymous, and Cocaine Anonymous) are just not enough.

We recognized that we were treating some patients who truly did not require hospitalization in an acute care setting, but no alternatives were available. Although the most restrictive, intensive, and expensive treatment options, inpatient detoxification and rehabilitation, were the norm, they were the only treatment fully reimbursed by Medicare, Medicaid, and the major insurance companies. Our awareness also grew of the increasingly large number of patients who had relapses in the first two weeks after discharge and who had never engaged in outpatient treatment.

Clinically and economically, this made no sense. The delivery system was off balance with hospitalization as the primary treatment. Admission to an inpatient acute care or residential setting must be available when clinically justified. This is, however, but one end of a continuum of patient services. Many patients do not require inpatient care; outpatient care is better for them. We felt that intensive outpatient services should be the centerpiece of addiction treatment. At the conclusion of two to three weeks of intensive outpatient services, the frequency of contact can be slowly decreased to weekly relapse prevention groups. Participation in Alcoholics Anonymous, Narcotics Anonymous, or Cocaine Anonymous should be encouraged.

MARKETING RESEARCH

We did secondary research in the form of an extensive literature review. The drug treatment studies we found were usually descriptive. There were also reports of how businesses are changing their approaches to the problem of substance abuse; however, little had been written about the difficulties encountered in implementing the changes. Because few studies have been done on drug addiction treatment, we also reviewed the ample and rigorous research on the treatment of alcoholism. The dynamics of alcoholism are similar to those of drug addiction.

The literature on alcoholism consistently demonstrates that inpatient treatment, while far more expensive than outpatient care, is not more effective. Annis (1986) looked at inpatient versus outpatient treatment and concluded that the outcomes are equivalent, but costs are less for outpatient care. Several advantages of outpatient or day treatment approaches were presented: outpatient care allows for a more valid assessment of factors leading to drinking urges, and it allows the patient to test new coping strategies while in the supportive framework of treatment.

Miller and Hester (1986) reviewed numerous studies and concluded that the majority of alcoholics did not need medical detoxification, and that fewer than 10% required hospital supervision. They found no case where inpatient care produced superior outcomes. Instead, they stated that all observed differences favored outpatient settings. A reasonably consistent trend showed that more severe alcoholics, who are less socially stable, do better in more intensive treatment. Less severe and more socially stable alcoholics have more favorable outcomes with less intensive treatment. Miller and Hester stated that society must address the fact that the policies of reimbursement for alcoholism treatment run counter to the findings of current research.

Washton (1987) asserted that outpatient care is the treatment of choice for the majority of cocaine abusers because it is more accessible, less disruptive to the patient's job and family, and avoids the stigma of hospitalization. Lee (1987) investigated the escalating use of psychiatric and substance abuse services from the perspective of corporate America—the payer of the bill in the form of providing health care insurance. Major corporations have responded to the substance abuse crisis by investing in day treatment programs. General Motors, Lockheed, and United Technologies are among the companies developing outpatient programs.

Clearly, there was growing awareness that costly and lengthy inpatient admissions are not the answer to providing care for addicted patients. The overwhelming and consistent finding in the literature is the move from inpatient treatment to multiple types of outpatient treatment that are equally or more effective and that always cost less.

MARKETING STRATEGIES

The purpose of PRS was to provide high-quality services to meet addicted *patients'* needs, not the health care system's needs, and to do this in a cost-effective way. We planned to accomplish this by developing and defining our products as patient management and consultation services and managed mental health care. A major challenge was to transform a plan on paper to actual patient care and management services.

After incorporating in October 1986, we needed revenue and a base of operations. To gain these, we decided to submit a proposal for managing inpatient addiction treatment services to the hospital where we worked. The executive vice president endorsed our plans. Our contract outlined our job responsibilities. In exchange for our salaries, the hospital was able to offer high-quality mental health services, thereby gaining an additional source of patients. We would admit patients who required such care to this facility. Later, the hospital would gain increased visibility from our outpatient treatment activities. This resolved for us the ethical conflict caused by our working for the hospital at the same time we were establishing our own business.

PRS was then able to focus on developing the specifics of a comprehensive outpatient addiction service. With supporting documentation from the literature, a clinical program was developed: managerial structures were clarified and costs identified. Our targeted market was addicted members of health maintenance organizations (HMOs). These organizations were experiencing high costs and discontinuity of services. We could provide cost-effective, needed services.

Getting contracts was difficult, because we had no existing program and no proven experience in outpatient substance abuse treatment. We called on area HMO administrators. They agreed that there was a need for our services, accepted the supporting documentation for our program, but were wary of our inexperience.

Without contracts with HMOs, we were unable to lease space, hire staff, and implement our plan, because we needed a larger revenue and client referral source.

We continued to manage our inpatient service and developed a weekly outpatient group. While doing this, we "beat the bushes" to achieve our goal. We presented our program proposal to referral sources, talked to colleagues, and attended professional meetings. Our reputation grew. Eventually our networking was successful: we learned that an HMO with 36,000 adult members was seeking proposals for inpatient mental health services.

Pricing services for an HMO is difficult because it is a capitated system. Payment to providers is set at a fixed dollar amount per member per month. The HMO had no data on outpatient utilization of services, but shared its data regarding number of addiction admissions, diagnosis, and length of stay. We then estimated the cost of these hospitalizations and deduced their annual cost to the HMO. We assumed that the number of HMO members who would use our services would increase by 10% the first year due to the promotional efforts of the HMO, although this figure was an educated guess. Expenses PRS had to cover were staff salaries and benefits, operational costs, and the price of inpatient care when necessary. We also needed to make a profit. Using the projected number of members who would seek treatment, and adding the annual expense, broken down to a member-per-month rate, to our program costs, we arrived at a price for our service and submitted a proposal. Negotiations were successful, and we were awarded the contract for addiction services beginning July, 1987.

In exchange for our fee per HMO member per month, the HMO's addicted members receive full outpatient services, including individual, group, and family counseling, 24-hour emergency telephone access, and inpatient services when needed. The HMO gained effective services with costs contained.

The ice was broken! A request for a proposal for outpatient mental health services was made by the same HMO. We were also awarded that contract. Several months later, we successfully concluded a contract for addiction treatment with a second, smaller HMO.

RESULTS AND EVALUATION

By the end of the first nine months, PRS had 59 members from the large HMO and 20 from the smaller one in active treatment. These numbers increased each month, and still have not topped out. Of these patients, two to three are admitted each month for inpatient care. Before contracting with us, the larger HMO had an average of 10 admissions a month.

Our short-term outpatient clinical results are as good as those of inpatient treatment. Because we have been providing outpatient addiction services for about one year, we have little hard data on long-term outcome. Most of the data are very subjective; half of our patients in active treatment say they are substance free. Patients seem to be benefiting from outpatient care.

Because the cost to the HMO was based on the previous year's expenditures for addiction services, the cost to the HMO has stabilized, while more patients are receiving care. The contract with PRS for addiction services is thus benefiting the HMOs; their costs have not increased, but have been contained. PRS continues to manage the addiction services at the hospital. This continues to work well for both PRS and the hospital.

Today PRS is providing managed care in mental health to a client group of over 40,000. In addition to the three principals, our staff includes a licensed clinical psychologist (PhD), eight masters-prepared clinicians, secretarial support, and a consulting internist. During the first year of operation, we refined our program. Our market niche is the delivery of comprehensive addiction treatment services in a center city location. We price our services to allow for a fair, reasonable profit, while remaining competitive. Because we are not seeking to expand the business at this time, our promotional efforts are directed toward maintaining satisfied patients, families, referring physicians, and the HMOs with whom we have contracts. By providing high-quality, comprehensive addiction services for reasonable, preset fees, we meet the needs of the patients, the HMOs, and the hospital with whom we have contracts.

REFERENCES

Annis, H.M. (1986). Is inpatient rehabilitation of the alcoholic cost-effective? *Advances in Alcohol and Substance Abuse, 5*, 175–190.

Lee, F.C. (1987). Purchasers address escalating psychiatric and substance abuse utilization. *Employee Benefits Journal, 12*(7), 9–13.

Miller, W.R., & Hester, R.K. (1986). Inpatient alcoholism treatment: Who benefits. *American Psychologist, 41*, 794–805.

Washton, A.M. (1987). Structured outpatient treatment of cocaine abuse. *Advances in Alcohol and Substance Abuse, 6*, 143–157.

Marketing Women's Health Care

Pamela Klauer Triolo, MSN, RN, CNM, ARNP
Associate Director of Nursing, Program Administration
The University of Iowa Hospitals and Clinics
Iowa City, IA

INTRODUCTION

Over the past 40 years, women's health care has gone through dramatic changes. The first change began in the early 1950s and championed choice and voice in childbirth. It resulted in what is called family-centered childbirth. Hospitals permitted fathers in the delivery room, allowed sibling visitation, developed birthing rooms, and treated the family as a whole with childbirth at the center. As the women's movement evolved and grew in the 1960s, emphasis continued to be on choice and alternatives. Preventive health care and women regaining control of their bodies were important issues of the 1970s. This philosophy is pervasive today, and has been the basis of thousands of women's health programs throughout the United States.

THE MARKETING SITUATION

We developed the Women's Health Day program at the University of Iowa Hospitals and Clinics to improve the health status of women staff members, boost morale, improve the quality of the work environment, and decrease ill and absent time, thereby increasing productivity. Promotion of the ob-gyn clinic to our employees was also a goal of the Health Day program. This program would meet the needs of women employees by providing free health education and services in a convenient place and in an efficient way.

The women's health market can be segmented into five groups: (1) traditional, (2) family-centered, (3) sports-oriented, (4) wellness/wholeness, and (5) avoiders (Harrell & Fors, 1985). Traditional women generally use an organized system of health care. They seek health care when they are sick or need a checkup; they are also generally compliant with the medical regimen. Family-centered women have the role of family health care decision-maker, and take pride in family health, enthusiastically supporting and promoting the family's well-being. Sports-oriented women are independent, competitive, and concerned about body performance. When ill health interferes with performance, they seek treatment. The wellness/wholeness segment tends to prefer alternative health care rather than traditional medical care whenever it is available. The approach of women in this segment is holistic; they are interested in nutrition, longevity, and in attaining the best state of health possible. Avoiders strive to minimize contact with the health care system. This can be due to distrust, fear, lack of money, or disinterest. Delay in seeking health care and self-prescription are characteristic of this segment.

We believed that the program would primarily attract women from the wellness/wholeness segment. However, we had no easy way to separate our women employees into these segments. Also, the goals of the program had broader implications than just satisfying the needs of a small segment. Consequently, this program was developed for all the women in our institution.

PROGRAM DEVELOPMENT

Development of the Women's Health Day program involved balancing the needs of the consumer with the needs and resources of the organization. In order to do this, we set up a multidisciplinary group. The chairman of the department of obstetrics and gynecology and the clinical director for nursing co-chaired the group. Members came from the medical, nursing, and hospital administration staffs.

Planning for the program was extensive. We planned a Women's Health Day for all members of the hospital staff. Wellness promotion, educational programs, and free health screening exams would be provided. Topics for the educational programs were women's health overview, breast disease, premenstrual syndrome, menopause, sexually transmitted diseases, osteoporosis, gynecologic exams and pap smears, and family planning. Each program was to be 30 minutes long. Nursing and medical staff would give the lectures. A history and physical examination, including urinalysis, stool guaiac, and pap smear, would be done.

This free event was planned for a Saturday. Nursing and medical staff would give their time. Hospital administration agreed to pay for all the costs for laboratory tests, food, printing, mailing, and any other miscellaneous items. The hospital would, after all, reap the benefits of the program.

We developed two forms for the health screening: a self-administered history and a short physical exam form. Consent forms were drafted by the hospital lawyers. In addition, we designed evaluation forms for the screening and educational programs. Integrated throughout these questionnaires were market research items. We wanted to know what the employee thought of the institution and its health services, which health care organization the employee preferred, what health care needs and wants the employee had, and what kind of service the employee preferred in having those needs and wants met (Snook & Zimmerman, 1987).

A brochure was designed and mailed to all 3,000 women employees. The cover letter was signed by the hospital administrator. It explained the purpose of the program, and invited recipients to participate in the program. They were asked to schedule a health screening appointment and to return a postcard indicating their preferences for educational program topics. A deadline for response was imposed.

On the day of the program, the participants registered at a central location and were given a map of the hospital with room locations for the educational programs and the clinic site. A snack of fruit, cheese, and vegetables was available to them.

RESULTS AND EVALUATION

Ten physicians and twelve nurses volunteered their time in the clinic. Eight additional nurses served as hostesses for the educational rooms and the clinic area, and three registered participants for the day's activities.

A total of 170 women registered for this program. They represented almost all hospital departments. In all, 83 women had health screening exams. Their ages ranged from 23 to 65 years of age. The most common age group using the service was 26 to 40. Of those who had the exams, 57% had a physician for ob-gyn care; 43% did not have a physician. During the prior two years, 51% of these women had not had a physical and 47% had not had a pap smear. At least 10 of the women had never had a pelvic examination. Because many of the women had not seen a physician for a number of years, a significant amount of pathology was identified. A staff physician followed up all abnormal results.

Of those women attending the educational sessions, the majority went to three to six programs. Most were in the 30–39 age group. The programs that had the highest attendance rates were those on osteoporosis, premenstrual syndrome, menopause, and gynecologic examination and pap smear.

The response to the day's program was dramatic. Comments ranged from "very pleasant atmosphere for a service that isn't always anticipated with pleasure," to "this is the nicest thing the hospital has ever done for us." Evaluations of the health screening were outstanding. Participants described the care as warm and courteous in a relaxed setting with a pleasant atmosphere. Many remarked that they would be willing to pay for such a service because there was no waiting and the atmosphere was relaxed.

For the multidisciplinary group that made this program possible, the Women's Health Day was a tremendous success. Because of the overwhelmingly positive response, the group, with the support of hospital administration, decided to hold another Women's Health Day program for university employees. The program was held six months later and had a similar response.

From evaluation of these two programs, we learned that primary barriers to using health care services were aspects of time and place: that is, inconvenience of scheduling, lack of proximity that increases travel time, and waiting time at the site. Clinic time scheduled and managed so that it meets the needs of working women is successful from both the organization's and the employee's vantage points. To meet the health care needs of our female employees, we established a monthly half-day well-women's clinic exclusively for staff members. A complete physical exam would be given by staff physicians and residents in a convenient place and in a expeditious manner.

Paying attention to the health needs and wants of women employees can benefit both the women and the organization. The women felt cared for and wanted by the organization, and the organization gained loyalty, goodwill, and increased productivity from the women. Our marketing plan was a success for providers and recipients of the service.

REFERENCES

Harrell, G.D., & Fors, M.F. (1985). Marketing ambulatory care to women: A segmentation approach. *Journal of Health Care Marketing, 5*(2), 19–28.

Snook, I.D., & Zimmerman, G.M. (1987). Market research tools for health care managers. *Health Care Supervisor, 5*(4), 31–42.

Marketing a Nursing Division

Joan Trofino, EdD, RN, CNAA
Vice President, Patient Care Services
Riverview Medical Center
Red Bank, NJ

THE MARKETING PROBLEM

Introduced in New Jersey in 1980 as a system to contain health care costs, prospective reimbursement based on diagnostic related groups (DRGs) has spurred the competitive instincts of the health care industry in this country. As a direct result of this change in reimbursement, most hospitals have adopted a marketing orientation in order to attain and retain that competitive edge. A marketing orientation focuses on satisfying the needs and desires of consumers, and represents an outward approach to conducting business.

Riverview is a 500-bed community medical center located in a suburban community in central New Jersey. A balance of "high-tech/high-touch" is its focus. The problem that began for us at Riverview Medical Center in 1980, with DRG reimbursement, was obtaining new patients while providing nursing service that would meet consumer expectations in a cost-effective way. This problem still exists.

Consumers have been swamped with hospital advertising on billboards, newspapers, radio, and television. Patients have found the hospital atmosphere changing from stark to inviting. Valet parking, gourmet meals, and same-day surgery attempt to respond to a convenience-oriented society. A recent survey of patients' opinions of area hospitals, conducted by a national marketing firm, placed Riverview 10 points ahead of any hospital in two counties with regard to the nurses and personalized care.

Nursing Organization

Internal analysis of the nursing division in 1974 identified a traditional, hierarchical organizational structure in crisis. Union elections for registered nurses were scheduled for two months after I arrived. A sincere commitment for change on the part of administration resulted in a vote in favor of the hospital, beginning a decade of much-needed internal reforms.

Participative management, with delegation of responsibility and authority to the clinical areas and first-line managers, promotes individual nurse autonomy, accountability, and retention. Staff satisfaction with governance, salary, scheduling, and psychological rewards are the best marketing tools available. Costly nurse turnover may be avoided by attending to the nursing organization structure. An environment that supports nurses in their practice gains internal and external credibility with all nurses.

It is essential to assess the nursing environment frequently. This may be done through written patient and nurse surveys, telephone interviews, and careful analysis of patient complaints, as well as exit interviews with nurses. A commitment to ongoing internal and external market research is essential for every nurse executive. Close working relationships with the public relations department, as well as with the nurse marketing and media committees (and sometimes hiring a marketing firm) helps the nurse executive to promote nursing and to satisfy all markets.

Marketing to Patients

Patients make their judgments about hospitals through direct contact, information gleaned from friends, associates, and family members, and newspaper advertising. Professional nursing practice uses patient needs as the basis of therapeutic relationships. Nursing care is not always perceived as such by patients. While patient needs may vary widely, the main themes relate to the need for state-of-the-art technology and the caring provided by nurses.

Early efforts to promote the expertise of nursing began in 1981 with a special article, describing the vital role of the emergency department triage nurse, in a local newspaper. Since then, one of our annual goals is to target a different nursing area for publicity and story coverage in both local and statewide newspapers.

A special patient booklet, *Today's Nurse,* was designed by staff nurses. This booklet is given to every inpatient. It describes contemporary nursing practice and provides the patient with a questionnaire with which to evaluate nursing care at discharge. This brave effort, initiated in 1982, provides us with an excellent monitor of nursing care from the patient's perspective. It has long been my belief that a happy nurse results in a happy patient, a happy physician, and a happy hospital.

Marketing to Nurses

The current nursing shortage has increased the need for hospitals to maintain a marketing approach in regard to nursing personnel. Health care must be viewed from at least two vantage points: the patient who exercises the option of choice and the nurse who responds to patients' needs with professional expertise. A hospital's mission reflects to a great extent the needs of the patient for nursing care. Advanced equipment and its data are monitored and interpreted by nurses. The caring involved with recovery or a dignified death is an essential part of nursing practice.

Establishing an organizational structure that fulfills professional and personal needs and promotes individual growth and expertise of nurses has been an ongoing challenge. From a strong sense of empowerment, and the sure knowledge that they are fairly and firmly represented at all levels of the hospital hierarchy, nurses will then represent the hospital to the consumer, with the same caring attitude that is directed toward them. Nurses meet patient needs daily; as the primary sales force of every hospital, they must feel that their needs are being met with regard to scheduling, salary, benefits, and genuine concern about them as individuals.

Marketing to Physicians

Another dimension added to the marketing problem is physicians. Hospitals clamor for their loyalty and admissions. Some physicians are increasing their office procedures and/or associations with free-standing clinics, surgery, maternity centers, and the like. While physicians continue to dominate the health care field, by virtue of their admitting privileges, a better informed public is playing a larger role in hospital selection by apprising physicians of their preferences, or even selecting physicians with admitting privileges at the hospital of their choice. Thus, the marketing problem for hospitals has become extremely complex. Acute care organizations now need to position themselves favorably with physicians and patients in order to attract their business. We see the development of joint ventures in the form of physician-hospital partnerships, and an effort on the part of hospitals to satisfy physician needs that range from special surgical equipment to expeditious communication systems.

MARKETING STRATEGIES

Planning

Our marketing plan for nurse recruitment and retention was developed and then clearly defined in our annual written goals and objectives. A marketing committee composed of staff and management has been responsible for guiding progress and responding to issues related to marketing. Planning strategies are a joint effort of the Nurse Marketing Committee, nurse recruiter, nursing administration, public relations, and a marketing consultant. All appropriate people were involved during planning. Realistic target dates for implementation were set.

Implementation

Once the plan was developed, implementation proceeded smoothly and quickly. Staff support was a key element in successful implementation of the marketing plan. All personnel understood that the well-being of the organization depended on successful market exchanges. A desire to be "close to the customer" permeated the organization. Customer relations programs were offered as required continuing education to all employees who had patient contact. Hotel chains have this expertise, and can serve as a good referral source for speakers.

Nurses and patients have an increasingly larger choice of jobs and health care services. It is the job of the nurse executive and of all the nurse managers to market effectively so that these customers (both nurses and patients) not only choose your organization but stay with it.

Marketing strategies are influenced by the amount of human and material resources the organization can invest. Strategies used by competitors, the political climate, and legislative restrictions for product acceptance should also be considered. Finally, science, technology, and organizational commitment will influence the choice of marketing strategies. Over the last 10 years, we have employed a wide variety of marketing strategies in our efforts to recruit and retain nursing personnel. I discuss our recruitment and retention program in this case study.

Leadership and Management Structure

Our commitment to participative management and shared governance for nurses has been ongoing. We continually seek opportunities to improve and enhance the nursing role within the organization. This nursing leadership approach is our strongest recruitment and retention tool. A reputation for caring about nurses has assisted in both local and distant recruitment. Our average retention rate is seven years for registered nurses, and eight years for licensed practical nurses. This attests to a caring atmosphere that has been sustained over time by nursing and hospital administration. Marketing strategies must honestly reflect what the nurse will find in the organization. Nurses gain their knowledge of an institution primarily from nurses already working there. Establishing credibility with the nursing community is paramount in successful recruitment and retention.

Nurse Recruiter

A well-organized program for nurse recruitment begins with the nurse recruiter. Careful selection of this individual is essential. The right recruiter will improve market position and increase recruitment. An experienced nurse with an attractive appearance, excellent interpersonal skills, and good follow-through should be included in your requirements.

I meet monthly with our nurse recruiter for updates on recruitment efforts, the changing expectations of nurses, and the results of exit interviews. This information helps me to keep benefits and rewards appropriate and to determine the need for organizational and management adjustments.

We take great care in the design and presentation of displays and brochures the recruiter uses at career days and job fairs. Frequently, a knowledgeable and articulate clinical nurse will accompany the recruiter. The nurse gives information directly to potential staff nurses and reports back to unit staff. These efforts raise staff morale and interest. Visible recruiting activities are especially helpful to the nurses on units with vacancies.

The nurse recruiter participates in our open house programs. These programs, accompanied by dinner or refreshments, describe and promote the nursing division. Nurse managers and staff nurses discuss their units and specialty. Guided tours of the units are given.

Public Relations Programs

Writing for Publication

Publication in professional journals yields important publicity; the authors and organization receive recognition. Writing for publication should be included as a goal of the nursing division. Nurse managers should support and encourage all nurses' efforts to publish. Our nurses have published articles in management and specialty journals. Along with spotlighting the division, writing skills are developed.

Nursing Newsletter

A special internal newsletter, developed by the nurses, provides important information about our division and nursing activities beyond the hospital's walls. Information regarding continuing education programs is included. Nursing's newsletter provides a vehicle for nurses to share information and to use and develop their writing skills. We encourage all nurses to submit articles, so that we can publish a variety of opinions. I submit an article reporting on my activities and special professional issues. The newsletter is sent out for printing and is published quarterly. It is widely circulated within the hospital to nursing staff, physicians, administration, other departments, and the board of trustees.

We distribute the newsletter at nursing school career days, to potential nurse employees, local legislators, and community members. It is essential that the newsletter contain current information about nurses and their professional activities. Also, its appearance is critical, because it portrays nursing to a variety of publics.

Logo and Slogan

We established a nursing identity through the development and use of a logo and slogan. This identity is used on brochures, advertisements of educational programs, nursing positions, and the like. We chose the slogan "Where Theory and Practice Come Together." The slogan must be credible to nurses both inside and outside of the organization. With an ever-increasing number of employers seeking nurses, easy recognition in advertisements and publicity can prove helpful in recruitment.

Professionally produced artwork is well worth the expense. It conveys an integrated image and assists in establishing the uniqueness of a nursing division. One or two professionally designed brochures describing the nursing division are more effective than a large number of the homemade variety. Reach for high quality in all marketing tools. While a professional is invaluable in design, at Riverview the nursing staff contributes the content and develops the specific message.

Educational Seminars

Most nursing divisions maintain a centralized staff development department, and most educational programs are conducted primarily for the nursing staff of the hospital. We have enhanced our programs, our reputation, and our finances by marketing programs to the nursing community at large. All our nurses are encouraged to participate in these programs as educators.

A very popular program, which highlighted our commitment to staff nurse participation in the nursing quality assurance program, was "Quality Assurance: A Concern for All Nurses." Another program, "Behind Closed Doors," was developed by our anesthesia, operating, and recovery room staffs, and focused on perioperative experiences. All monies collected from educational programs becomes part of the nursing seminar budget, and is used by our nurses to attend continuing education programs at other agencies.

Distinguished Speakers

Inviting nurse leaders to speak provides many nurses with the opportunity to meet and learn from those who have made an impact on our profession. Topics are identified by surveying nursing staff. We have also co-sponsored speakers with local college nursing programs. An added benefit is that we thereby interest students in working in our hospital.

Public Speaking and Testimony

The nurse executive of an organization can lead a public speaking effort by accepting invitations to speak at nursing seminars or graduations, and by giving testimony regarding nursing and health issues. However, this approach to promoting the nursing division should not be limited to the nurse executive. All members of the nursing staff can participate.

In 1986 and 1987, a staff nurse, the chairperson of our professional practice committee, prepared and gave testimony to a New Jersey Assembly health care committee and to the New Jersey Rate Setting Commission, regarding the effects of nursing shortages and low salaries on nurses and patient care. Coming from a direct care provider, it had great impact on the legislators and commission members. This nurse was also interviewed on the evening television news. We gained publicity while doing a service.

Our speaking program has had positive results. With encouragement and support from the nurse executive and management staff, the level of achievement for all staff has increased. It is an effective way to promote your division.

Television and Radio

We seek and accept invitations to appear on television and radio shows. Many nurses are dissatisfied with the public image of nursing; I believe it is up to nurses to change that image. Professional presentations and positive stories about nursing will go far to change our image. We have a proud history and are currently achieving many wonderful results with older and sicker patients, so take opportunities to talk about successes. Nurses can be the best marketers of our profession. We do ourselves a disservice when we fail to promote the profession and its many opportunities, challenges, and achievements. Horror stories will not result in a positive image or in recruited nurses.

Excellence in Nursing Award

We established the Excellence in Nursing Award in 1983. This award, a specially designed 14-karat gold pin, is given annually by the hospital to an outstanding clinical nurse. Recipients are nominated by any member of the nursing staff and are selected by blind peer review. The hospital Nurses Fund contributes a cash award of $200. A picture and a plaque with the name of the nurse is permanently hung in the nursing office.

This special event is an excellent way to promote nursing at Riverview Medical Center. Hospital administration, the board of trustees, and medical staff are invited, as well as the nursing staff. Frequently, recipients proudly invite their families and friends. Local and state newspapers are always invited; they generally cover the story with pictures and copy. Positive publicity is gained by the profession, the division, and the hospital.

Annual Meeting

The annual meeting gives the nursing staff an opportunity to publicly report their activities. Consumers have been poorly informed about nursing, in part because we have been reticent to promote ourselves and our successes. All the nurses, administration, board members, deans of nursing schools, community leaders, state and local legislators, and media are invited.

I chair the meeting. Audiovisual aids are used to present the accomplishments of nursing during the past year. The chief executive officer and I address the nurses and give recognition for their professional contributions to the organization. Local newspapers generally run stories on the meeting.

Special Programs

Over the years, selected programs have been established and are conducted annually. These programs are directed toward recruitment to nursing, job enhancement, and nurse recognition and reward.

In the "Shadow a Nurse" program, high school students are invited to spend a day with an experienced professional nurse. Students, nurses, and clinical areas are selected with care. A pre- and post-conference completes this experience. Such efforts help students with career choices, and also enhance the image of the hospital and nursing.

We have two summer programs for baccalaureate nursing students. While the programs satisfy students' needs for clinical experience, they enhance our reputation and also give us many well-oriented new graduate recruits.

The fellowship program is open to senior students who are interested in gaining experience in nursing management, staff development, or any other area. They work with professional nurse experts in their area of choice. Begun in 1982, the extern program provides junior students with a work-study program. This annual program is eagerly sought out by students.

Nursing Research

An annual program presented by our Nursing Research Committee is "Nursing Research: Alive and Well in a Community Medical Center." Identifying problems and developing a study is an exciting adventure for nurses. Many of our nurses have become interested in research. Affiliations with colleges and universities in the tri-state area have brought us graduate students who are interested and eager to do nursing research. Data collection for my doctoral research was assisted and supported by staff nurses at Riverview and at five other hospitals in New Jersey.

Potential recruits to a nursing staff are interested in wages and scheduling. However, they are also interested in evidence of professionalism within the division. Scientific inquiry should be included in any professional nursing model. It is also an effective marketing tool for nurse recruitment.

RESULTS AND EVALUATION

The effectiveness of our recruitment and retention program is demonstrated in a retention rate that is three times higher than state and national averages. This is particularly significant because we are a nonteaching, community medical center in a heavily regulated state. We use this information in advertising by including pictures and testimonials from our nurses.

While nursing satisfaction is reflected in retention rates, patient perceptions are evaluated with surveys. Our patient questionnaires regarding nursing care continue to reflect a satisfaction level of good to excellent by 98% of the patients surveyed. An independent marketing survey of community members identified Riverview nurses as the best in two counties.

We are constantly looking for new ways to improve and enhance nursing practice and the resultant patient care. A survey of staff nurses recently was developed to give information to enable us to enhance job design.

All indicators point to a future in which health care marketing is not only necessary for success but also a prerequisite for survival. The nursing division is a primary factor in the work of every hospital. Nurse managers must constantly seek new ways to enhance satisfaction in the exchange relationships of the health care marketplace. Marketing nursing can be an exciting experience, resulting in measurable rewards and image building for our profession.

Marketing an Eating Disorder Program

Ernestine B. Ware, BSN, RN
Head Nurse, Eating Disorder Program
Washington Hospital Center
Washington, DC

THE MARKETING SITUATION

In response to the changing economic environment, with its increased competition for scarce resources, the Washington Hospital Center turned to the marketing process for direction. This hospital is an 821-bed tertiary care provider in Washington, DC. While it is not a university hospital, it competes for staff and patients with nationally and internationally known institutions such as Johns Hopkins, Georgetown University Hospital, and George Washington Hospital.

We needed to make the most of what we already offered and to develop new products and services. Our goal was to attract patients. In order to make the decisions necessary to achieve this goal, the hospital considered many options. Marketing research was the first step. Based on the outcome of the research, we decided to add an eating disorders treatment unit to our services. This case study discusses the process by which we arrived at the decision and how the program has developed.

MARKETING RESEARCH

Secondary Research

Anorexia nervosa was first reported in the 1700s by Morton (Drossman, 1988). Sir William Gull described the disorder in 1868 and 1874. According to Russell, Gull concluded that the "want of appetite is due to a morbid mental state" (Russell, 1982, p. 1379). Anorexia used to be considered a rare disease; however, since the 1930s there has been an increase in its occurrence. The incidence of new cases ranges from 0.6 to 1.6 per 100,000 of the whole population. People as young as 10 and as old as 50 are affected. Among high-risk groups, schoolgirls and young women, incidence may be as high as 1 of 250 (Romeo, 1984; Russell, 1982).

Bulimia is a chronic phase of anorexia nervosa. Articles in the medical literature during the early 1980s estimated the incidence to be as high as 20% among young

389

women. Some writers suggested that as many as 50% of college women were bulimic. However, in the first national study done, Drewnowski, Hopkins, and Kessler (1988) found that only 1% of all college women had bulimia, and only 0.2% of college men had the disease. Undergraduate women living in group housing on campus was the group with the highest incidence. This study supports Schotte and Stunkard (1987), who found that 1.3% of women and 0.1% of men at the University of Pennsylvania had bulimia.

Studies Done

Because our secondary market research showed that there might be a need for inpatient treatment of eating disorders, the hospital hired a firm to conduct primary marketing research. The results showed that people with eating disorders were either not being treated, or that they were in treatment that did not deal with the origins of their problems. There was one other treatment program in our community. In their practices, our attending physicians saw few or no patients with eating disorders.

MARKETING STRATEGIES

Based on our analysis, we decided to open an 18-bed, inpatient eating disorder treatment unit as part of our Department of Psychiatry. Our management team was composed of a medical director, head nurse, clinical psychologist, and program manager. Each was committed to making the program clinically strong and a financial success.

Marketing to Patients

A controlled environment, in the form of hospital admission, is the only way of restoring normal nutrition once severe loss of weight has occurred. Patients should not be forced to enter a program, however, because their cooperation is necessary throughout the course of the illness. Nursing care is an essential part of the treatment of anorectic and bulimic patients; in fact, it is the major reason for admission (Russell, 1982). We would be providing a service to these patients that they could not purchase elsewhere in our community.

After ascertaining our costs, we decided to charge the same rates as patients paid in the rest of the hospital. Most insurance programs do reimburse for treatment of eating disorders, as part of their coverage for mental and nervous disorders. Some insurance companies require precertification and recertification at intervals ranging from 72 hours to 7 days.

Since the physicians could not be a referral source, because of their dearth of eating disorder patients, the nursing staff was responsible for finding patients. We had to promote our program aggressively in order to attract patients. Our success depended on our ability to attract patients to inquire about the program, and then to convince them to choose our program for treatment. Marketing strategies helped us with this.

We established a 24-hour telephone inquiry line that people could call for information. When a person telephones on this line, a staff nurse talks with them. Immediate difficulties are dealt with and support is given, but patients in crisis are referred to an emergency department. Most admissions are elective, except in the case of anorectic patients with electrolyte imbalance or syncope. The caller is invited to visit the unit. This visit provides an opportunity to speak with a nurse about the eating disorder, see our treatment setting, and gather information that helps the client make an informed decision. Using a comprehensive interview form, a nurse does the preadmission screening. After the interview, we have a conference with the medical director and decide whether hospitalization is needed. Those people who do not require hospitalization are given information and other assistance as requested. Arrangements for admission are made for those who would benefit from inpatient treatment. Medical care after admission is usually under the direction of one of the six staff psychiatrists.

Several promotional strategies were developed. An early promotional activity was an open house. Later, we invited hospital staff and the community. We then made informational presentations to high schools, colleges, and universities, to referral sources such as private practitioners, and to other interested groups. We also participated in health fairs, shopping mall events, workshops, and conferences. Direct mailings were sent to area psychologists and social workers. The mailings included a letter, an indexed telephone card, and a brochure describing our treatment approach and facilities, as well as a profile of anorectic and bulimic symptoms. Other promotional activities included newspaper ads, radio commercials, and participation on radio talk shows.

Supporting Nursing Staff

My responsibilities as head nurse of the unit included planning, organizing, communicating, monitoring unit activities, and controlling resources to ensure safe, high-quality care. In addition, I had to create an atmosphere that encouraged revenue-generating activities. This I accomplished by supporting the nurses and building on their value systems. I had regular meetings with the nurses. Initially, I focused on the unit's mission, philosophy, goals, and objectives. We examined and defined our role in relation to the other professionals and to the organization. I encouraged staff to verbalize their fears, perceptions, and concerns. They were helped to support one another and to articulate their role as members of this unit, staff, and team.

A major problem for the nurses was dealing with the direct influence their decisions had on hospital income. We had to convert telephone inquires into admissions. The nurses were most uncomfortable during the preadmission interview when payment and reimbursement were discussed. Insurance programs pay for less than half the cost; patients must pay for the uncovered portion. By emphasizing three important benefits of the interview, I was able to help the nurses accept responsibility for discussion of payment. These benefits were: (1) the patient can plan better for hospitalization; school, family, job, and financial responsibilities can be managed more easily; (2) the health care team can plan and implement treatment more effectively if it knows the patient's planned length of stay; and (3) the discharge plan is begun early.

The nursing staff and other professionals met at regularly scheduled meetings. These meetings led to mutual understanding, helped resolve conflicts, and fostered more cooperative attitudes. Group lunches and off-unit activities enhanced collegiality. This open communication has been the key to development of a strong treatment program. A strength of our multidisciplinary treatment team has been that we are able to communicate effectively among ourselves. We evaluate program goals and outcomes regularly. Needed changes are implemented in a timely fashion. As head nurse, I listen to the team members for content and for feeling tone. We are able to exchange ideas freely. A positive result of this has been personal growth for the staff in their role as primary nurses.

RESULTS AND EVALUATION

We implemented our program in 1984. Over 50% of our patients are self-referrals. Many of the others are referred by psychologists, social workers, and employee assistance programs. Usually they call our telephone inquiry line after seeing or hearing one of our promotional activities. About 40% of our patients have anorexia and remain an average of 60 days, while the 60% who are bulimic stay about 30 days. We have been able to maintain our census at levels required for financial viability. Patient surveys are conducted to evaluate our performance. We constantly evaluate and modify our efforts to satisfy patient needs and wants. Changes, made as needed to provide high-quality care, are an integral part of our program. Twelve weeks of outpatient treatment is offered without additional cost after discharge.

Despite much trepidation, the nursing staff became expert in assessing the potential patient for appropriateness of treatment in our unit, in describing the program to the person, and in helping those needing inpatient treatment make this commitment. A clearly defined marketing approach led to increased census and revenue, while accomplishing clinical goals. Nurses are the mainstay of this program. They are the salespeople and the chief providers of the service. In short, without them the program would not exist.

Using marketing has helped the hospital achieve increased census and income, and enhanced its image in the community by satisfying patient needs and wants with high-quality care. Retention of nurses has increased. Their contributions are recognized by hospital administration and by the physicians and other professionals with whom they work. This unit requires that nurses use their professional skills for the good of the patient and that all professionals work collaboratively. The image of nursing has become more positive. Marketing has enabled us to use our resources to best advantage.

REFERENCES

Drewnowski, A., Hopkins, S.A., & Kessler, R.C. (1988). The prevalence of bulimia nervosa in the US college student population. *American Journal of Public Health, 78,* 1322–1325.

Drossman, D.A. (1988). The eating disorders. In J.B. Wyngaarden & L.H. Smith (Eds.), *Cecil textbook of medicine* (18th ed.) (pp. 1215–1219). Philadelphia, PA: W.B. Saunders.

Romeo, F.F. (1984). Adolescence, sexual conflict, and anorexia nervosa. *Adolescence, 19,* 551–555.

Russell, G.F.M. (1982). Anorexia nervosa. In J.B. Wyngaarden & L.H. Smith (Eds.), *Cecil textbook of medicine* (16th ed.) (pp. 1379–1382). Philadelphia, PA: W.B. Saunders.

Schotte, D.E., & Stunkard, A.J. (1987). Bulimia vs bulimic behaviors on a college campus. *Journal of the American Medical Association, 258,* 1213–1215.

Marketing by Nurse Entrepreneurs: Launching a Magazine

Constance M. Berg, MBA, RN
Executive Editor, *Today's Executive Nurse Magazine*
Principal, CMB CONSULTING
San Francisco, CA

Eileen O'Riordan, MS, MBA, RN
Managing Editor, *Today's Executive Nurse Magazine*
Systems Manager, Washington Hospital
Fremont, CA

THE MARKETING SITUATION

The idea for a joint venture began during a casual conversation. We were two self-employed, entrepreneurial nurse businesswomen who were interested in developing and launching a new product. Exploratory meetings were immediately scheduled to pursue further some of the ideas that had surfaced. Our primary goal was to identify a new product idea that would address the business needs of executive nurses on a large scale and to which we could respond through our given skills and expertise.

First, we evaluated our own resources and capabilities to determine a direction. We explored possible consulting areas such as nursing productivity, marketing, financial management, educational conferences, and information systems. We targeted the nurse executive market as the one that could benefit the most from our skills and expertise.

We believed that a carefully prepared business plan was essential to help us identify our need for capital as well as potential sources of capital. The business plan also provided us with a tool that promoted effective planning of all phases of the business undertaking. It enabled us to delineate some major tasks that needed to be accomplished to achieve our goals. These tasks included market research, marketing goals and objectives, an organizational and operational plan, and a financial plan.

MARKET RESEARCH

Secondary Research

Primary and secondary research methods helped us to explore product ideas. We began with secondary research. Our search of the literature included articles in the popular press as well as professional literature. One theme running through the articles from the popular press was the nursing shortage; another was the negative image of nursing.

As we conducted our literature search, we targeted the nurse executive. Nurse executives manage large organizations and multimillion dollar budgets that are as complex and challenging as any in the business world. They may have up to 50% of the hospital's staff reporting directly or indirectly to them. Furthermore, health care organizations are in a state of flux, as they strive to contain costs, comply with changing regulations, and deal effectively with prospective reimbursement and increased competition. All these factors add to the complexity of the nurse executive role. The nurse executive is required to be an effective, humanistic manager and an expert strategist to make the most of opportunities in areas of finance, program planning, marketing, human resources, and technology. Nurse executives must direct all these functions to provide a given standard of patient care. They are recognized in health care as key organizational executives, and are rewarded accordingly. The average base salary for nurse executives increased by 20.5% between 1987 and 1988 (Cole & Sizing, 1988). This increase was 6.3% greater than that received by CEOs, the group which had the next highest increase.

To assist them in their high-level management role, nurse executives need ready access to current nursing, management, and technology information. Some professional journals are directed more to middle-level managers. Few publications provide nurse executives with the level or quality of business information their role demands. We reached a conclusion that we could develop and launch a magazine that would be attractive to nurse executives, so we began exploring this idea.

Primary Research: Focus Group Interviews

The next step was to do primary market research in the form of focus groups. According to Warshaw (1985), the focus group method of qualitative research inquires into the emotional content of individual responses from a small group of consumers. It explores why one likes or dislikes something, how strongly each feels, and what forces could alter that feeling. The focus group process can serve as a powerful marketing research tool. The energy that the group both produces and draws upon can lead to positive results. We concluded, therefore, that the personal contact with a group of nurse executives would either help us to confirm the need for our new product idea or possibly generate other ideas with greater promise.

We first defined the purpose of our focus group. It was to serve as a vehicle to help us determine: (1) if there was a need for an upscale, image-enhancing publication targeted for nurse executives; (2) what topics would be of interest; and (3) the appropriate image for the magazine.

Ten participants for the focus group were recruited by calling vice presidents for nursing in Northern California. We described our project, and invited them to participate. Most readily agreed. One vice president even flew in from midstate to participate. Although focus group participants are generally paid for their time, we did not do this. Instead, we stressed the opportunity to meet with peers and share ideas.

The focus group process, which was moderated by one of us, was very successful. Participating nurse executives were very interested in our proposed publication and saw a need for it. We explored desired characteristics of the magazine, such as subjects for articles, advertising, length, frequency of publication, and its quality and image. In order to meet the professional needs of nurse executives, and to build on the positive image aspects of the nursing profession, we found that content should include strategic, long-term and short-term planning, marketing, business, and technological information, as well as physical fitness, fashion, and personal money management ideas.

To enhance and validate the data obtained from the focus group interviews, we extended our qualitative research effort through telephone interviews with vice presidents for nursing in hospitals in Chicago, Philadelphia, Los Angeles, and New York. We also surveyed influential health care executives, nursing professors, representatives from health care industry vendors, and consultants from the major health care management firms. The overall results confirmed that we were indeed on the right path. Publishing a magazine for nurse executives was an appropriate goal.

MARKETING STRATEGIES

Implementation Schedule

Recognizing the magnitude of the task we were about to undertake, namely, development of a professional magazine, we identified the critical need for a well-planned implementation schedule. The plan enabled us to delineate and synchronize all the steps necessary to successfully implement our project. Responsibilities were assigned and realistic completion dates were set. We used this schedule as an effective management tool. We reviewed it at each management meeting to track the project and to keep us apprised of its status.

The Name

One of the first marketing strategies delineated on our implementation schedule was to establish a name for our new product. Creating an appropriate name for the magazine required free-flowing brainstorming as well as focused thinking. Through brainstorming, we came up with 35 possible titles, each of which was reviewed and discussed in terms of appropriateness, its attention-grabbing qualities, and the purpose of the magazine. Through this process, we selected 10 names for the semifinal list that was sent to each focus group and telephone interview participant. The participants were asked to vote for one name or to enter a name of their own. Ninety-eight percent of recipients replied. *Magazine for Today's Executive Nurse (TEN)* received the majority of votes, and was officially adopted as the project and publication name.

The Operational Plan

Having defined and selected a name, our next strategy was to outline a plan that would help us determine needed resources. We recognized the need for a publisher and designer, and selected a seasoned magazine publisher and an award-winning designer who were involved in all remaining project phases. We next projected minimum first-year costs for launching the magazine. Because promotion is so important for a new product, these costs were defined in detail. We evaluated multiple promotional strategies. A market test was planned to further evaluate product viability. Likewise, development of an overall promotion campaign was identified as an important strategy.

A direct-mail market test of interest is advised before doing a full-fledged launch (Friefeld, 1988). Therefore, we planned two test mailings to a total of 22,000 potential subscribers. The mailing lists include hospital vice presidents of nursing, associate and assistant directors of nursing, deans of academic nursing programs, and other nurses in leadership positions who provide service to nurse executives, such as consultants and information systems specialists. To project costs of the direct mailing, an itemized list was developed. The list included the development and design of a prototype magazine, a one-page cover letter, subscription cards, return franked envelopes, mailing envelopes, mailing labels, and mail house charges. Other operational and promotional costs include telephone service with a toll-free number, a bulk-rate mail permit, printing and mailing costs, trade show advertising and other promotional activities, salaries, equipment, overhead, and miscellaneous costs.

Organizational Structure

Designing the organizational structure for management of our new magazine was both challenging and rewarding. We first needed to identify two other important groups, namely, the contributing editors and the advisory board. We also had to define specific roles and responsibilities for each group. We agreed that the contributing editors would be expected to write articles periodically and to provide ideas or topics for articles. Advisory board members would advise us regarding trends and topics for *TEN*.

Because several of the focus group participants had expressed an interest, they were later invited to serve as contributing editors or advisory board members. Our personal and professional networks enabled us to identify others to participate. We received a 95% positive response rate to our invitations. The main reason given by those who refused were that they were already overcommitted.

A table of organization was then developed to help us assign responsibility for coordination and management of all activities, including operations management, subscription and circulation, budget, promotion, advertising, and liaisons with our contributing editors and advisory board.

Financial Plan

The operational plan, which was previously developed, was used to help us establish first-year cost estimates. From these cost estimates, we determined how much money we needed to start publication and the overall cash flow required to maintain viability of the magazine. The estimates helped us determine the amount of sponsorship funds needed. To provide for a large part of our initial funding, we decided to pursue major corporations for sponsorship and advertising. Having made this decision, we developed a substantial list of potential sponsors. The list included select companies from *Business Week's* top 1,000 companies and health care vendors, such as drug and information systems companies, consulting firms, and hospital suppliers.

Sponsors were necessary to help us launch the magazine before we had income from subscribers and advertisers. Two sponsorship levels were defined. Companies receive benefits through sponsoring the magazine by becoming either major or contributing sponsors. Each potential sponsor needed a specifically designed solicitation letter. Numerous follow-up telephone calls were required to get sponsorship commitment. The response, on the whole, has been very encouraging and has kept us moving forward.

RESULTS AND EVALUATION

Persistent efforts to achieve our goal have brought us to the point where our dream is about to be realized. Systematic application of marketing techniques has been the key factor in moving forward. The results of our marketing strategies are summarized below.

1. *Identification of a product for a specific target market.* We used research to ascertain that there was a market for a product that would enhance the nurse executive's ability as a business leader through provision of timely management, financial, and technological information.

2. *Visualization and identification of the product.* We determined that an upscale, professional magazine would address the need of nurse executives for ready access to high-level information for their role.

3. *Verification of both the need and the product through market research.* Focus group and individual interviews by telephone confirmed the need for, and the attraction of, the proposed product.

4. *Product development.* Management techniques, networking, and fund raising resulted in the development of the magazine prototype. Content for the first year's issues has been defined. Initial articles are being written by the contributing editors.

5. *Market test of magazine.* We are preparing for our marketing test. Our goal is to reach 22,000 potential subscribers through this process.

6. *Promotion to a sample of the potential readership.* Plans for this market testing are underway. We anticipate sending copies of the prototype to a limited number of our potential subscribers.

7. *Full scale product launch.* Several preparatory steps have been taken, such as acquiring mailing lists, soliciting advertising, and hiring magazine staff. We estimate it will take eight months before regular publication begins.

During the development process, we experienced two significant obstacles. First, a solid financial base was required to support such a major venture. Our efforts began with a shoestring budget. As we moved along, we became painfully aware of the expenses involved. Much research and many phone calls were needed to attain required financial backing. The responses we elicited from many potential sponsors were not very palatable; in fact, we were shocked that some major health care corporations did not see the value of their company's supporting a business magazine for executive nurses. These responses caused momentary discouragement and forced us at times to ask ourselves if we should proceed.

The second obstacle was our inability to devote our full-time efforts to the project, because we had other work that demanded attention. This led to great frustration and impatience as we strove to keep the project on track. It was at times like these that the results of our marketing research and support from nurse colleagues across the country bolstered our courage. These results helped to remind us that our business venture had been supported by the target market. This renewed our energy and commitment so that we could persist in achieving our goal.

By using the marketing management process, we are on track and are currently writing and accepting articles for *TEN,* as well as focusing on the financial needs of this exciting project. Of course, the success of our marketing efforts must still be proven. A satisfied readership will be the conclusive evidence. According to Goethe, "Whatever you can do, or dream you can, begin it; boldness has genius, power, and magic in it." This served as our motivating force throughout the process.

REFERENCES

Cole, B.S., & Sizing, M. (1988). Compensation survey. *Modern Healthcare, 18*(44), 41–58.

Friefeld, K. (1988, March). Cashing in on the newsletter business. *New Woman,* pp. 120–123, 126.

Warshaw, R. (1985, November). Market experts. *Ms Magazine,* pp. 44–48.

GLOSSARY

Advertising: any paid form of nonpersonal sales message, including space or time in newspapers, magazines, radio, television, direct mail, and billboards.

Available market: a subset of consumers who are interested, able to engage in an exchange, and who have access to a specific market offer.

Brochure: a publication that is often multipaged or folded; also called *flyer, folder,* or *pamphlet.*

Business plan: a written document that describes in narrative and financial detail the nature and expectations of the new product.

Channel: a conduit that brings together a seller and a buyer/consumer to facilitate an exchange.

Concentrated marketing: targeting one segment for a major effort.

Consumer: end user of goods or services.

Consumerism: an organized movement of citizens and government to strengthen the rights and power of buyers in relation to sellers.

Corporate identity media: those things that influence and establish an image or perception of an organization. Included are visual items such as stationery, brochures, signs, logos, business forms, buildings, and uniforms, as well as ambience.

Cost recovery: recouping of most or a reasonable part of costs.

Customer: buyer of goods or services.

Customer/Consumer orientation: energy is focused on identifying the needs and wants of primary customers and on delivering services that satisfy them; also known as *marketing orientation.*

Demarketing: a planned marketing effort to decrease consumption or use of a product.

Demographics: vital and social statistics, such as age, births, deaths, diseases, or marriages of populations.

Diagnostic related groups (DRGs): a medical classification system used as the basis for prospective payment.

Differentiated marketing: targeting at least two segments by focusing on the unique needs and characteristics of each segment.

Dumping: selling a product below cost in order to increase market share.

401

Environmentalism: an organized movement of citizens and government to protect and improve the environment.

Ethics: a system of moral principles; the rules of conduct recognized in respect to a particular class of human actions or a group or culture; the branch of philosophy dealing with values pertaining to human conduct with respect to rightness and wrongness of certain actions and to the goodness and badness of the motives and ends of such actions.

Fixed costs: overhead; the expenses that must be paid each month regardless of use or production rates.

Focus groups: a qualitative research technique using small groups, selected from a target market, who are paid to share their feelings, opinions, and attitudes on a marketing topic.

Gatekeeper: a person or organization that limits options available but does not make the final decision for the consumer. (Examples in health care: third-party payers, physicians, nurses, and social workers.)

Gross national product (GNP): the total of all goods and services produced in a nation.

Incentive: something of value added to an offer to encourage purchase.

Individual depth interview: a qualitative research technique using one-on-one interviewing.

Intrapreneurs: entrepreneurs within an organization.

Logo: a symbol, letter, or sign used to represent an entire organization or profession.

Market: the set of potential or actual buyers and users of goods, services, and ideas; the place where the exchange of goods and services is negotiated.

Marketing mix: the individualized blend of marketing strategies used to achieve marketing goals and objectives.

Marketing orientation: energy is focused on identifying the needs and wants of primary customers and on delivering services that satisfy them; also known as *customer/consumer orientation.*

Market research: a systematic process of designing the study of a specific marketing problem, collecting and analyzing the data, and reporting findings.

Market share: the percentage of the total market for a product that is captured by one producer or vendor.

Market testing: evaluating a product offer and its marketing program in the actual marketplace.

Megamarketing: the individualized blend of marketing strategies used to attract markets that are blocked or protected by third parties.

Morality: conformity to the rules of right conduct.

Newsletter: a periodic publication prepared by or for a group or institution, such as a company, charitable or membership organization, or government agency, to provide information to employees, contributors, members, stockholders, the press, and general public.

News release: a piece written by a company to give its view and provide information about an event to media such as newspapers or news programs. It is done in the hope of gaining positive publicity; also called *press release.*

Niche: a small, potentially attractive market segment.

Nominal group process: a qualitative research technique used to reach consensus on issues and specific group decisions.

Oligopoly: a market with few sellers.

Oligopsony: a market with few buyers.

Organizational culture: the implicit and explicit shared beliefs, values, and norms that shape the work environment.

Penetrated market: a subset of qualified available consumers who are actually using the product.

Place: how products are made available and accessible to consumers. *Distribution* is, perhaps, a more accurate term.

Positioning: the process of developing and communicating the attractive characteristics of a product.

Potential market: a subset of consumers with some interest in a specific market offer.

Press kit: a collection of background material reporters need to develop a story; may include photos, illustrations, data, and news releases.

Press release: a piece written by a company to give its view and provide information about an event to media such as newspapers or news programs. It is done in the hope of gaining positive publicity; also called *news release.*

Price: the sum or amount of money or its equivalent for which anything is offered for sale, bought, or sold; the total values consumers exchange for the use of a product or service.

Product: goods, services, or ideas offered to a market for use, consumption, acquisition, or attention in order to satisfy needs or desires.

Production orientation: energy is focused on the efficient output and distribution of the product or service.

Product life cycle: the four stages of a product's progress through introduction, growth, maturity, and decline.

Product line: a group of products that are closely related by function, customer use, distribution channels, or price.

Product line management (PLM): a system of planning, organizing, directing, and controlling a group of related products from development through delivery to consumers.

Product mix: the set of all products that an organization or individual offers to consumers.

Product orientation: energy is focused on providing goods and services that the provider thinks are good for the consumer, regardless of the consumer's opinion.

Promotion: those marketing mix strategies that tell people about the product and persuade them to buy it.

Prospective payment: reimbursement that is determined before services are rendered.

Public: of, or pertaining to, or affecting the people as a whole, or of a community, state, or country (general usage); a group that has a potential or actual interest in, or an effect on, an organization (marketing usage).

Publicity: public attention resulting from unpaid mention in the print or electronic media, or through any other medium or means of communication, including word of mouth.

Public relations: activities that are carried out to earn and maintain favorable publicity for a company. The management function includes evaluation of the public's attitudes, identification of an individual or organization with the public interest, and planning and implementing a program to gain public understanding and acceptance.

Public service announcement (PSA):   television or radio spots that inform the public and give the sponsoring organization publicity.

Qualified available market: a subset of consumers who are interested, able to engage in an exchange, and who have access to, and qualify for, the specific market offer.

Sales orientation: energy is focused on stimulating interest in services presently offered, through ads, public relations, and personal selling.

Segmentation: the process of dividing a market into groups that share certain characteristics.

Served market: a subset of the qualified market that the organization is attracting and serving.

Service: an intangible activity or benefit that is offered to another party without resulting in ownership of the product.

Social marketing: programs designed, implemented, and controlled to increase the acceptability of an idea, cause, or practice.

Societal marketing orientation: energy is focused on determining the needs and desires of actual and potential markets and on delivering goods and services that foster individual and societal well-being.

Strategic business unit (SBU):   a decentralized organizational unit with its own mission, goals, and objectives that varies in size from a division or department to a unit or product line.

Strategic planning: long-range planning based on assessments of present and projected external and internal environments.

Survey research: a quantitative research approach that asks individuals a series of questions about their attitudes, behaviors, characteristics, and preferences.

Targeting: the process of selecting one or more market segments for a directed marketing effort.

Total costs: fixed and variable costs combined.

Undifferentiated marketing (mass marketing): marketing uniform products to all customers, focusing on common needs and characteristics.

Utility: the principle and end of utilitarian ethics; that which will bring about happiness and well-being for the greatest number (philosophy); the ability of a commodity or a service to satisfy some human want (economics).

Value: an operational belief; an ideal, custom, or institution of a society or group toward which the members of the group have an affective regard; any object or quality desirable as a means or as an end in itself; in exchange theory, the benefits received through an exchange minus the price paid in return.

Variable costs: the expenses that fluctuate directly with the amount of service provided or goods produced.

INDEX